Jay Chhablani
Parthopratim Dutta Majumder
J. Fernando Arevalo
Editors

Retinal and Choroidal Imaging in Systemic Diseases

Springer

Editors
Jay Chhablani
L.V. Prasad Eye Institute
Hyderabad
India

Parthopratim Dutta Majumder
Sankara Nethralaya
Chennai
India

J. Fernando Arevalo
The Johns Hopkins University
Baltimore, MD
USA

ISBN 978-981-10-5459-4 ISBN 978-981-10-5461-7 (eBook)
https://doi.org/10.1007/978-981-10-5461-7

Library of Congress Control Number: 2017956569

Printed on acid-free paper

This Springer imprint is published by Springer Nature
The registered company is Springer Nature Singapore Pte Ltd.
The registered company address is: 152 Beach Road, #21-01/04 Gateway East, Singapore 189721, Singapore

Retinal and Choroidal Imaging in Systemic Diseases

Foreword

Who needs another book? More pictures? New technology? Is there anything else to learn?

The answers to these questions are very simple. Working backwards, one appreciates the fact that learning never stops. It is our objective as physicians to continually learn so as to better ourselves and therefore improve the care we provide to our patients. While there are many ways of learning, someone must always be a student and someone must always be the teacher. Is there new technology? Of course there is and it is our obligation as students of ophthalmology to learn that technology, relying on good teachers to help us understand that which is new and different. We are fortunate in that we are witness to incredible advances in technology in our lifetimes, but we must be committed to not letting the technology get away from us. Therefore we look to proven methods of teaching, provided by good teachers and educators, to enlighten us and keep us up to date on the newest technologies in our field. And who is it that said that a picture is worth a thousand words? As we know that most of us learn from pictures and a well-illustrated document, with concise and well-organized writing, to explain those illustrations which helps enormously in the learning process. Pattern recognition is key to our profession and thus imaging is key to what we do every day. And finally one must ask, do we need another book? And the answer is unquestionably, yes. And the reason for that is simple. The best way to keep up with new technology is through a well-illustrated text that serves as a reference and provides a well-organized, meticulously scripted, heavily referenced document. The textbook does exactly that.

We, the students, are fortunate in that doctors Jay Chhablani, Parthopratim Majumdar, and J. Fernando Arevalo are superb teachers who have assembled a list of experts to address a variety of systemic conditions. By using various imaging modalities they are able to illustrate and better define these conditions. By focusing these modern imaging technologies on selected systemic conditions, we have an unusual format for the learning process. Whether we are ophthalmologists who specialize in retinal diseases, general ophthalmologists, uveitis specialists, ocular oncologists, internists, or family physicians interested in understanding the language of imaging technology in ophthalmology, these teachers instruct us as never before. Beautifully illustrated and beautifully written, this textbook will undoubtedly become a mainstay of the practicing physician as well as medical students and residents alike. This text will become a first resource for so many individuals trying to understand the complexity of the many systemic diseases which are demonstrated through ophthalmic imaging.

We must compliment and acknowledge the editors of this extremely important text for their efforts and their successful accomplishments in bringing to the readership this very valuable text.

Alexander J. Brucker
Scheie Eye Institute
University of Pennsylvania
Philadelphia, PA
USA

Preface

Various systemic diseases involve the eyes, and in few diseases, the eyes could provide the first clue for the systemic disease. Retinal findings on clinical examination have been reported previously in systemic diseases. Advancement of posterior segment imaging has significantly improved the understanding of pathophysiology and has become an essential part in management strategy of posterior segment diseases. Advanced imaging techniques such as enhanced depth imaging, oximetry, adaptive optics, and retinal blood flowmetry are now being explored in subjects with systemic diseases. With improved understanding on such imaging techniques in various systemic diseases, the knowledge about pathomechanism, early diagnosis, and more targeted therapeutic approaches has improved.

In this book, we focus on findings with various imaging modalities in various systemic conditions. Systemic conditions included, but are not limited to, neurological diseases such as Alzheimer's disease, multiple sclerosis, Parkinson's disease, schizophrenia, and migraine; systemic vasculitis such as Behçet's disease; systemic lupus erythematosus; ocular toxicity secondary to systemic drugs; blood dyscrasias such as sickle cell disease and hematologic disorders; renal diseases; trauma-related conditions such as Purtscher-like retinopathy, whiplash retinopathy, and shaken-baby syndrome; intracranial hypertension; cancer-associated retinopathy; gastrointestinal diseases; immunologic diseases such as autoimmune retinopathy and sarcoidosis; systemic infectious diseases such as tuberculosis and choroidal and retinal metastasis; oculoneurocutaneous syndromes; Vogt-Koyanagi-Harada disease; pregnancy; systemic hypertension; and Valsalva retinopathy.

This book, entitled *Retina and Choroidal Imaging in Systemic Diseases*, is the first attempt to provide information on retinal and choroidal findings using advanced imaging technologies in systemic diseases. This book is intended for ophthalmologists, retina specialists, uveitis specialists, ocular oncologists, and internal medicine specialists.

We wish that this book improves the current understanding about the imaging findings in systemic diseases which helps for early diagnosis and management of these conditions.

We would like to thank all the authors who shared their experience and valuable time and effort for the book. We would like to thank the Springer staff, who guided us to make this book happen. At the end, we would like to thank our patients, colleagues, and families who supported us to bring this book in a timely manner.

Hyderabad, India Jay Chhablani
Chennai, India Parthopratim Dutta Majumder
Baltimore, MD, USA J. Fernando Arevalo

Contents

About the Editors

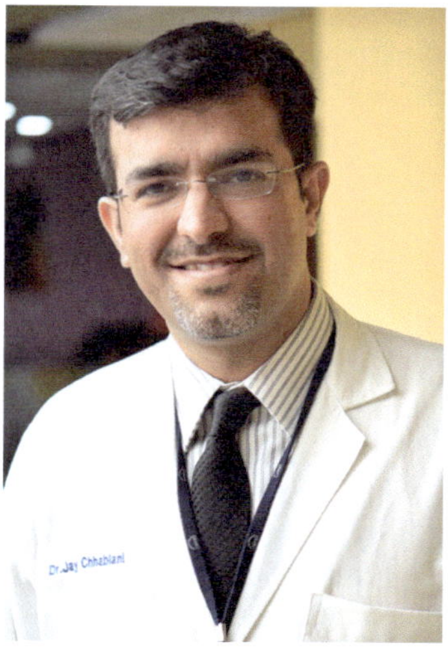

Dr. Jay Chhablani completed his clinical vitreoretinal fellowship at Sankara Nethralaya, Chennai. He was an International Council of Ophthalmology (ICO) fellow at Jules Gonin Eye Hospital, Switzerland, in 2009 and a clinical instructor at the Jacobs Retina Center at Shiley Eye Center, University of California, San Diego, USA (from 2010 to 2012), before he joined L. V. Prasad Eye Institute, Hyderabad, India, as faculty. His areas of interest are macular disorders and recent imaging techniques. He has published several articles in peer-reviewed journals with specific emphasis on the field of choroid. He is on the reviewing and editorial boards of many high-impact ophthalmology journals. He is member of global ONE network committee of the American Academy of Ophthalmology. He has won several national and international awards. He has delivered the inaugural Ian Constable Lecture at the Asia-Pacific Vitreo-retina Society on his work on intravitreal ziv-aflibercept therapy.

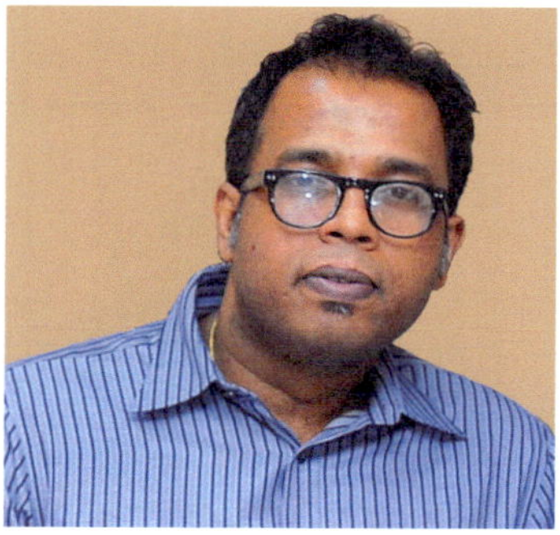

Dr. Parthopratim Dutta Majumder completed his graduation and post-graduation at Silchar Medical College and Hospital, Assam University. He completed his fellowship in medical retina and uvea at Sankara Nethralaya and joined the Department of Uvea and Intraocular Inflammation. He was awarded with the Dr. T. L. K. Row Endowment Award for the best associate consultant for 2010–2011. He had received the Dr. Nataraja Pillai Award and Dr. K. R. Dutta Award for best paper. He has attended and presented papers in various national and international conferences. His areas of interest include medical management of uveitis and scleritis, uveitis in autoimmune disorders, and phacoemulsification in uveitic cataracts. He is now working as consultant in the Department of Uvea and Intraocular Inflammation, Sankara Nethralaya, Chennai. He has published many articles in various peer-reviewed and non-peer-reviewed journals. He is the editor of *INSIGHT*, the scientific journal of medical and vision research foundation. He is the founder cum chief editor of the popular ophthalmology portal www.eophtha.com.

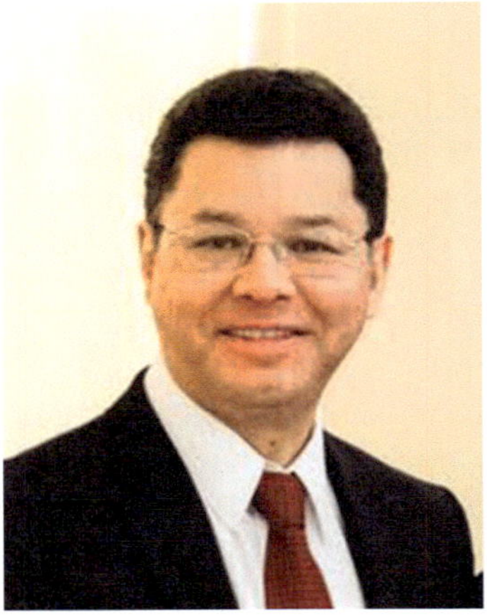

J. Fernando Arevalo, MD, FACS has been recognized as one of the leading ophthalmologists in South America and worldwide and, in 2001, founded the Arevalo-Coutinho Foundation for Research in Ophthalmology.

In 2011, Dr. Arevalo was invited by Johns Hopkins University (JHU) in Baltimore to work as a professor of ophthalmology and the chief of the Retina Division of the King Khaled Eye Specialist Hospital (KKESH) in Riyadh, Saudi Arabia, for a 4-year tenure (July 2011–2015), followed by an appointment at the Wilmer Eye Institute of the Johns Hopkins University School of Medicine as the Edmund F. and Virginia B. Ball professor of ophthalmology in the Retina Division and an appointment as chief of ophthalmology at Johns Hopkins Bayview Medical Center in 2015. As a clinical scientist, Dr. Arevalo has more than 900 scientific publications (more than 250 on MEDLINE), 12 books, more than 700 scientific paper presentations, and more than 1100 invited lecture presentations in North America, South America, Central America, Europe, Africa, and Asia that have led to international recognition and awards. Dr. Arevalo is the current president-elect of the Pan-American Association of Ophthalmology (PAAO).

Contributors

Aniruddha Agarwal Department of Ophthalmology, Advanced Eye Center, Post Graduate Institute of Medical Education and Research (PGIMER), Chandigarh, India

Ocular Imaging Research and Reading Center (OIRRC), Menlo Park, CA, USA

Stanley M. Truhlsen Eye Institute, University of Nebraska Medical Center, Omaha, NE, USA

Michael T. Andreoli Department of Ophthalmology and Visual Sciences, University of Illinois at Chicago, Chicago, IL, USA

J. Fernando Arevalo Department of Ophthalmology, Johns Hopkins Bayview Medical Center, Baltimore, MD, USA

Retina Division, Wilmer Eye Institute, The Johns Hopkins University School of Medicine, Baltimore, MD, USA

Mary E. Aronow Department of Ophthalmology, Retina Division, Wilmer Eye Institute, Johns Hopkins University School of Medicine, Baltimore, MD, USA

Francesco Bandello Department of Ophthalmology, University Vita-Salute, Scientific Institute San Raffaele, Milan, Italy

Giulio Barteselli Genentech Inc., South San Francisco, CA, USA

Department of Ophthalmology, Shiley Eye Institute, University of California San Diego, La Jolla, CA, USA

Catalina Becerra Fundación Oftalmológica Nacional, Bogotá, DC, Colombia

Lucia Benatti Department of Ophthalmology, University Vita-Salute, Scientific Institute San Raffaele, Milan, Italy

Judy J. Chen Department of Ophthalmology, University of Illinois at Chicago, Chicago, IL, USA

Preeti Patil Chhablani Jasti V Ramanamma Children's Eye Care Centre, L. V. Prasad Eye Institute, Hyderabad, Andhra Pradesh, India

Jay Chhablani Smt. Kanuri Santhamma Retina Vitreous Centre, L. V. Prasad Eye Institute, Hyderabad, India

Maria Vittoria Cicinelli Department of Ophthalmology, University Vita-Salute, Scientific Institute San Raffaele, Milan, Italy

Fatemeh Darvizeh Department of Ophthalmology, University Vita-Salute, Scientific Institute San Raffaele, Milan, Italy

Laura Dell'Arti Ophthalmological Unit, Department of Clinical Sciences and Community Health, Ca' Granda Foundation-Ospedale Maggiore Policlinico, University of Milan, Milan, Italy

David Ehmann Wills Eye Hospital, Philadelphia, PA, USA

David Fell Stony Brook School of Medicine, Stony Brook University, New York, NY, USA

María Cristina Gabela Fundación Oftalmológica Nacional, Escuela de Medicina y Ciencias de la Salud, Universidad del Rosario, Bogotá, DC, Colombia

Uppal Gandhi Jasti V Ramanamma Children's Eye Care Centre, L. V. Prasad Eye Institute, Hyderabad, Andhra Pradesh, India

Sunir Garg Wills Eye Hospital, Philadelphia, PA, USA

Vishali Gupta Department of Ophthalmology, Advanced Eye Center, Post Graduate Institute of Medical Education and Research (PGIMER), Chandigarh, India

Alessandro Invernizzi Eye Clinic, Department of Biomedical and Clinical Science "Luigi Sacco", Luigi Sacco Hospital, University of Milan, Milan, Italy

Swathi Kaliki The Operation Eyesight Universal Institute for Eye Cancer, L V Prasad Eye Institute, Hyderabad, India

Irfan Khan Wilmer Eye Institute, Johns Hopkins University, Baltimore, MD, USA

Parthopratim Dutta Majumder Department of Uvea and Intraocular inflammation, Sankara Nethralaya, Chennai, India

Andrea Mazzaferro Department of Ophthalmology, University Vita-Salute, Scientific Institute San Raffaele, Milan, Italy

William F. Mieler Department of Ophthalmology and Visual Sciences, University of Illinois at Chicago, Chicago, IL, USA

Department of Ophthalmology, University of Illinois at Chicago, Chicago, IL, USA

Manabu Mochizuki Department of Ophthalmology and Visual Science, Tokyo Medical and Dental University Graduate School of Medicine, Tokyo, Japan

Akshay G. Nair Ophthalmic Plastic Surgery and Ocular Oncology Services, Advanced Eye Hospital and Institute, Navi Mumbai, India

Akshay Gopinathan Nair Ophthalmic Plastic Surgery and Ocular Oncology Services, Advanced Eye Hospital and Institute, Navi Mumbai, India

Maura Di Nicola Ophthalmological Unit, Department of Clinical Sciences and Community Health, Ca' Granda Foundation-Ospedale Maggiore Policlinico, University of Milan, Milan, Italy

Remya Mareen Paulose Little Flower Hospital and Research Centre, Angamaly, Kerala, India

Smt.Kanuri Santhamma Retina Vitreous Centre, L. V. Prasad Eye Institute, Hyderabad, Andhra Pradesh, India

Lea Querques Department of Ophthalmology, University Vita-Salute, Scientific Institute San Raffaele, Milan, Italy

Giuseppe Querques Department of Ophthalmology, University Vita-Salute, Scientific Institute San Raffaele, Milan, Italy

Nishant Radke Shri Ganesh Vinayak Eye Hospital, Raipur, India

Sherief Raouf Stony Brook School of Medicine, Stony Brook University, New York, NY, USA

Ashvini Reddy Wilmer Eye Institute, Johns Hopkins University, Baltimore, MD, USA

Francisco J. Rodríguez Fundación Oftalmológica Nacional, Escuela de Medicina y Ciencias de la Salud, Universidad del Rosario, Bogotá, DC, Colombia

Fundacion Oftalmologica Nacional, Bogota, DC, Colombia

Hitesh Sharma Department of Uvea and Intraocular inflammation, Sankara Nethralaya, Chennai, India

Carol L. Shields Ocular Oncology Service, Wills Eye Hospital, Thomas Jefferson University, Philadelphia, PA, USA

Ilaria Zucchiatti Department of Ophthalmology, University Vita-Salute, Scientific Institute San Raffaele, Milan, Italy

Authors' Biography

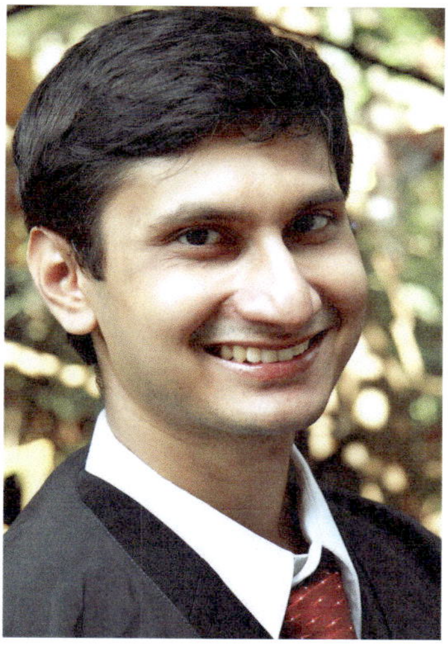

Aniruddha Agarwal is currently working as a clinical vitreoretinal fellow in the Department of Ophthalmology, Postgraduate Institute of Medical Education and Research (PGIMER), Chandigarh, India. He has completed his clinical research fellowship (subspecialty of vitreoretina and uveitis) in the Ocular Imaging Research and Reading Center, Stanley M. Truhlsen Eye Institute, Omaha, Nebraska, USA. He did his ophthalmology residency at PGIMER, Chandigarh, India. He has authored more than 112 publications and 25 book chapters. His areas of interest include surgical diseases of the retina, diabetes, and uveitis.

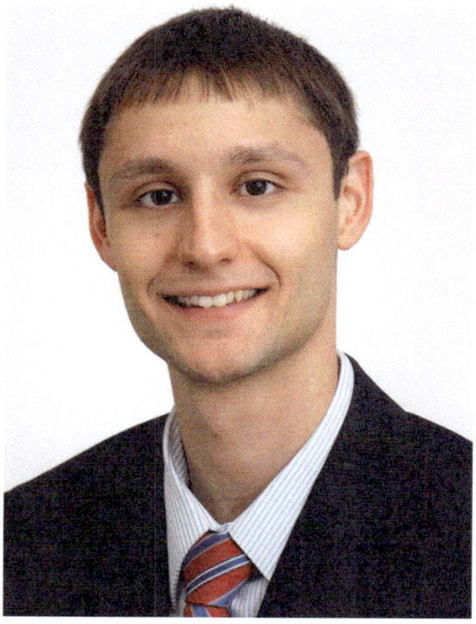

Dr. Michael Andreoli was born and raised in Wheaton, Illinois. He completed his ophthalmology residency and vitreoretinal surgery fellowship at the University of Illinois at Chicago. He plans to continue his research and clinical practice in vitreoretinal surgery and ocular oncology.

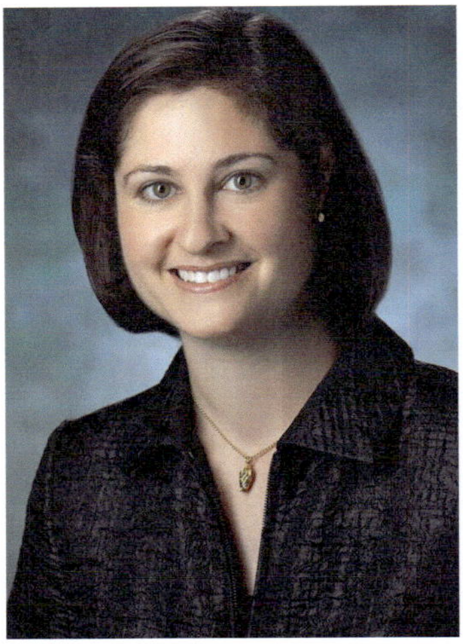

Mary E. Aronow, MD is an assistant professor of ophthalmology at the Wilmer Eye Institute, Johns Hopkins University School of Medicine. She specializes in the full range of adult and pediatric eye cancer and the medical management of vitreoretinal diseases. Dr. Aronow received her medical degree from the Yale University School of Medicine. Following an internship in internal medicine at Brigham and Women's Hospital at Harvard, she completed her ophthalmology residency at the Cole Eye Institute at the Cleveland Clinic. Her subspecialty fellowship training in ophthalmic oncology was at the Cole Eye Institute at the Cleveland Clinic. She then completed a fellowship in medical retina at the National Eye Institute, National Institutes of Health.

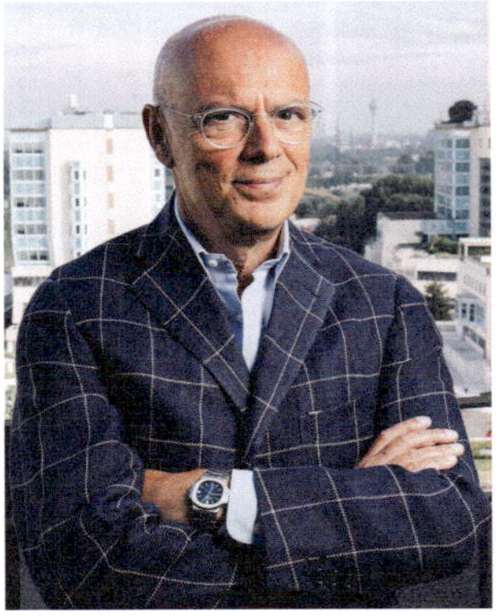

Francesco Bandello is Full Professor and Chairman at the Department of Ophthalmology at University Vita-Salute, Scientific Institute San Raffaele, Milan, Italy. He is Academic Dean of "Corso di Laurea Specialistica/Magistrale in Medicina e Chirurgia" at the same University.

Professor Bandello is Past President of EURETINA, President of Academia Ophthalmologica Europea and Vice-President of EuroLam.

Prof. Bandello is Co-Editor of the *European Journal of Ophthalmology* and former board member of the Club Jules Gonin and Macula Society. He is member of Executive Board of ESASO Foundation (European School for Advanced Studies in Ophthalmology), member of the Academia Ophthalmologica Internationalis and the Accademia Nazionale di Medicina.

Prof. Bandello is co-author of 11 books and he serves as a peer reviewer for grant applications for the NEI. He has authored or co-authored of 447 articles on PubMed Journals and he served as trained Principal Investigator in several clinical trials performed following ICH/GCP and mainly concerning retinal diseases.

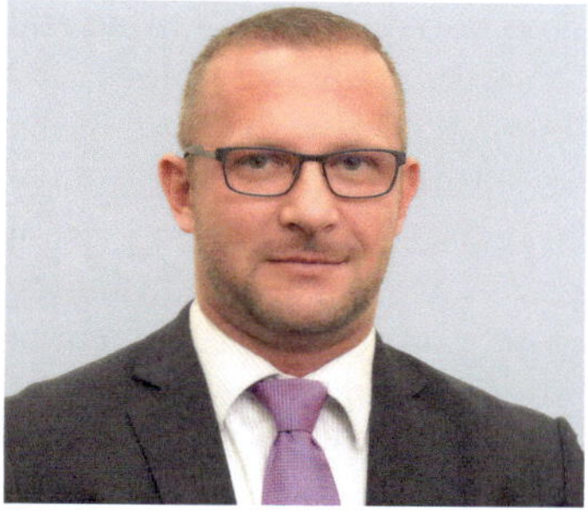

Dr. Giulio Barteselli is Associate Medical Director at the Ophthalmology Department at Genentech Inc., South San Francisco, CA, USA. He also serves as Assistant Professor of Ophthalmology at the University of California San Diego, La Jolla, CA. He has previously worked as retina specialist at the Ca' Granda Foundation, Milan, Italy. His research interest is primarily in clinical trials and new molecules or treatment options for ophthalmology indications. He has published more than 50 peer-reviewed articles, and he's an active reviewer for multiple ophthalmology journals.

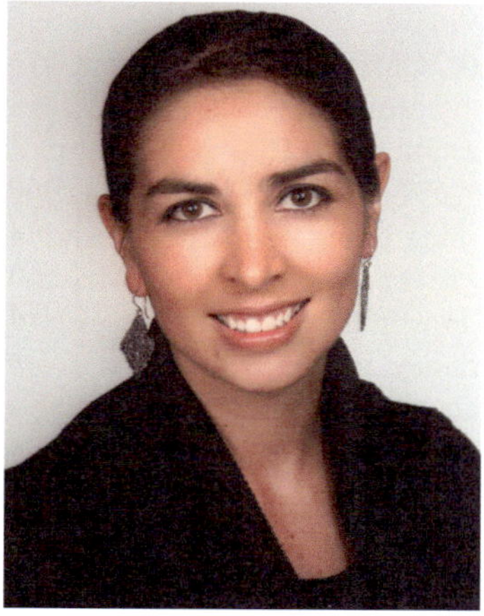

Catalina Becerra, MD Medical degree from Universidad Nacional de Colombia, Ophthalmology Residency Program at Pontificia Universidad Javeriana, Bogota, Colombia, Ocular ultrasonography fellowship at Asociación para Evitar la Ceguera en México – Universidad Nacional Autonoma de México, Assistant professor, Department of Ocular Ultrasound at Asociación para Evitar la Ceguera en México

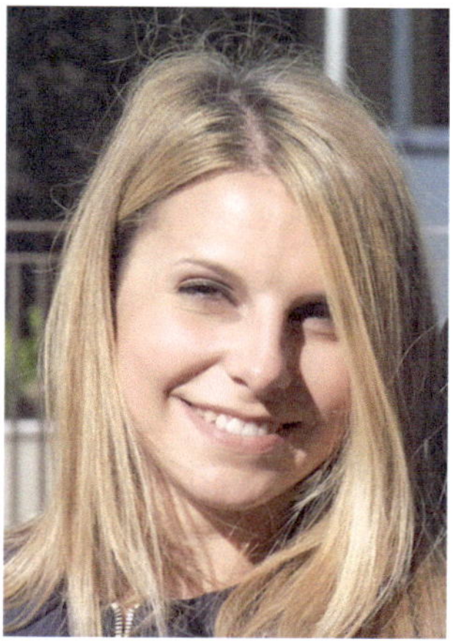

Lucia Benatti, MD is a first-year Resident in Ophthalmology at Parma University. She earned her medical degree from Vita-Salute San Raffaele University in Milan in 2015. She has attended the department of Opthalmology at University Vita-Salute, IRCCS Ospedale San Raffaele, Milan. She authored and co-authored several papers in Medical Retina, concerning Retinal Vein Occlusion, Diabetic Retinopathy and Central Serous Chorioretinopathy.

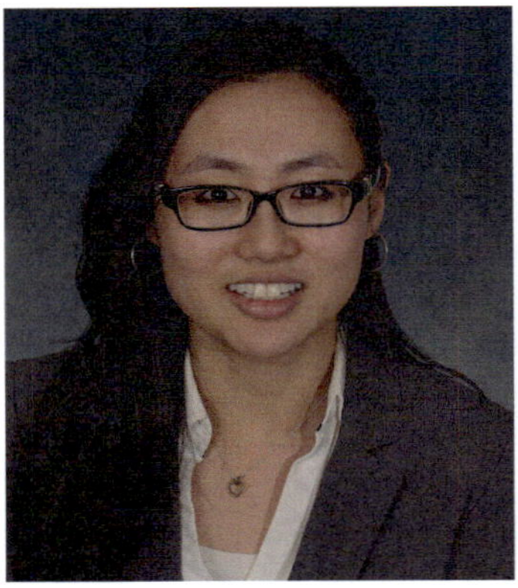

Judy J. Chen was born in Taipei, Taiwan and chose to pursue a career in ophthalmology, and ultimately vitreoretinal surgery, because of the field's innovative advancements in technology and the profound impact that improving vision can have on patients' lives. While contributing to the textbook, Judy was a senior resident at the University of Illinois at Chicago (UIC). She is now a surgical vitreoretinal fellow with the West Coast Retina Medical group in the San Francisco bay area. In the future, she hopes to combine her interests in clinical medicine, research, and teaching into a fulfilling career.

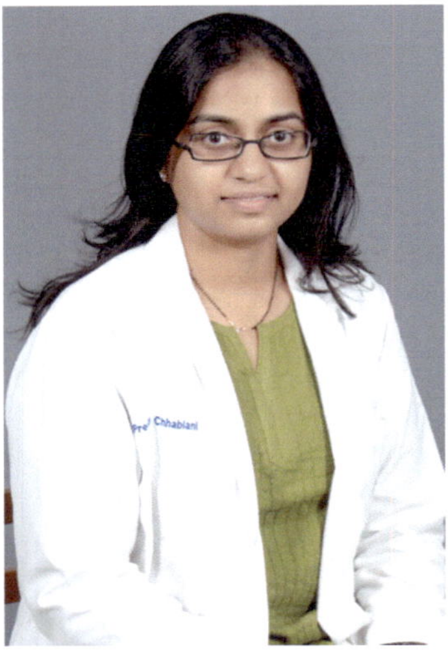

Dr. Preeti Patil Chhablani is currently a consultant ophthalmologist at the Jasti V. Ramanamma Children's Eye Care Centre, L V Prasad Eye Institute, Hyderabad, India. She completed her undergraduate medical training from Lokmanya Tilak Municipal Medical College, Sion Hospital, Mumbai. She completed her residency in Ophthalmology from Sankara Nethralaya in Chennai (2006–2009) and was awarded the "Best Outgoing Postgraduate Student" award by the Medical Research Foundation, Sankara Nethralaya. She also received the prestigious "Dr G Venkataswamy Gold Medal for Ophthalmology" (June 2009) for standing first in Ophthalmology in India in the Diplomate of National Board (DNB) Examinations. She then went on to do a fellowship in Pediatric Ophthalmology and Strabismus from Sankara Nethralaya (2009–2010). She was also a visiting fellow in Neuro-ophthalmology and Pediatric Ophthalmology and Strabismus at the University of California, San Diego, California, USA (2011–2012), before she joined LVPEI. Her areas of interest include pediatric and adult neuro-ophthalmology, pediatric cataract surgery, and strabismus.

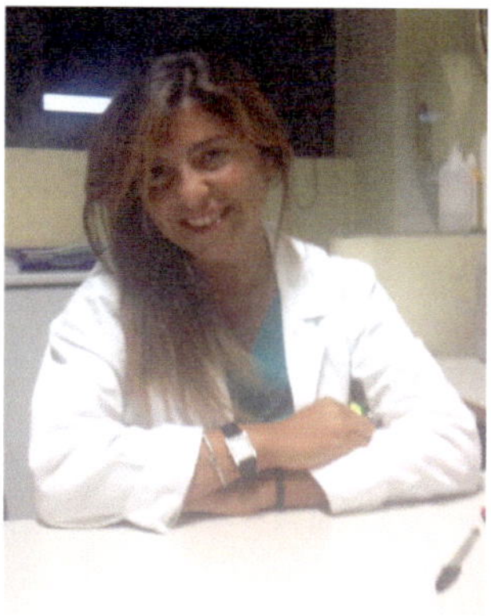

Maria Vittoria Cicinelli, MD is a medical resident in Opththalmology at University Vita-Salute, IRCCS Ospedale San Raffaele, Milan, Italy. Her main topics of interest are Medical Retina, Epidemiology and Oculoplastic Surgery. She is a fellow of the Global Vision Database (GVD) and she has completed a short-term fellowship in Oculoplastic Surgery at L V Prasad Eye Hospital, Hyderabad (India). Dr Cicinelli has contributed to more than 50 peer-reviewed articles and book chapters published mainly in the areas of Medical Retina (age-related macular degeneration, retinal vascular diseases, hereditary retinal diseases, vitreoretinal surgery) and Epidemiology of Eye Diseases (as member of the Vision Loss Expert Group of the Global Burden of Disease Study). She is editorial assistant of "*Ophthalmology – Point of Care*" (editor in chief Prof. Giuseppe Querques) and reviewer for major peer-reviewed journals.

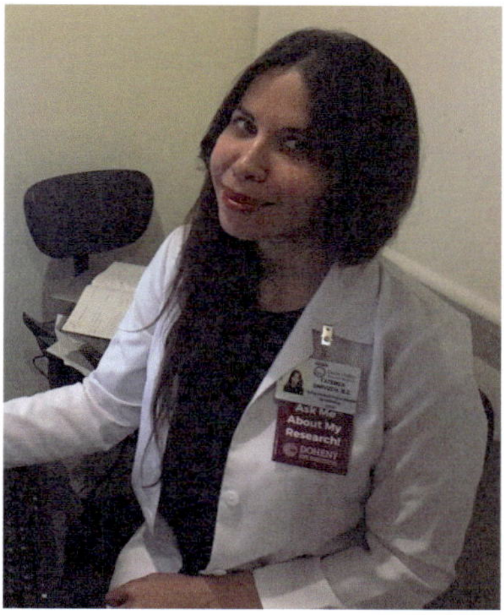

Fatemeh Darvizeh, MSc, MD has obtained her master in Analytical Chemistry (Chemometrics) from Sharif University of Technology, Tehran, Iran, 2010.

She has graduated from Medical School in 2016 with honors from University Vita-Salute San Raffaele, Milano, Italy. Dr Darvizeh has given an effective contribution in medical research projects mainly in the field of Viteroretinal diseases and Neuro-ophthalmology. She has worked as a Research Doctor at IRCCS Ospedale San Raffaele, Milano, Italy and Doheny Eye Center, Los Angeles, CA, USA.

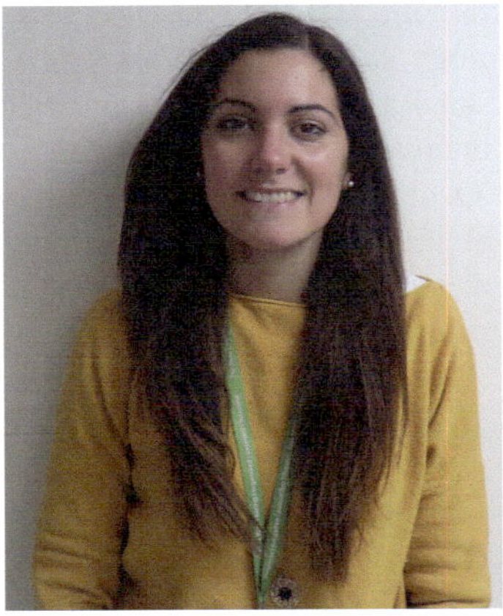

Dr. Laura Dell'Arti received her medical degree at the University of Milan (Milan, Italy) in 2010, where also she completed her ophthalmology residency in 2016. She is currently a fellow in neuro-ophthalmology at the Moorfields Eye Hospital (London, UK). She has been a Fellow of the European Board of Ophthalmologists since 2016.

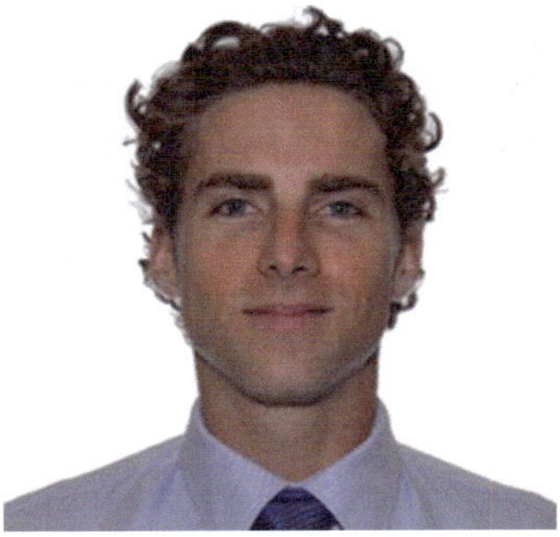

David Ehmann, BSc, MD, FRCSC is a second-year vitreoretinal surgical fellow at Wills Eye Hospital, Philadelphia, PA, USA.

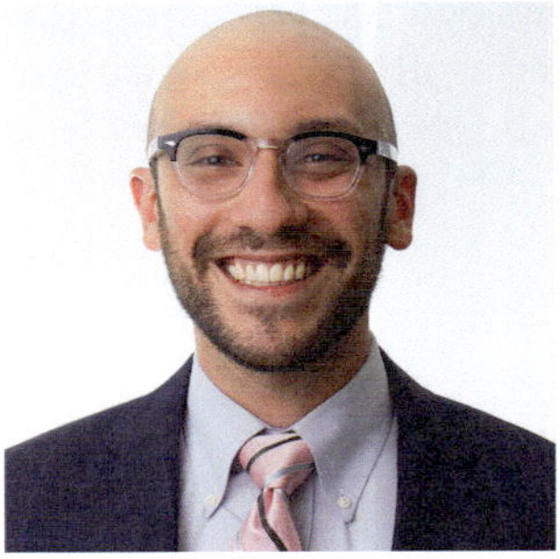

David Fell is a medical student at the State University of New York (SUNY) in Stony Brook, Long Island. After completing his undergraduate studies in music at New York University, David went on to work as an ophthalmic technician while he completed his pre-medical coursework at Hunter College in Manhattan. He will begin his residency training in ophthalmology in the summer of 2019.

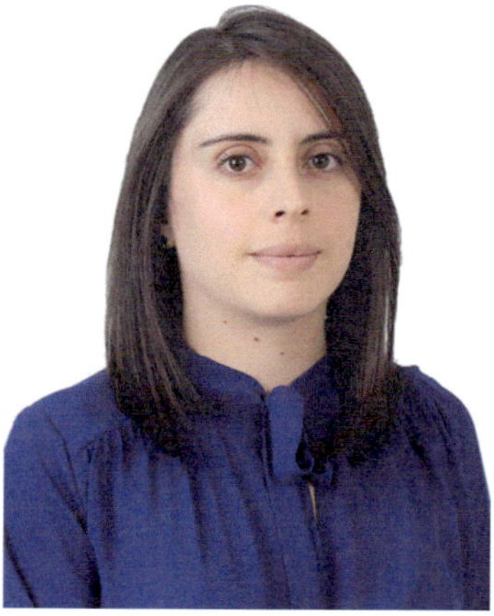

Maria Cristina Gabela-Gabela, MD Medical degree from Universidad San Francisco, Quito, Ecuador, Ophthalmology residency program at Fundación Oftalmologica Nacional, Bogota, Colombia, Retina fellow at Fundación Oftalmologica Nacional, Bogota, Colombia.

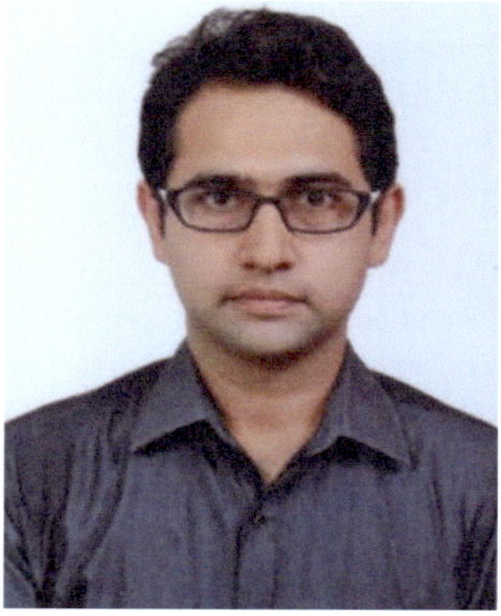

Uppal V. Gandhi is currently doing his fellowship in Pediatric ophthalmology, Strabismus and Neuroophthalmology.

His research interest is primarily in nystagmus, imaging in optic disc disorders and few special types of strabismus like MED and TED. He has 2 publications so far.

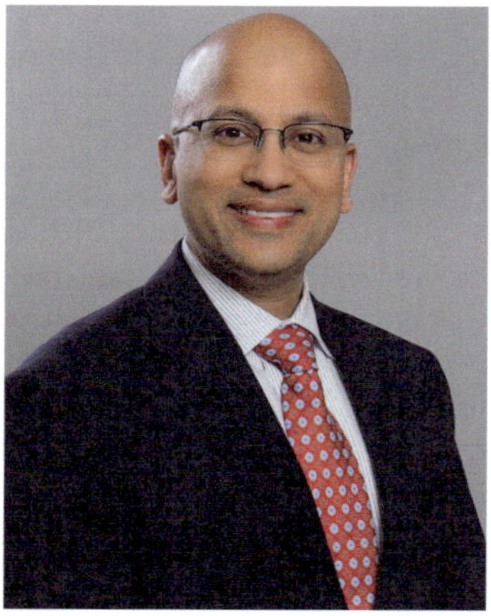

Sunir Garg, MD, FACS is professor of ophthalmology on the Retina Service of Wills Eye Hospital, Thomas Jefferson University, Philadelphia, Pennsylvania. He is a member of the Retina Society, the Macula Society, and the American Society of Retina Specialists.

His research interest is primarily in macular degeneration, diabetic retinopathy, uveitis, and vitreoretinal surgery

He has published over 200 peer-reviewed and non-peer-reviewed papers and is editor or co-editor of three textbooks. He is the editor-in-chief for *Retina Times*, the official publication of the American Society of Retina Specialists. He has received an Achievement Award from the American Academy of Ophthalmology and a Senior Honor Award from the American Society of Retina Specialists.

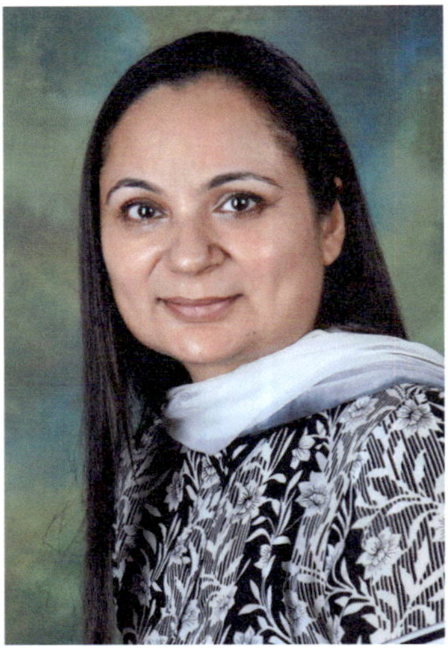

Dr. Vishali Gupta is a Professor in Ophthalmology in the Retina and Uveitis Services of Advanced Eye Center, Post Graduate Institute of Medical Education and Research (PGIMER), Chandigarh, India. She runs a busy uveitis clinic where nearly 300 uveitis patients are examined per week. Her research interests include addressing the diagnostic challenges involving intraocular tuberculosis, application of molecular biology techniques to diagnose intraocular tuberculosis, describing the phenotypic expression of the disease and the management strategies. Dr. Gupta has over 194 indexed publications and authored more than 76 chapters and 3 books. She is a much sought-after international speaker and delivered several keynote lectures. Prof. Gupta is currently the Vice President of the Uveitis Society of India and the Principal Investigator of the Collaborative Ocular Tuberculosis Study Group (COTS) with over 25 international centers participating in the study.

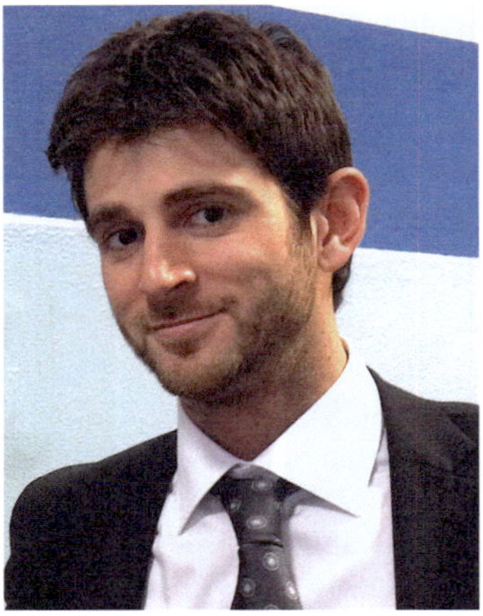

Dr. Alessandro Invernizzi graduated in medicine in 2007 and completed his specialization in ophthalmology in 2012 at the University of Milan. Since his last years of residency, he developed special interest in imaging, medical retina, and uveitis. He spent about 1 year in India, at the PGIMER institute (Chandigarh), in order to increase his knowledge on infectious and tropical diseases. Since 2013 he works as a consultant for the Retina Unit at the Eye Clinic of Luigi Sacco Hospital in Milan, and he is in charge of the Uveitis Service. Alessandro is part of international research groups such as the Collaborative Ocular Tuberculosis Study Group, and he has published more than 40 papers on peer-reviewed journals. Since June 2016, Alessandro is assistant professor at the Eye Clinic at the Department of Biomedical and Clinical Science "Luigi Sacco," University of Milan.

His research is mainly focused on imaging, medical retina, and uveitis.

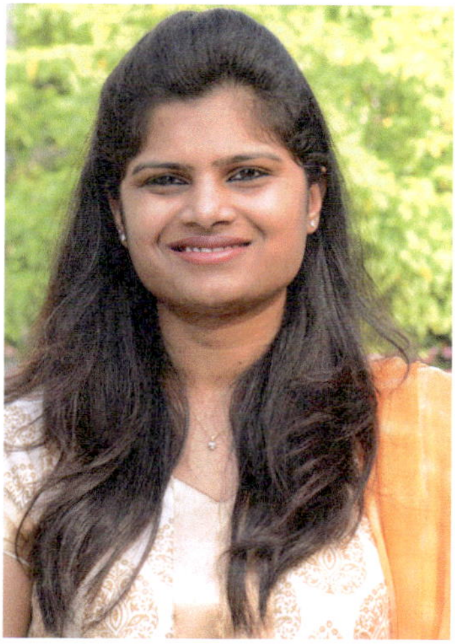

Swathi Kaliki, MD is a trained ocular oncologist and currently heads the Ocular Oncology Unit at the Operation Eyesight Universal Institute for Eye Cancer at the reputed L. V. Prasad Eye Institute, Hyderabad, India. She has lectured at various prestigious national and international forums and has published extensively on various ocular and adnexal tumors including eyelid sebaceous gland carcinoma, ocular surface squamous neoplasia, retinoblastoma, ocular melanoma, and various other eye tumors.

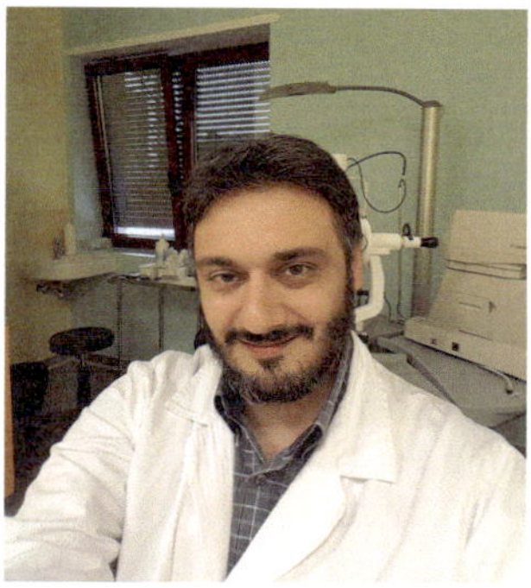

Andrea Mazzaferro is an ophthalmologist who is practicing at the Policlinico San Pietro (Ponte San Pietro, Bergamo, Italy) with particular interest in general ophthalmology, medical retina, and surgery of the anterior segment.

He graduated at the University of Messina and specialized with honors at the University of Palermo. He attended a fellowship in Medical Retina with Prof. Giuseppe Querques at the San Raffaele Hospital in Milan, headed by Prof. Bandello.

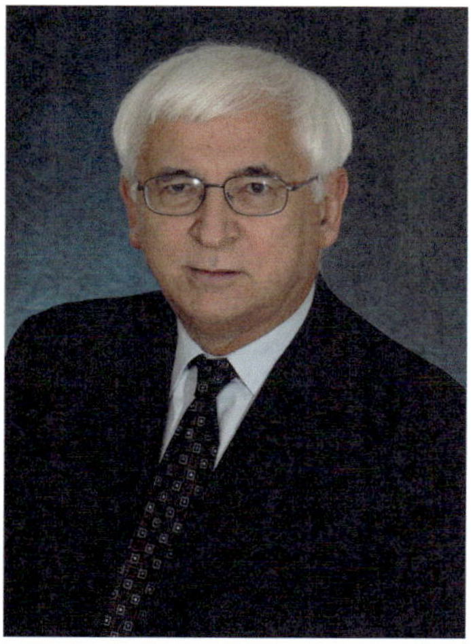

Dr. William F. Mieler is the Cless Family professor of ophthalmology and vice-chairman for education in the Department of Ophthalmology and Visual Sciences at the University of Illinois at Chicago (UIC), Chicago, IL. He also serves as the residency program director and as the director of vitreoretinal fellowship training. Dr. Mieler recently received the UIC 2016 College of Medicine Faculty of the Year Award. His specialty areas include diseases and surgery of the retina and vitreous, along with ocular oncology.

Dr. Mieler received his doctorate of medicine degree at the University of Wisconsin-Madison School of Medicine (1979). After completion of his internship at Mercy Hospital and Medical Center in San Diego, CA (1980), he completed his 3-year ophthalmology residency at the Bascom Palmer Eye Institute, University of Miami, Miami, FL (1980–1983). This was followed by a 1-year vitreoretinal fellowship at the Eye Institute, Medical College of Wisconsin, Milwaukee, WI (1983–1984). He then returned to the Bascom Palmer Eye Institute where he served as chief resident and clinical instructor (1984–1985). Dr. Mieler then completed a second fellowship in ocular oncology at Wills Eye Hospital, Thomas Jefferson University, Philadelphia, PA (1985). In 1985, he joined the full-time faculty at the Medical College of Wisconsin, where he became professor of ophthalmology (1992) and was awarded the Jack A. and Elaine D. Klieger chair in ophthalmology (1998). Dr. Mieler then joined the faculty at the Baylor College of Medicine, in Houston, TX, as professor of ophthalmology (1999–2004). He then accepted the position of professor and chairman of the Department of Ophthalmology at the University of Chicago (2004–2008), prior to his current position at the University of Illinois at Chicago (2008–present).

Dr. Mieler has authored or co-authored 350 scientific papers, 85 book chapters, and 7 textbooks, including *The Retinal Atlas*, 2nd edition (2017), along with presenting 25 named lectures. He is/has been the principal investigator or co-investigator of more than 60 scientific grants and collaborative studies. He has served the American Board of Ophthalmology (ABO) as a board director (1998–2005), as chairman of the board (2005), as associate executive director (2006), and as emeritus director (2006–present). He also served on several committees with the American Board of Medical Specialties (ABMS). Dr. Mieler is also the past president of the Macula Society (2003–2004), and he received the Gass Medal (2013). He has served on the executive committees of the Retina Society and the American Society of Retina Specialists (ASRS). In 2011, he was named recipient of the Founders Award by the ASRS. He is a past member of the Pan-American Board of Directors (2001–2008), and he has chaired the PAAO Foundation Grants Committee (2006–2011). Dr. Mieler has served on the ARVO Board of Trustees (2010–2016), representing the Retina Section, and was president of ARVO (2014–2015). He received the Distinguished Service Award from ARVO (2016). He has served on the editorial board of the *Archives of Ophthalmology, RETINA*, and *Current Eye Research* and currently serves on the editorial board of the *Asia-Pacific Journal of Ophthalmology* and the *American Journal of Ophthalmology Case Reports.* He also serves as a scientific reviewer for 34 additional scientific journals. From the American Academy of Ophthalmology (AAO), he has received the Honor Award (1992), the Lifelong Education for the Ophthalmologist Award (2000), the Senior Honor Award (2001), and the Life Achievement Honor Award (2011). He also has served as a member of the AAO Council (2001–2008) and the EyeNet Editorial Advisory Board (2003–2007) and is the chair of the Schepens Award (2007–2010). He also has served the AAO as a media spokesman, as a member of the CME Committee, and as associate secretary for the AAO Subspecialty Day programs (2011–2015). Most recently, he was elected to serve on the AAO Board of Trustees (2017–2020).

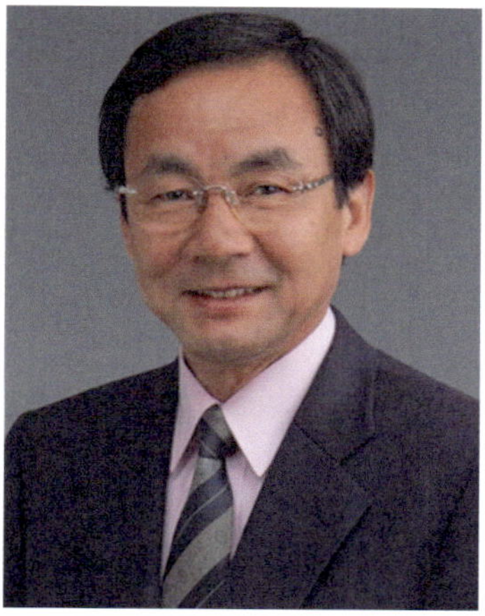

Dr. Manabu Mochizuki, MD, PhD was born in 1947 and completed his medical education at Kyushu University School of Medicine in 1973 and residency in ophthalmology at Tokyo University Hospital (1973–1974). He was assigned associate professor of the Department of Ophthalmology at Tokyo University (1986–1990), professor and chairman of the Department of Ophthalmology at Kurume University (1990–1998), professor and chairman of the Department of Ophthalmology and Visual Science at Tokyo Medical and Dental University (TMDU) (1990–2013), and emeritus professor of TMUD (2013–present).

Dr. Mochizuki is an internationally well-recognized expert in ocular inflammation, immunology, infection, and pharmacology. He is author and co-author of over 600 scientific publications and gave many named lectures and symposia. He organized the 3rd International Ocular Inflammation Society (IOIS) Congress in 1994 in Fukuoka, Japan.

He was the president of the Japanese Ocular Inflammation Society (2007–2013), the president of the Japanese Ocular Pharmacological Society (2008–2010) and Council of Japan Ophthalmological Society (1995–2017), a founding member and general secretary of the International Ocular Inflammation Society (IOIS) (1994–1998; 2011–2015), an ARVO gold fellow since 2010, an ARVO program committee member (2010–2012), and a member of the International Uveitis Study Group (IUSG), American Uveitis Society, International Society for Eye Research (ISER), and many other international scientific societies.

Dr. Mochizuki is co-editor of the *Japanese Journal of Ophthalmology* (2009–2014), member of the editorial board of the *Journal of Ophthalmic Inflammation and Infection* and *Ocular Immunology and Inflammation* and advisory board member of *Progress in Retinal and Eye Research*.

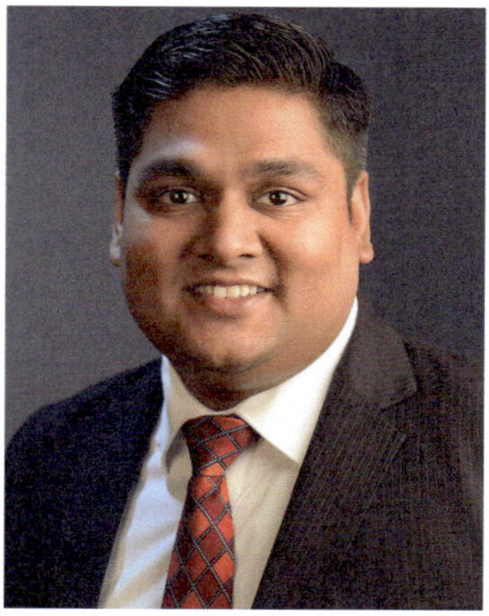

Akshay Gopinathan Nair received his medical degree from Maharashtra University of Health Sciences in 2007 and completed his residency training in ophthalmology from Sankara Nethralaya in Chennai, India. Following this, he underwent fellowship training in ophthalmic plastic surgery, ocular oncology, and facial aesthetics at L. V. Prasad Eye Institute, Hyderabad. Dr. Nair also completed his ICO fellowship in oculoplastic surgery at the New York Eye and Ear Infirmary of Mount Sinai, USA.

Dr. Nair has over 60 peer-reviewed publications in indexed journals and 9 book chapters and has delivered over 70 presentations at various scientific meets and forums. He has been awarded the best paper in neuro-ophthalmology at the All India Ophthalmological Conference in 2011, the Kanthimathinathan Gold Medal for the best graduating resident, and the best poster award at the American Academy of Ophthalmology Meet in 2013 at New Orleans. His areas of special interest are ocular surface and eyelid tumors, ocular trauma, ophthalmic imaging, and neuroimaging.

Dr. Nair is a faculty member at Lokmanya Tilak Municipal Medical College, Mumbai, India, and is also affiliated with Advanced Eye Hospital and Institute in Navi Mumbai and Aditya Jyot Eye Hospital in Mumbai.

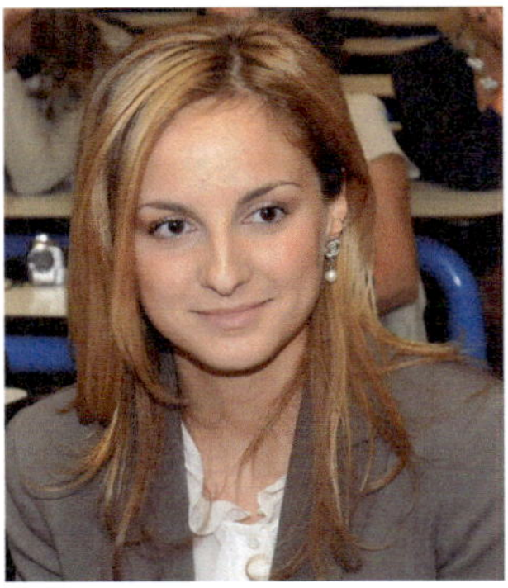

Maura Di Nicola, MD is a senior resident at Università degli Studi di Milano in Milan, Italy. She received her medical degree from Vita-Salute San Raffaele University in Milan, Italy. She has completed an Ocular Oncology Fellowship at Wills Eye Hospital under the direction of Drs. Carol and Jerry Shields in 2017. Her main clinical and research interests include ocular oncology and medical retina.

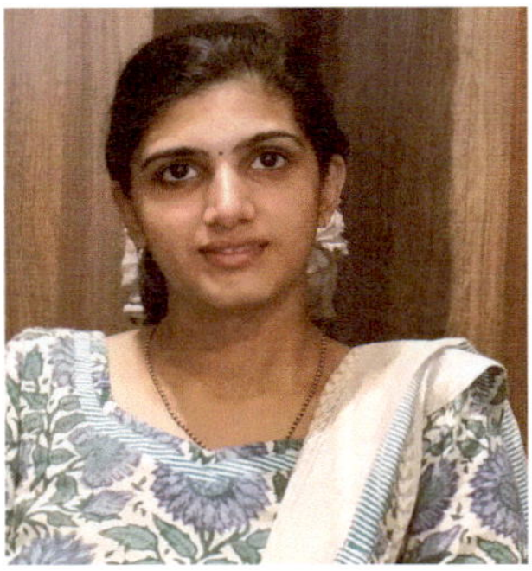

Dr. Remya Mareen Paulose is Consultant Vitreo- Retina surgeon in Little Flower Hospital and Research Center, Angamaly, Kerala, India.She has published 5 research papers in indexed journals.

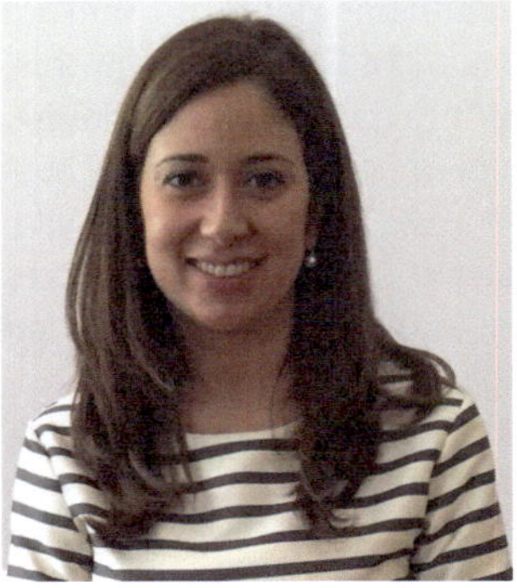

Lea Querques, MD is a Medical Retina Ophthalmologist at University Vita-Salute, IRCCS Ospedale San Raffaele, Milan, Italy. Her main topic of interest is Medical Retina. She has a been resident at the same University and has trained in Creteil, Paris (France) during her residency. Doctor Querques has contributed to more than 90 peer-reviewed articles and various book chapters published mainly in the areas of Medical Retina (age-related macular degeneration, retinal vascular diseases, hereditary retinal diseases, vitreoretinal surgery).

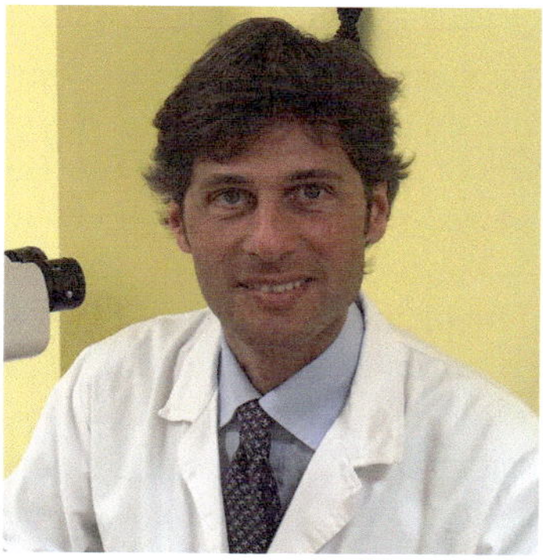

Giuseppe Querques, MD, PhD is associate professor at Vita-Salute San Raffaele University, IRCCS Ospedale San Raffaele, Milan, Italy. His main topics are medical retina and ophthalmic surgery (retina and cataract). Dr. Querques has contributed to more than 300 peer-reviewed articles published mainly in the areas of medical retina (age-related macular degeneration, retinal vascular diseases, hereditary retinal diseases, ophthalmic genetics). His current main area of both clinical and laboratory research is focusing on the diagnosis (imaging) and treatment of age-related macular degeneration, retinal vascular diseases, and hereditary retinal diseases. Dr. Querques is a member of the Italian Society of Ophthalmology (SOI), the French Society of Ophthalmology (SFO), the European Society of Retina Specialists (EURETINA), the American Academy of Ophthalmology (AAO), the Association for Research in Vision and Ophthalmology (ARVO), the Retina Society, the Club Jules Gonin, and the Macula Society.

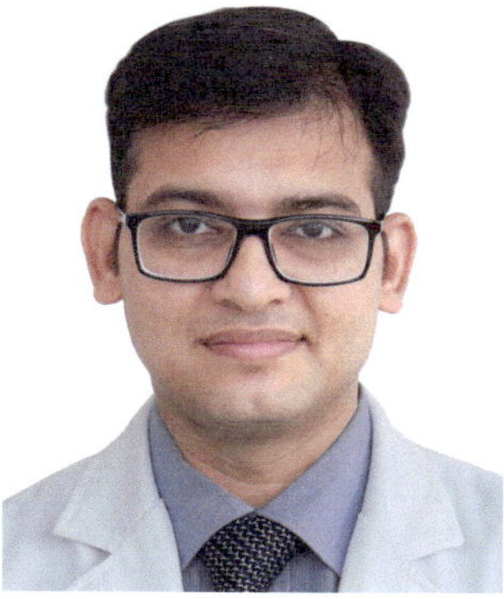

Nishant Radke is a Senior Consultant and International Faculty, Department of Retina and Vitreous Services at C-MER (Shenzhen) Dennis Lam Eye Hospital at present. He has done his Master's from the WHO Upgraded Regional Institute of Ophthalmology, Raipur. Thereafter, he completed his clinical fellowship in Retina and Vitreous at Shri Bhagwan Mahavir Vitreoretinal services, Sankara Nethralaya, Chennai. He has presented 17 Papers at State, National, and International conferences and 10 Posters as the chief author. Besides this, he has been a co-author for 3 other paper presentations at the National conferences. He has 18 Indexed publications and 4 non-indexed publications so far. He has received the Best Free paper by Resident award in 2007 in the annual state conference and was the winner of the Trauma session at AIOC 2009. He has been a runner-up in the poster competition held by SN-ARVO in 2011 and has also received Certificate of Appreciation from International Society of Ophthalmology at Hong Kong 2012. He is a life member of AIOS, ROS, VRSI, OTSI, DOS, USI, Sankara Nethralaya Alumni, CGOS, and RDOS.

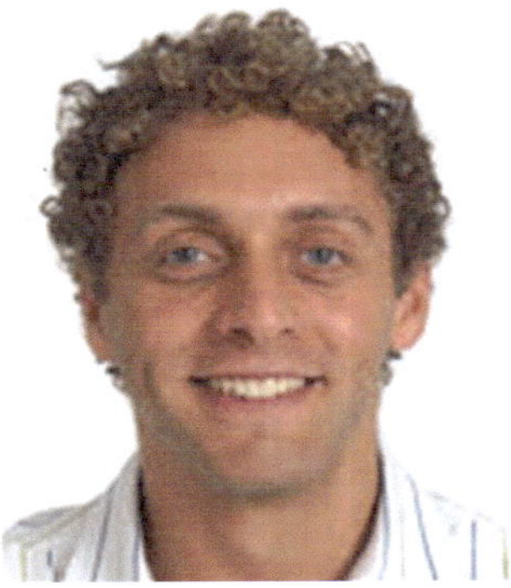

Sherief Raouf received his Bachelor of Arts and Sciences Degree from Swarthmore College and subsequently completed his medical degree from Stony Brook University School of Medicine in 2017. He will complete his residency training in Ophthalmology at the North Shore University Hospital of the Hofstra Northwell School of Medicine.

Dr. Raouf has contributed to over a dozen peer-reviewed publications, scientific book chapters and presentations at academic conferences in Ophthalmology. He was awarded the 2016 Best Poster in Neuro-ophthalmology at the annual conference of the American Academy of Ophthalmology in Chicago, Illinois. Thus far, his areas of particular interest are vitreoretinal vascular pathology and neuro-ophthalmologic imaging.

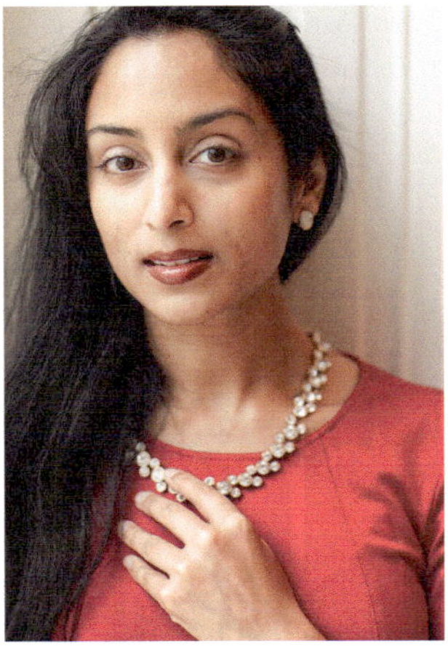

Dr. Ashvini Reddy is an assistant professor of ophthalmology at the Wilmer Eye Institute. Her specialties include ocular immunology, such as uveitis and ocular inflammatory diseases, and the medical treatment of retinal diseases. Dr. Reddy's research interests include autoimmune retinal diseases, outer retinopathies, intraocular lymphoma and infectious uveitis.

In her spare time, she also contributes to the general press and has developed articles on evolving ethical issues in ophthalmology as an editor of the American Medical Association's official ethics journals, Virtual Mentor and the Journal of Ethics. Dr. Reddy currently serves on the American Academy of Ophthalmology's Online Education Committee and is a member of multiple medical societies, including the American Uveitis Society and American Society of Retina Specialists.

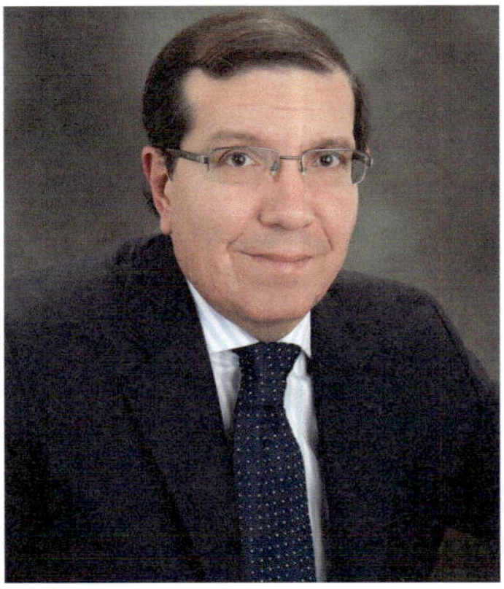

Francisco J. Rodriguez, MD Chairman, Fundación Oftalmologica Nacional, Director, Department of Ophthalmology, Universidad del Rosario – School of Medicine, Bogota, Colombia.

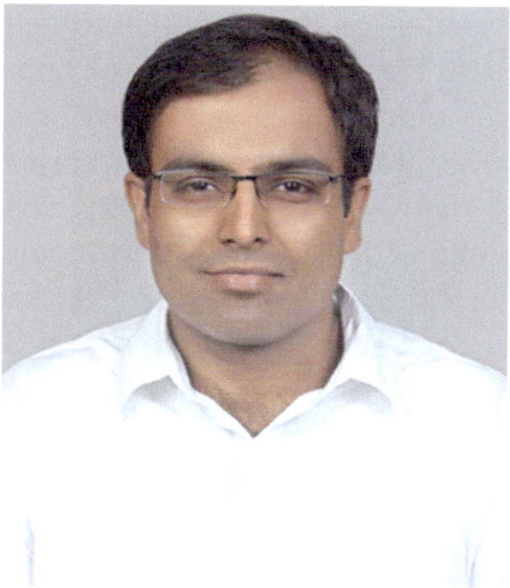

Dr. Hitesh R. Sharma has done his M.S. in ophthalmology at the Institute of Medical Sciences, Banaras Hindu University, located at Varanasi, India. He has done his fellowship in medical retina and uvea at the renowned Sankara Nethralaya, Chennai. He has some good publications to his credit and has written a few chapters in ophthalmology textbooks. He has presented various papers and posters at conferences. He has special interest in ocular tuberculosis and Vogt-Koyanagi-Harada disease. He is currently attached to Aditya Jyot Eye Hospital at Mumbai as a medical retina and uvea expert.

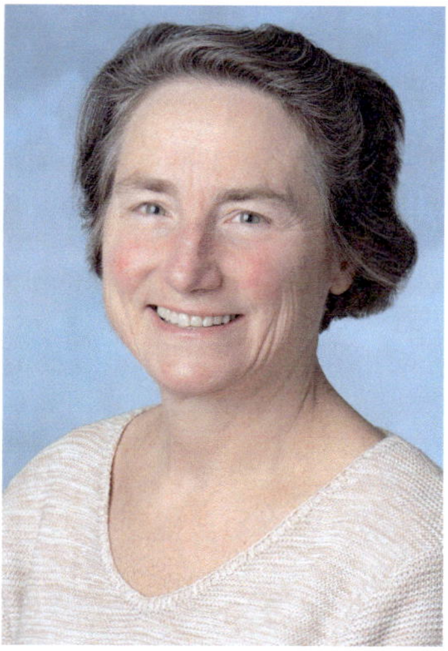

Carol L. Shields, MD Born in Sharon, Pennsylvania, Dr. Carol Shields attended the University of Notre Dame for undergraduate pre-medical studies and played 4 years of Varsity basketball on the Women's basketball team, serving as captain for 3 years. She completed her medical school at the University of Pittsburgh and residency in ophthalmology at Wills Eye Hospital in Philadelphia in 1987. She subsequently completed fellowship training in ocular oncology, oculoplastic surgery, and ophthalmic pathology.

Dr. Carol Shields is currently the Director of the Oncology Service, Wills Eye Hospital, and Professor of Ophthalmology at Thomas Jefferson University in Philadelphia.

Dr. Carol Shields has authored or coauthored 12 textbooks, over 1600 articles in major peer-reviewed journals, over 320 textbook chapters, given over 800 lectureships, and has received numerous professional awards. Some of her awards include The Byron Kanaley Award (1979) given to the top student-athlete at the University of Notre Dame (she was the first woman to receive this award) and The Donders Award (2003) given by the Netherlands Ophthalmological Society every 5 years to an ophthalmologist worldwide who has contributed extensively to the field of ophthalmology. She received an Honorary Doctorate of Science Degree from the University of Notre Dame (2005) and Catholic University (2011). She was bestowed the American Academy of Ophthalmology Life Achievement Honor Award (2011) and induction into the Academic All-American Hall of Fame (2011) for lifetime success in athleticism and career. She was the President of the International Society of Ocular Oncology (2013–2015)—this is the largest international society for study of ocular tumors. She was the first elected

President of this society. Dr. Shields has also been cited on the Ophthalmology Power List—nominated by peers as one of the top 100 leaders in the field of ophthalmology in 2014 and 2016. She is a member of numerous ocular oncology, pathology, and retina societies and has delivered 52 named lectures in America and abroad. She has been active in the American Academy of Ophthalmology. She serves on the editorial board of several journals including JAMA Ophthalmology, Retina, Journal of Pediatric Ophthalmology and Strabismus, Ophthalmic Plastic and Reconstructive Surgery, and International Journal of Clinical Oncology.

Dr. Carol Shields practices ocular oncology on a full-time basis with her husband, Dr. Jerry Shields and associates on the Oncology Service at Wills Eye Hospital. She and her husband Jerry are the parents of 7 children, ranging from ages 17 to 29 years.

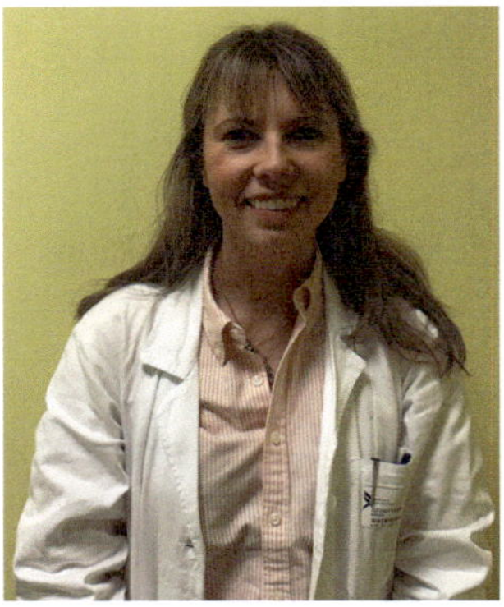

Ilaria Zucchiatti is consultant in Medical Retina & Imaging Unit of the Department of Ophthalmology, University Vita-Salute, Scientific Institute San Raffaele (Milan, Italy). She obtained her medical degree at the Università degli Studi di Padova (Italy) and her specialization in Ophthalmology at the Department of Ophthalmology, University Vita-Salute, Scientific Institute San Raffaele (Milan, Italy). Dr Zucchiatti published 34 articles on Pub-Med journals mainly related to retinal diseases and is co-author of two books. She had experience as study coordinator, visual acuity examiner, OCT operator and injecting physician in several clinical trials performed following ICH/GCP and mainly concerning Age Related Macular Degeneration and Diabetic Retinopathy.

Neurological Diseases

1

Uppal Gandhi, Preeti Patil Chhablani, Akshay G. Nair, and Jay Chhablani

Abstract

Imaging has become an integral part of the management of retinal diseases. Being window to the brain, imaging of the posterior segment is useful in evaluating neurological diseases. These imaging findings are used for early diagnosis to correlate with severity of the disease and to monitor progression. This chapter describes important findings on imaging modalities in neurological disease and their clinical implications.

1.1 Introduction

The eyes are the windows to the brain. Various neurological diseases affect eyes, and in many of them, they provide the first clue to the systemic disease. In many, other than clinical follow-up, there is no marker for severity of the disease.

The understanding of individual layers of the retina and choroid has been improved significantly with advanced imaging modalities. Optical coherence tomography (OCT) is now able to provide in vivo histological images of the retina

U. Gandhi • P.P. Chhablani (✉)
Jasti V Ramanamma Children's Eye Care Centre, L. V. Prasad Eye Institute, Kallam Anji Reddy Campus, L.V. Prasad Marg, Banjara Hills, Hyderabad 500 034, Andhra Pradesh, India
e-mail: drpreetipatil@gmail.com

A.G. Nair
Ophthalmic Plastic Surgery and Ocular Oncology Services, Advanced Eye Hospital and Institute, Navi Mumbai, India

J. Chhablani
Smt.Kanuri Santhamma Retina Vitreous Centre, L. V. Prasad Eye Institute, Kallam Anji Reddy Campus, L.V. Prasad Marg, Banjara Hills, Hyderabad 500 034, Andhra Pradesh, India

J. Chhablani et al. (eds.), *Retinal and Choroidal Imaging in Systemic Diseases*,
https://doi.org/10.1007/978-981-10-5461-7_1

and choroid. There are multiple reports on OCT findings in these neurological diseases ranging from the commonly occurring diseases like Parkinson's disease and Alzheimer's disease to the rarer disorders like schizophrenia. OCT findings have been reported to be beneficial in early diagnosis of neurological diseases as well as to understand and follow the course of these diseases.

This chapter summarizes the important and useful OCT findings of the retina reported in various neurological diseases and their clinical applications.

1.1.1 Alzheimer's Disease

Alzheimer's disease (AD) is the most common cause of dementia among the numerous causes, and its incidence increases exponentially with age. AD is primarily a disease of the brain. Besides cognitive abnormalities, various visual function impairments are noted including color perception, depth perception, contrast sensitivity, and visual field measures, these being the common complaints which have shown to decrease the quality of life of the patients even at the early stage of the disease [1]. Earlier these were believed to be due to the malfunction of the central visual pathways [2, 3]; however, Hinton et al. [4] showed that these changes could be due to the axonal degeneration of optic nerves in patients with AD.

It is a well-known fact that the retina is an extension of the brain, derived from the neural tube like other structures of the brain [5], and various studies have shown the eye especially the retina to be involved in AD [4, 6, 7].

Accumulation of intracellular neurofibrillary tangles of hyperphosphorylated tau protein and extracellular amyloid β protein deposits (Aβ) trigger inflammation in the brain. This inflammation could cause thinning of retinal ganglion layer, as the retina and brain share similar responses to inflammation [8]. Such stress situations are particularly relevant to the exposed and metabolically sensitive retinal ganglion cells (RGC) and photoreceptor cells. Interestingly, in 2008, both the retinal and choroidal vascular Aβ deposits were reported in animal models of AD [9]. This lead to the use of optical coherence tomography to study these changes in the retina in patients with AD.

Iseri et al. demonstrated a relation between reduction in macular volume and the severity of cognitive impairment using time-domain OCT [7]. Due to limitations of the device, changes in the individual layer were not possible to be evaluated. Few studies found this thinning of inner layers as diffuse or localized (superior or both superior and inferior quadrants) [10, 11]. While correlating thinning of the retinal nerve fiber layer (RNFL) with cognitive impairment, Kromer et al. [12] showed that the global thinning of RNFL had fairly low MMSE (mini-mental state examination (MMSE) or Folstein test) scores ranging from 11 to 19 and from 8 to 28. MMSE score greater than 27 out of 30 suggests normal cognition. However, Berisha et al. reported MMSE scores between 17 and 30 in subjects with RNFL thinning only in the superior sector. Furthermore, the superior sector could be used to discriminate between mild cognitive impairment and severe Alzheimer's disease [12], while there was no significant difference found between the RNFL thickness of mild cognitive impairment and mild Alzheimer's disease patients.

Histologic studies showed 52% decrease in neuronal density in Alzheimer's disease [13]. Bayhan et al. reported thinning of the ganglion cell thickness in individuals with Alzheimer's disease leading to thinning of the macular thickness with no significant change in outer retinal thickness [14]. In this study, the scan was performed primarily on the temporal part of the fovea to achieve more information, which is the most commonly involved area in Alzheimer's disease. They also found a significant correlation between the macular ganglion cell thickness and MMSE scores. In regard to retinal function, Berisha et al. showed a correlation between the RNFL thickness and a number of pattern-electroretinogram characteristics, especially with the P50-N95 amplitude, but not with visual-evoked potentials [15].

Marziani et al. used two instruments (RT-Vue® and Spectralis®) to evaluate RNFL in Alzheimer's disease. RT-Vue® measures RNFL and ganglion cell layer (GCL) together and the Spectralis® permits the quantification of the RNFL separately [16]. They reported reduction in only the inner layers (RNFL and RNFL and GCL combined) in Alzheimer's disease. However, they were unable to determine which layer either RNFL or GCL was most affected in Alzheimer's disease.

Larrosa et al. evaluated diagnostic ability of standard OCT parameters using linear discriminant functions (LDFs), and logistic regression statistical analysis, to detect the presence of Alzheimer's disease [17]. LDFs had two parts: retinal LDF were obtained using information from the nine early treatment diabetic retinopathy study (ETDRS) area thicknesses. Peripapillary LDFs were obtained using 768 points in peripapillary scan (grouped to obtain 24 uniformly divided locations). They reported that the retina LDFs had only moderate diagnostic accuracy, while the RNFL LDFs were a very useful and precise tool for diagnosis of Alzheimer's disease. The LDFs were sensitive and specific as the methods currently used for Alzheimer's disease diagnosis.

To sum up, many studies have reported a significant decrease in the mean overall RNFL thickness in patients with AD, and some have reported significant reductions in the individual quadrants. The superior and inferior quadrants demonstrating the greatest thinning in patients with AD compared with healthy controls in most studies, whereas the nasal and temporal quadrants are only found to be significantly thinner in few studies [18].

A meta-analysis done in 2015, based on 11 studies, suggested that AD patients are likely to have a reduced RNFL thickness as assessed by OCT. This reduction in RNFL thickness, as observed in most studies on AD patients, was significantly greater than that observed in the age-matched controls and thus cannot be exclusively ascribed to aging [19]. Further, the analysis showed a uniform significant decrease in RNFL thickness in each of the four retinal quadrants, suggesting that whatever factors that cause the degenerative process in AD progression affects the entire retinal layer.

Thus to conclude, the OCT technique for measurement of the peripapillary RNFL and macular thickness is useful for the potential correlation with the severity of the disease which in turn could help in early diagnosis of the disease.

1.1.2 Parkinson's Disease

Parkinson's disease (PD) is a degenerative disorder of the central nervous system, secondary to death of pigmented dopamine neurons in the substantia nigra of the midbrain, caused by the accumulation of the protein alpha-synuclein in neuronal Lewy bodies [20]. Parkinson's disease is also associated with loss of dopaminergic neurons such as retinal amacrine cells leading to thinning of retinal ganglion cells. It also leads to loss of similar neurons in the higher visual areas (e.g., lateral geniculate nucleus, cholinergic nucleus basalis of Meynert, and visual cortex) [21]. Levodopa, a dopamine precursor, is released by human retinal pigment epithelial (RPE) cells [22, 23]. Looking at it differently, the dopamine loss in patients with PD may be in part because of the thinning of the RPE [24].

Motor-related problems are the usual features seen in the early disease and cognitive and behavioral ailments occurring in the late stages. Affected foveal vision with decreased contrast sensitivity and color vision and altered visual-evoked potentials in patients with PD have been described previously. These have been attributed to the dysfunction of the intraretinal dopaminergic circuitry and final retinal output to the brain [25, 26].

These changes in the retinal layers are thought to be of help in early diagnosing of a case of PD. Multiple studies have reported RNFL changes in PD [24, 27–29].

Using time-domain OCT, La Morgia et al. reported significantly thinner temporal RNFL in patients with PD compared to controls [30]. Using spectral domain (SD)-OCT, Aaker et al. reported significant thinning in macular thickness [31]. However, there was no significant reduction in peripapillary RNFL and inner retinal layer thickness between PD patients and controls. In contrast, Garcia-Martin et al. showed a reduction in both macular and RNFL measurements [32].

Garcia-Martin et al. used "Nsite Axonal Analytics" application of Heidelberg to detect changes due to PD [33]. As reported previously in Alzheimer's disease and multiple sclerosis, they formulated retinal LDF, which had sensitivity of 89.5%. They reported that the likelihood ratio value of 4.59 for retinal LDF rules out the chances of having PD. They recommended SD-OCT as a reliable diagnostic tool for subclinical PD diagnosis.

In conclusion, PD is still a commonly encountered disease among aging population, but the accuracy of the clinical diagnosis of PD is still limited. Especially in the early stages, when cardinal symptoms are not conclusive, diagnosis can be delayed as structural neuroimaging methods such as CCT or MRI do not provide characteristic features that allow the diagnosis of this chronic neurodegenerative disorder [34]. Apart from the early diagnosis of PD, serial RNFL recordings can be done to monitor the progression of the disease as well. Recently in a meta-analysis of 13 case-control studies done by Ji-guo Yu et al. in 2016, it was concluded that the RNFL thickness decreased in all quadrants in PD patients compared with the healthy control group and that the OCT can be useful in monitoring the disease progression [35].

1.1.3 Migraine

Migraine is a widely encountered condition in the general population. According to data from the American Migraine Prevalence and Prevention study, the cumulative lifetime incidence of migraine was reported to be 43% in women and 18% in men [36].

Ophthalmologists are often the first to evaluate the patients with migraine due to the accompanying ocular complaints like periorbital pain, photophobia, and other visual disturbances.

Although there are a considerable number of studies and theories on the pathophysiology of migraine, the exact nature of the condition is still considered to be unknown [37]. Currently, migraine is accepted as a neurovascular syndrome resulting from the activation of the nociceptors that innervate the meningeal blood vessels.

Recent reports have demonstrated direct electrophysiological evidence for the activation of trigeminovascular neurons during a migraine attack. The dura mater is largely innervated by the sensory nerve fibers originating from the trigeminal ganglion. Sensorial innervation of the eye is also supplied by the trigeminal nerve. Long and short ciliary nerves, which originate from the ophthalmic division of the trigeminal nerve, innervate various structures in the eye Short ciliary nerves also carry autonomic nerve fibers, which innervate the choroidal vasculature [38, 39].

Tan et al. reported no reduction in RNFL thickness in migraine patients with or without aura compared to healthy individuals [40]. Martinez et al. reported no difference in mean RNFL thickness between patients with migraine and healthy controls except in the temporal quadrant [41]. Gippono et al. found no difference in the foveal thickness and macular volume in females with migraine compared to healthy women but found that there was a significant thinning in the RNFL thickness in the upper quadrant [42]. Recently, Ekinci et al. reported significant thinning in RNFL and GCL in patients with migraine with aura in comparison to migraine patients without aura and the healthy controls [43].

In another recent study, Zeynep Dadaci et al. found that in patients with unilateral headaches, the choroidal thickness measurements obtained during the attack period were significantly increased only in the eyes on the headache side compared to basal levels. At the fovea, the choroidal thickness measured in the pain-free interval was 373.45 ± 76.47 μm (mean ± SD), which increased to 408.80 ± 77.70 μm during the attack period ($p < 0.001$).

The findings obtained from the various abovementioned studies can be valuable in understanding the pathophysiology of migraine and its association with normal tension glaucoma, better keeping in mind the common innervation of the meninges and the eye by the trigeminal nerve.

1.1.4 Schizophrenia

Schizophrenia is among the top ten leading causes of disease-related disability in the world because of the pervasiveness of associated deficits and frequently lifelong course.

It is a chronic and relapsing illness with generally incomplete remissions. It is characterized by an admixture of positive, negative, cognitive and mood symptoms [44]. Schizophrenia has been associated with deficits in visual perception and processing [45, 46]. Dopamine is established to be a major neurotransmitter and modulator in the retina by Djamgoz et al. [47] and may be responsible for these visual changes in neurodegenerative diseases. But unlike Parkinson's disease wherein dopamine levels are reduced, in schizophrenia these levels are raised. Possibly excess glutamate leading to neural excitotoxicity could be contributory to the neurodegenerative process of schizophrenia [48]. Glutamate has been shown to act as a neurotoxin, which exerts its toxic effect causing destruction of retinal ganglion cells [49]. Retina lacks myelin; hence, any changes in retina reflect axonal damage following any brain tissue damage [44].

Putting all this together, structural changes in the retina specifically RNFL changes are expected in these patients. Only few studies have been done in schizophrenic patients to evaluate the RNFL changes so far.

The first study done in 2010 by Francisco J. et al. reported that schizophrenic patients showed a statistically significant reduction of the overall RNFL thickness (95 ± 13 μm) compared with those values observed in control eyes (103 ± 8 μm) and also observed reduced peripapillary RNFL thickness in nasal quadrant (75 ± 17 μm) when compared with controls (84 ± 10 μm). The remaining peripapillary RNFL quadrants, macular thickness, and volume did not reveal differences between both groups.

Another study by Chu EM et al. performed OCT in 38 schizophrenia, 11 schizoaffective disorder, and 40 matched healthy controls and found out that patients and controls had similar whole retina RNFL thickness ($p = 0.86$) and macular volume (MV) ($p = 0.64$), but RNFL in the right nasal quadrant of the schizoaffective group was thinner than in the schizophrenia group ($p = 0.02$).

Lee et al. studied the structural OCT parameters especially RNFL changes in schizophrenia patients in comparison to age-matched controls [44]. They looked at patients with variable duration of illness and found that chronic (2–10 years) and long-term chronic (>10 years) schizophrenic patients have a significant peripapillary RNFL thinning, macular thinning, and reduction of macula volume when compared to controls ($P < 0.001$), and these features correlated with the duration of illness. They advised that OCT can play a major role in detecting worsening of neuronal degeneration by measuring the RNFL thickness.

In conclusion, OCT can have a major role in detecting worsening of neuronal degeneration by measuring the RNFL thickness especially when used in correlation with MRI since the latter is an established method to know the progression of the disease by measuring the volumetric brain volume reduction. With more researches in the future, it is hoped that OCT can be a useful investigative tool in schizophrenia and can be used to monitor the progression of disease.

1.1.5 Multiple Sclerosis

Multiple sclerosis presents commonly as optic neuritis characterized by recent vision loss associated with visual field loss, color desaturation, and pain with eye movement. Most of the patients recover to normal visual acuity levels; however, the quality of the vision is affected.

Inner retinal layers have been evaluated extensively using OCT in multiple sclerosis. Walter et al. reported that multiple sclerosis eyes had significant thinning of the inner retinal layers RNFL, GCL, and IPL (inner plexiform layer) compared with disease-free control eyes. They also found the degree of thinning is much greater in eyes with optic neuritis compared to non-optic neuritis eyes [50] (Fig. 1). Additionally, they reported that the retinal GCL, IPL, and RNFL thinning in multiple sclerosis patients was strongly correlated with visual function, quality of

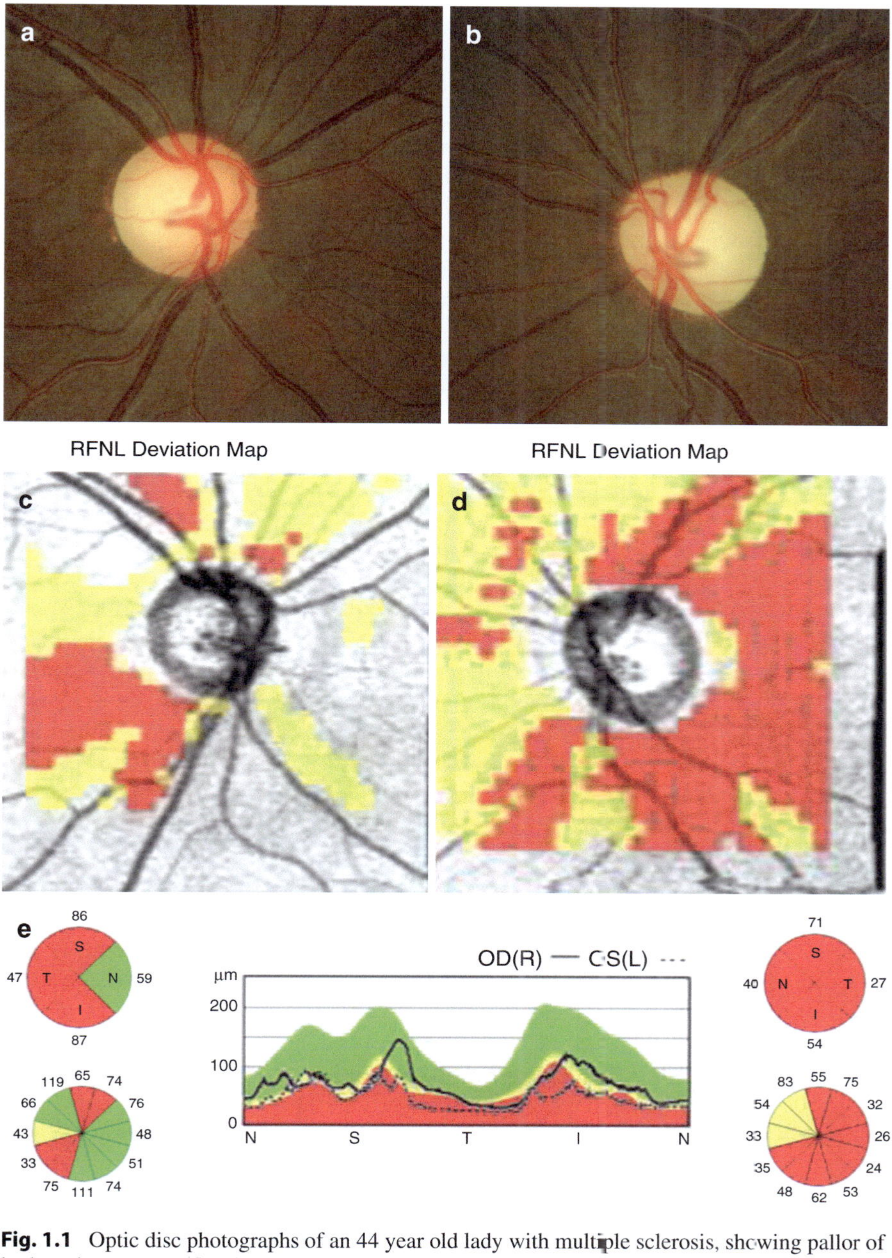

Fig. 1.1 Optic disc photographs of an 44 year old lady with multiple sclerosis, showing pallor of both optic nerves (**a**, **b**). OCT scans show advanced changes on the RNFL deviation maps (**c**, **d**) and severe RNFL thinning (**e**, **f**)

life, and disability tests such as high-contrast visual acuity (VA), low-contrast letter acuity (LCLA), National Eye Institute Visual Function Questionnaire (NEI-VFQ 25), and ten-item Neuro-Ophthalmic Supplement composite score [50]. Similarly, previous studies have shown significant peripapillary RNFL dropout in multiple sclerosis non-optic neuritis eyes [51–53].

Furthermore, non-optic neuritis eyes showed significant thinning of the macular RNFL with no difference in GCL, IPL, and other retinal layers when compared to controls. This could be due to subclinical episodes of optic neuritis or due to axonal loss with relative sparing of the retinal GCL [54, 55]. They suggested that GCL and IPL thickness measurement act as a potential structural marker of patient-reported visual disability. The literature suggests that thinning of GCL on OCT is similar to gray matter atrophy on magnetic resonance imaging (MRI) as the ganglion cells in the retina are analogous to gray matter in the brain [56, 57].

Burgansky-Eliash et al. reported a LDF using combinations of RNFL parameters obtained from Stratus OCT to evaluate the detection of perimetric glaucoma [58]. Similarly, Garcia-Martin et al. formulated LDF using peripapillary RNFL thickness parameters obtained from Spectralis® OCT system for the detection of multiple sclerosis [59]. They reported that the formulated LDF has the highest sensitivity (83.02%) and specificity compared to single RNFL parameter in detection of multiple sclerosis compared to controls. A likelihood ratio of higher than 3.14 for the LDF (cutoff point for 95% specificity) virtually rules out the chance of patient having multiple sclerosis.

Another additional tool was proposed by the same group using artificial neural networks (ANN) for RNFL parameters obtained by OCT. ANN are machine-learning algorithms that perform nonlinear classifications based on the representative and adequately large training data set. This approach produces robust classifiers which are insensitive to noise and outliers in the data [60]. They reported a combination of these RNFL thickness measurements from 24 locations in the peripapillary area. ANN technique offers better ability to detect RNFL damage than any single RNFL parameter. These techniques including LDF and ANN in combination with the other parameters and clinical explorations could be helpful with an early diagnosis or a no definitive multiple sclerosis diagnosis; however, further evaluation is warranted.

Overall, measurement of GCL and RNFL thicknesses by OCT may be a better way than brain MRI to detect and monitor axonal loss in multiple sclerosis, due to its easier acquisition, better resolution, and better correlation with visual functions [60].

1.2 Idiopathic Intracranial Hypertension

Idiopathic intracranial hypertension (IIH), also known as pseudotumor cerebri (PTC), is a clinical entity that presents with elevated intracranial pressure (ICP), usually seen in obese women of child-bearing age along with signs and symptoms of headaches, pulsatile tinnitus, visual changes, and papilledema [61]. Papilledema

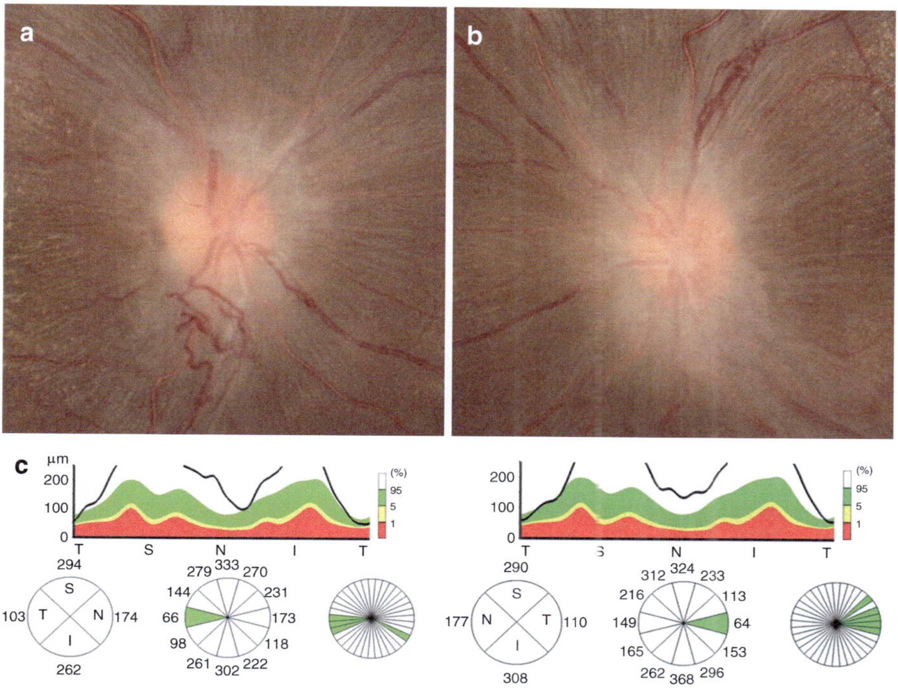

Fig. 1.2 Optic disc photo graphs showing disc edema (**a**, **b**) with blurring of the peripapillary retinal nerve fibre layer (RNFL), in a 19 year old lady, diagnosed with IIH with normal vision and color vision . The corresponding RNFL OCT (**c**) scan shows increased RNFL thickness

associated with subsequent visual field loss is a dreaded consequence, and this clinical presentation determines the management and outcome of IIH [62]. However, clinical evaluation of the disk and subjective evaluation using Frisen scale to evaluate longitudinal changes may be challenging [63].

The Frisen scale is a noncontinuous ordinal grading based on specific features described in fundus photographs or on ophthalmoscopy to assess and monitor the disk changes in papilledema [64]. However, this scale reportedly lacked sensitivity to small changes in the degree of disk edema and the interpretation varies among observers [65, 66]. OCT, on the other hand, quantitatively assesses the multiple layers of the retina, allowing objective measurement of the RNFL thickness, and thereby helps with evaluation of longitudinal changes (Figs. 2 and 3). Additionally, OCT offers several advantages over conventional photographic imaging such as ability to image eyes with small pupils and cataracts [66]. Patients with newly diagnosed IIH show RNFL thickening when compared to healthy controls. This RNFL thickness decreased over time with treatment of IIH. Therefore, RNFL thickness could be a potential longitudinal measure in the management of IIH [62, 67]. Wang et al. developed an automated method for the quantification of volumetric optic disk swelling on SD-OCT imaging in individuals with papilledema [68]. They further

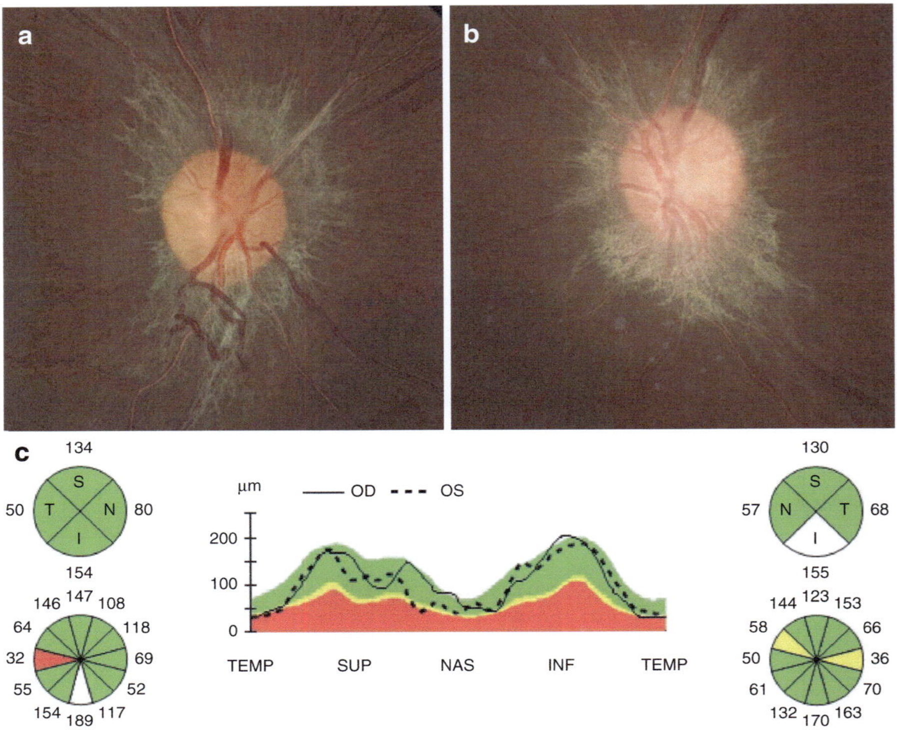

Fig. 1.3 Optic disc photo graphs (**a**, **b**) of the same patient showing a reduction disc edema with peripapillary gliosis, after 4 months of oral acetazolamide therapy. OCT (**c**) of the same patient shows a significant decrease in the RNFL thickness as compared to the earlier scan (Fig. 1) and is now within the normal range

investigated for correlation of volumetric measurements with Frisen scale grades (from fundus photographs) and two-dimensional RNFL and total retinal thickness measurements from SD-OCT. Their results suggested that volumetric measurements of the degree of disk swelling in individuals with papilledema appeared to be roughly linearly correlated to the Frisen scale grade [69]. Other reports have also concurred that in newly diagnosed IIH, OCT demonstrated alterations of the peripapillary retina and optic nerve head (ONH) correlate with Frisen grading scale, but not with clinical features or visual dysfunction [70].

Increased peripapillary retinal thickness measured by OCT is associated with increased ICP in newly diagnosed IIH patients [69]. However, in long-standing IIH patients who have been previously treated, OCT appears to be of limited value in predicting ICP. Similarly, Rebolleda and Muñoz-Negrete reported that RNFL thickness abnormalities assessed by OCT in patients with mild papilledema were quantitatively correlated with visual field sensitivity losses as determined by automated perimetry. However, the drawback with OCT is that, when the thickness is decreasing, it is not possible to distinguish whether it is the effect of treatment or there is actual loss of nerve fibers [71]. In such a setting, GCL analysis may provide more accurate information than RNFL analysis, and it might be an early structural indicator of irreversible neuronal loss [72]. One must always rule out other possible causes of vision loss such as submacular fluid, choroidal folds, or any other concurrent maculopathy.

To overcome the above-discussed drawbacks, Kaufhold et al. proposed a new custom segmentation algorithm using an extension of the RPE through the ONH as reference line, which enabled them to automatically assess ONH volume and shape in IIH patients that could be applicable in diseases with elevated ICP and optic disk swelling [62]. Their pilot study found that their proposed 3D parameters – optic nerve head volume (ONHV) and optic nerve head height (ONHH) – were able to discriminate between controls, treated and untreated patients. Both ONHV and ONHH measures were related to levels of intracranial pressure (ICP) [62]. Hence, SD-OCT can be used as a tool to differentiate between papilledema and pseudopapilledema; further strengthening the view, it can be used in the assessment and monitoring of the optic disk in IIH [73].

Another current advance in OCT technology is phase contrast OCT, which allows visualization of capillaries and quantification of blood flow within the capillary bed without the use of contrast agents [63].

In summary, there is growing evidence that suggests the use of OCT as a noninvasive quantitative method of monitoring the amount and evolution of papilledema as disk volume that correlates with RNFL and peripapillary total retinal thickness [62, 63]. Therefore, OCT may obviate the need for repeated lumbar punctures to measure the opening pressure to assess papilledema progression. At present, the most beneficial OCT-derived features pertinent to papilledema are measurement of disk volume, thickness of retinal GCL, and appearance of subretinal fluid. Furthermore, OCT can help differentiate causes of visual loss in IIH and predict the outcome [62, 63, 72].

References

1. Tzekov R, Mullan M. Vision function abnormalities in Alzheimer disease. Surv Ophthalmol. 2014;59(4):414–33.
2. Cronin-Golomb A, Corkin S, Rizzo JF, Cohen J, Growdon JH, Banks KS. Visual dysfunction in Alzheimer's disease: relation to normal aging. Ann Neurol. 1991;29(1):41–52.
3. Morrison JH, Hof PR, Bouras C. An anatomic substrate for visual disconnection in Alzheimer's disease. Ann N Y Acad Sci. 1991;640:36–43.
4. Hinton DR, Sadun AA, Blanks JC, Miller CA. Optic-nerve degeneration in Alzheimer's disease. N Engl J Med. 1986;315(8):485–7.
5. Muller F, O'Rahilly R. The development of the human brain from a closed neural tube at stage 13. Anat Embryol. 1988;177(3):203–24.
6. Berisha F, Feke GT, Trempe CL, McMeel JW, Schepens CL. Retinal abnormalities in early Alzheimer's disease. Invest Ophthalmol Vis Sci. 2007;48(5):2285–9.
7. Iseri PK, Altinas O, Tokay T, Yuksel N. Relationship between cognitive impairment and retinal morphological and visual functional abnormalities in Alzheimer disease. J Neuroophthalmol. 2006;26(1):18–24.

8. Lee YS, Amadi-Obi A, Yu CR, Egwuagu CE. Retinal cells suppress intraocular inflammation (uveitis) through production of interleukin-27 and interleukin-10. Immunology. 2011;132(4):492–502.
9. Ning A, Cui J, To E, Ashe KH, Matsubara J. Amyloid-beta deposits lead to retinal degeneration in a mouse model of Alzheimer disease. Invest Ophthalmol Vis Sci. 2008;49(11):5136–43.
10. Paquet C, Boissonnot M, Roger F, Dighiero P, Gil R, Hugon J. Abnormal retinal thickness in patients with mild cognitive impairment and Alzheimer's disease. Neurosci Lett. 2007;420(2):97–9.
11. Kesler A, Vakhapova V, Korczyn AD, Naftaliev E, Neudorfer M. Retinal thickness in patients with mild cognitive impairment and Alzheimer's disease. Clin Neurol Neurosurg. 2011;113(7):523–6.
12. Kromer R, Serbecic N, Hausner L, Froelich L, Aboul-Enein F, Beutelspacher SC. Detection of retinal nerve fiber layer defects in Alzheimer's disease using SD-OCT. Front Psych. 2014;5:22.
13. Blanks JC, Torigoe Y, Hinton DR, Blanks RH. Retinal pathology in Alzheimer's disease. I. Ganglion cell loss in foveal/parafoveal retina. Neurobiol Aging. 1996;17(3):377–84.
14. Bayhan HA, Aslan Bayhan S, Celikbilek A, Tanik N, Gurdal C. Evaluation of the chorioretinal thickness changes in Alzheimer's disease using spectral-domain optical coherence tomography. Clin Exp Ophthalmol. 2015;43(2):145–51.
15. Kromer R, Serbecic N, Hausner L, Froelich L, Beutelspacher SC. Comparison of visual evoked potentials and retinal nerve fiber layer thickness in Alzheimer's disease. Front Neurol. 2013;4:203.
16. Marziani E, Pomati S, Ramolfo P, Cigada M, Giani A, Mariani C, et al. Evaluation of retinal nerve fiber layer and ganglion cell layer thickness in Alzheimer's disease using spectral-domain optical coherence tomography. Invest Ophthalmol Vis Sci. 2013;54(9):5953–8.
17. Larrosa JM, Garcia-Martin E, Bambo MP, Pinilla J, Polo V, Otin S, et al. Potential new diagnostic tool for Alzheimer's disease using a linear discriminant function for Fourier domain optical coherence tomography. Invest Ophthalmol Vis Sci. 2014;55(5):3043–51.
18. Thomson KL, Yeo JM, Waddell B, Cameron JR, Pal S. A systematic review and meta-analysis of retinal nerve fiber layer change in dementia, using optical coherence tomography. Alzheimer's Dementia. 2015;1(2):136–43.
19. Coppola G, Di Renzo A, Ziccardi L, Martelli F, Fadda A, Manni G, et al. Optical coherence tomography in Alzheimer's disease: a meta-analysis. PLoS One. 2015;10(8):e0134750.
20. Braak H, Del Tredici K, Bratzke H, Hamm-Clement J, Sandmann-Keil D, Rub U. Staging of the intracerebral inclusion body pathology associated with idiopathic Parkinson's disease (preclinical and clinical stages). J Neurol. 2002;249(Suppl 3):1–5.
21. Archibald NK, Clarke MP, Mosimann UP, Burn DJ. The retina in Parkinson's disease. Brain. 2009;132(Pt 5):1128–45.
22. Schraermeyer U, Kopitz J, Peters S, Henke-Fahle S, Blitgen-Heinecke P, Kokkinou D, et al. Tyrosinase biosynthesis in adult mammalian retinal pigment epithelial cells. Exp Eye Res. 2006;83(2):315–21.
23. Hajee ME, March WF, Lazzaro DR, Wolintz AH, Shrier EM, Glazman S, et al. Inner retinal layer thinning in Parkinson disease. Arch Ophthalmol. 2009;127(6):737–41.
24. Altintas O, Iseri P, Ozkan B, Caglar Y. Correlation between retinal morphological and functional findings and clinical severity in Parkinson's disease. Adv Ophthalmol. 2008;116(2):137–46.
25. Bodis-Wollner I. Retinopathy in Parkinson disease. J Neural Transm. 2009;116(11):1493–501.
26. Price MJ, Feldman RG, Adelberg D, Kayne H. Abnormalities in color vision and contrast sensitivity in Parkinson's disease. Neurology. 1992;42(4):887–90.
27. Albrecht P, Muller AK, Sudmeyer M, Ferrea S, Ringelstein M, Cohn E, et al. Optical coherence tomography in parkinsonian syndromes. PLoS One. 2012;7(4):e34891.
28. Moschos MM, Tagaris G, Markopoulos I, Margetis I, Tsapakis S, Kanakis M, et al. Morphologic changes and functional retinal impairment in patients with Parkinson disease without visual loss. Eur J Ophthalmol. 2011;21(1):24–9.
29. Archibald NK, Clarke MP, Mosimann UP, Burn DJ. Retinal thickness in Parkinson's disease. Parkinsonism Relat Disord. 2011;17(6):431–6.

30. La Morgia C, Barboni P, Rizzo G, Carbonelli M, Savini G, Scaglione C, et al. Loss of temporal retinal nerve fibers in Parkinson disease: a mitochondrial pattern? Eur J Neurol. 2013;20(1):198–201.
31. Aaker GD, Myung JS, Ehrlich JR, Mohammed M, Henchcliffe C, Kiss S. Detection of retinal changes in Parkinson's disease with spectral-domain optical coherence tomography. Clin Ophthalmol. 2010;4:1427–32.
32. Garcia-Martin E, Satue M, Otin S, Fuertes I, Alarcia R, Larrosa JM, et al. Retina measurements for diagnosis of Parkinson disease. Retina. 2014;34(5):971–80.
33. Garcia-Martin E, Satue M, Fuertes I, Otin S, Alarcia R, Herrero R, et al. Ability and reproducibility of Fourier-domain optical coherence tomography to detect retinal nerve fiber layer atrophy in Parkinson's disease. Ophthalmology. 2012;119(10):2161–7.
34. Gaenslen A, Berg D. Early diagnosis of Parkinson's disease. Int Rev. Neurobiol. 2010;90: 81–92.
35. Yu J-G, Feng Y-F, Xiang Y, Huang J-H, Savini G, Parisi V, et al. Retinal nerve fiber layer thickness changes in Parkinson disease: a meta-analysis. PLoS One. 2014;9(1):e85718.
36. Stewart WF, Wood C, Reed ML, Roy J, Lipton RB. Cumulative lifetime migraine incidence in women and men. Cephalalgia. 2008;28(11):1170–8.
37. Tedeschi G, Russo A, Conte F, Salemi F, Tessitore A. The role of BOLD-fMRI in elucidating migraine pathophysiology. Neurol Sci. 2013;34(Suppl 1):S47–50.
38. Zhang XC, Levy D, Kainz V, Noseda R, Jakubowski M, Burstein R. Activation of central trigeminovascular neurons by cortical spreading depression. Ann Neurol. 2011;69(5):855–65.
39. Neuhuber W, Schrodl F. Autonomic control of the eye and the iris. Autonom Neurosci. 2011;165(1):67–79.
40. Tan FU, Akarsu C, Gullu R. Retinal nerve fiber layer thickness is unaffected in migraine patients. Acta Neurol Scand. 2005;112(1):19–23.
41. Martinez A, Proupim N, Sanchez M. Retinal nerve fibre layer thickness measurements using optical coherence tomography in migraine patients. Br J Ophthalmol. 2008;92(8): 1069–75.
42. Gipponi S, Scaroni N, Venturelli E, Forbice E, Rao R, Liberini P, et al. Reduction in retinal nerve fiber layer thickness in migraine patients. Neurol Sci. 2013;34(6):841–5.
43. Ekinci M, Ceylan E, Cagatay HH, Keles S, Huseyinoglu N, Tanyildiz B, et al. Retinal nerve fibre layer, ganglion cell layer and choroid thinning in migraine with aura. BMC Ophthalmol. 2014;14:75.
44. Lee WW, Tajunisah I, Sharmilla K, Peyman M, Subrayan V. Retinal nerve fiber layer structure abnormalities in schizophrenia and its relationship to disease state: evidence from optical coherence tomographyrnfl structure in schizophrenia. Invest Ophthalmol Vis Sci. 2013;54(12):7785–92.
45. Yeap S, Kelly SP, Reilly RB, Thakore JH, Foxe JJ. Visual sensory processing deficits in patients with bipolar disorder revealed through high-density electrical mapping. J Psychiatry Neurosci. 2009;34(6):459–64.
46. Butler PD, Javitt DC. Early-stage visual processing deficits in schizophrenia. Curr Opin Psychiat. 2005;18(2):151–7.
47. Miri S, Shrier EM, Glazman S, Ding Y, Selesnick I, Kozlowski PB, et al. The avascular zone and neuronal remodeling of the fovea in Parkinson disease. Ann Clin Transl Neurol. 2015;2(2):196–201.
48. Deutsch SI, Rosse RB, Schwartz BL, Mastropaolo J. A revised excitotoxic hypothesis of schizophrenia: therapeutic implications. Clin Neuropharmacol. 2001;24(1):43–9.
49. Sucher NJ, Lipton SA, Dreyer EB. Molecular basis of glutamate toxicity in retinal ganglion cells. Vis Res. 1997;37(24):3483–93.
50. Walter SD, Ishikawa H, Galetta KM, Sakai RE, Feller DJ, Henderson SB, et al. Ganglion cell loss in relation to visual disability in multiple sclerosis. Ophthalmology. 2012;119(6):1250–7.
51. Galetta KM, Calabresi PA, Frohman EM, Balcer LJ. Optical coherence tomography (OCT): imaging the visual pathway as a model for neurodegeneration. Neurotherapeutics. 2011;8(1): 117–32.

52. Syc SB, Warner CV, Hiremath GS, Farrell SK, Ratchford JN, Conger A, et al. Reproducibility of high-resolution optical coherence tomography in multiple sclerosis. Mult Scler. 2010;16(7):829–39.
53. Cettomai D, Pulicken M, Gordon-Lipkin E, Salter A, Frohman TC, Conger A, et al. Reproducibility of optical coherence tomography in multiple sclerosis. Arch Neurol. 2008; 65(9):1218–22.
54. Su KG, Banker G, Bourdette D, Forte M. Axonal degeneration in multiple sclerosis: the mitochondrial hypothesis. Current Neurol Neurosci Rep. 2009;9(5):411–7.
55. Zheng J, Bizzozero OA. Decreased activity of the 20S proteasome in the brain white matter and gray matter of patients with multiple sclerosis. J Neurochem. 2011;117(1):143–53.
56. Fisher E, Lee JC, Nakamura K, Rudick RA. Gray matter atrophy in multiple sclerosis: a longitudinal study. Ann Neurol. 2008;64(3):255–65.
57. Fisniku LK, Chard DT, Jackson JS, Anderson VM, Altmann DR, Miszkiel KA, et al. Gray matter atrophy is related to long-term disability in multiple sclerosis. Ann Neurol. 2008;64(3):247–54.
58. Burgansky-Eliash Z, Wollstein G, Chu T, Ramsey JD, Glymour C, Noecker RJ, et al. Optical coherence tomography machine learning classifiers for glaucoma detection: a preliminary study. Invest Ophthalmol Vis Sci. 2005;46(11):4147–52.
59. Garcia-Martin E, Pablo LE, Herrero R, Satue M, Polo V, Larrosa JM, et al. Diagnostic ability of a linear discriminant function for spectral-domain optical coherence tomography in patients with multiple sclerosis. Ophthalmology. 2012;119(8):1705–11.
60. Lamirel C, Newman NJ, Biousse V. Optical coherence tomography (OCT) in optic neuritis and multiple sclerosis. Rev Neurol. 2010;166(12):978–86.
61. Heidary G, Rizzo JF. Use of optical coherence tomography to evaluate papilledema and Pseudopapilledema. Semin Ophthalmol. 2010;25(5–6):198–205.
62. Kaufhold F, Kadas EM, Schmidt C, Kunte H, Hoffmann J, Zimmermann H, et al. Optic nerve head quantification in idiopathic intracranial hypertension by spectral domain OCT. PLoS One. 2012;7(5):e36965.
63. Kardon R. Optical coherence tomography in papilledema: what am I missing? J Neuroophthalmol. 2014;34(Suppl):S10–7.
64. Frisen L. Swelling of the optic nerve head: a staging scheme. J Neurol Neurosurg Psychiatry. 1982;45(1):13–8.
65. Scott CJ, Kardon RH, Lee AG, Frisen L, Wall M. Diagnosis and grading of papilledema in patients with raised intracranial pressure using optical coherence tomography vs clinical expert assessment using a clinical staging scale. Arch Ophthalmol. 2010;128(6): 705–11.
66. Sinclair AJ, Burdon MA, Nightingale PG, Matthews TD, Jacks A, Lawden M, et al. Rating papilloedema: an evaluation of the Frisen classification in idiopathic intracranial hypertension. J Neurol. 2012;259(7):1406–12.
67. Yri HM, Wegener M, Sander B, Jensen R. Idiopathic intracranial hypertension is not benign: a long-term outcome study. J Neurol. 2012;259(5):886–94.
68. Wang JK, Kardon RH, Kupersmith MJ, Garvin MK. Automated quantification of volumetric optic disc swelling in papilledema using spectral-domain optical coherence tomography. Invest Ophthalmol Vis Sci. 2012;53(7):4069–75.
69. Skau M, Sander B, Milea D, Jensen R. Disease activity in idiopathic intracranial hypertension: a 3-month follow-up study. J Neurol. 2011;258(2):277–83.
70. Group OCTS-SCfNIIHS, Auinger P, Durbin M, Feldon S, Garvin M, Kardon R, et al. Baseline OCT measurements in the idiopathic intracranial hypertension treatment trial, part II: correlations and relationship to clinical features. Invest Ophthalmol Vis Sci. 2014;55(12):8173–9.
71. Rebolleda G, Munoz-Negrete FJ. Follow-up of mild papilledema in idiopathic intracranial hypertension with optical coherence tomography. Invest Ophthalmol Vis Sci. 2009;50(11):5197–200.
72. Rebolleda G, Diez-Alvarez L, Casado A, Sanchez-Sanchez C, de Dompablo E, Gonzalez-Lopez JJ, et al. OCT: new perspectives in neuro-ophthalmology. Saudi J Ophthalmol. 2015;29(1):9–25.
73. Bassi ST, Mohana KP. Optical coherence tomography in papilledema and pseudopapilledema with and without optic nerve head drusen. Indian J Ophthalmol. 2014;62(12):1146–51.

2 Retinal Vasculitis in Systemic Disease

Irfan Khan and Ashvini Reddy

Abstract

Retinal vasculitis may be associated with various systemic vasculitides. It can result in cystoid macular edema, retinal ischemia, and occlusive disease and resultant sight-threatening sequelae such as neovascularization, vitreous hemorrhage, and neovascular glaucoma. The purpose of this chapter is to discuss the more common systemic diseases associated with retinal vasculitis, including Behçet's disease, systemic lupus erythematosus, Susac's syndrome, and ANCA-associated vasculitides. The diagnostic criteria of these multisystem disorders will be reviewed, as well as their ocular manifestations and presentations. Attention will be given to various imaging modalities including fluorescein angiography and optical coherence tomography to evaluate their utility and describe typical clinical findings.

2.1 Introduction

Vasculitis can affect the arteries, capillaries, and veins of any organ system; therefore, manifestations vary based on the site affected. For example, palpable purpura may be evident in individuals with cutaneous vasculitis, fluid retention and hematuria may occur in individuals with renal involvement, and focal neurologic deficits may manifest in those with central nervous system disease. While infectious causes of vasculitis exist, the majority appear to be autoimmune. The available evidence suggests that the dysfunction caused by vasculitis is the result of leukocyte-mediated alterations in blood vessel structure and function.

I. Khan • A. Reddy (✉)
Wilmer Eye Institute, Johns Hopkins University, Baltimore, MD 21218, USA
e-mail: areddy16@jhmi.edu

J. Chhablani et al. (eds.), *Retinal and Choroidal Imaging in Systemic Diseases*,
https://doi.org/10.1007/978-981-10-5461-7_2

Table 2.1 Predominant vessel type involved in various forms of ocular inflammation

Arteritis	Systemic lupus erythematosus, acute retinal necrosis syndrome, polyarteritis nodosa, granulomatosis with polyangiitis, idiopathic retinal vasculitis, aneurysms, and neuroretinitis syndrome (IRVAN), Susac's syndrome
Phlebitis	Behçet's disease, sarcoidosis, multiple sclerosis

The International Chapel Hill Consensus Conference on the Nomenclature of Systemic Vasculitides (CHCC2012) published their consensus on the nomenclature of vasculitides in 2012. Their system included groups of disease characterized by the size of vessel affected and groups such as single-organ vasculitis, vasculitis associated with systemic disease, and vasculitis associated with a probable etiology [1].

Vasculitis affecting the retinal blood vessels may occur in isolation or be associated with systemic diseases and infectious processes affecting the eye. Clinically, this vasculitis can manifest as sheathing of the blood vessels, retinal hemorrhages, cotton wool spots, vascular occlusion, and neovascularization of the retina. Together these inflammatory changes can result in vision loss, cystoid macular edema, and structural complications such as vitreous hemorrhage and retinal detachment. The primary site of retinal vascular inflammation (arteritis versus phlebitis; proximal versus distal) may narrow the differential diagnosis of retinal vasculitis (Table 2.1).

The scope of this chapter will include a summary of some of the systemic diseases that may feature vasculitis affecting the retinal and choroidal vasculature.

2.2 Behçet's Disease

Adamantiades-Behçet's disease (Behçet's disease) is a chronic, relapsing inflammatory disorder classically characterized by the presence of oral and genital aphthous ulcers, ocular inflammation, and characteristic skin lesions.

While Behçet's disease has a worldwide distribution, there are certain regions in which the incidence and prevalence are much higher. Turkey has the highest prevalence of Behçet's disease, with 420 cases per 100,000 population. The prevalence in Japan, Korea, China, Iran, and Saudi Arabia ranges from 13.5 to 22 cases per 100,000 population. The prevalence in North America and Europe is much less, with one case per 15,000–500,000 population [2].

The sex prevalence varies geographically, though the most severe manifestations of the disease including pulmonary aneurysms, uveitis, thrombophlebitis, and neurologic disease are all more common in males. Behçet's disease is most common in persons aged 20–40 years with a mean age at onset of 25–30 years [2].

The diagnosis of Behçet's disease is based on clinical findings, with the most widely used criteria published by the Research Committee of Japan and the International Study Group [3]. The clinical manifestations of the disease are broken down into major and minor criteria, and patients may only manifest a subset of these findings (Table 2.2).

Table 2.2 Research committee of Japan clinical criteria for the diagnosis of Behçet's disease

Major criteria
• Recurrent oral aphthous ulcers
• Skin lesions (erythema nodosum, acneiform pustules, folliculitis)
• Recurrent genital ulcers
• Ocular inflammatory disease
Minor criteria
• Arthritis
• Gastrointestinal ulceration
• Epididymitis
Behçet's disease classification
• Complete (four major criteria)
• Incomplete (three major criteria or ocular involvement with one other major criterion)
• Suspect (two major criteria with no ocular involvement)
• Possible (one major criterion)

Oral aphthous ulceration is the most prevalent manifestation of Behçet's disease in most series. These painful lesions have a high recurrence rate and typically appear as a cluster or crop of lesions.

Recurrent ulcerative genital lesions can occur on the scrotum and penile shaft in males and the labia, vagina, and perineum in females. Other skin manifestations include erythema nodosum and acneiform papulopustular lesions on the face, trunk, and extremities.

The disease can also affect other organ systems such as the brain (memory/recall, behavioral changes, meningoencephalitis, cerebral vasculitis), large blood vessels (pulmonary artery aneurysms, coronary vasculitis/thrombosis), and the GI system (deep intestinal ulceration).

Ocular involvement manifests in approximately 70% of patients who have Behçet's disease. In most instances, oral and genital ulceration precedes eye inflammation, though ocular disease has been observed as the initial manifestation as well. Behçet's uveitis typically consists of recurrent episodes of severe inflammation. In one series, anterior uveitis was present in 59% of cases, posterior uveitis was present in 76% of cases, and panuveitis was present in 88.1% of cases. While inflammation may present unilaterally, in most cases it progresses to involve both eyes. The classic anterior uveitis with shifting hypopyon is estimated to be present in less than one-third of patients [4].

Retinal vascular disease is the most serious complication of Behçet's uveitis with severe inflammatory arteritis and phlebitis. The initial manifestations of retinal arteritis and phlebitis may include cystoid macular edema and vascular occlusion, both of which may result in profound vision loss. Later manifestations may include secondary ischemia-induced neovascularization of the retina and optic disk. Neovascular glaucoma has been reported in eyes afflicted with severe occlusive vasculitis (Figs. 2.1 and 2.2).

The treatment for Behçet's disease is immunosuppression, particularly when ocular involvement is noted. Previous studies have demonstrated the benefit granted by

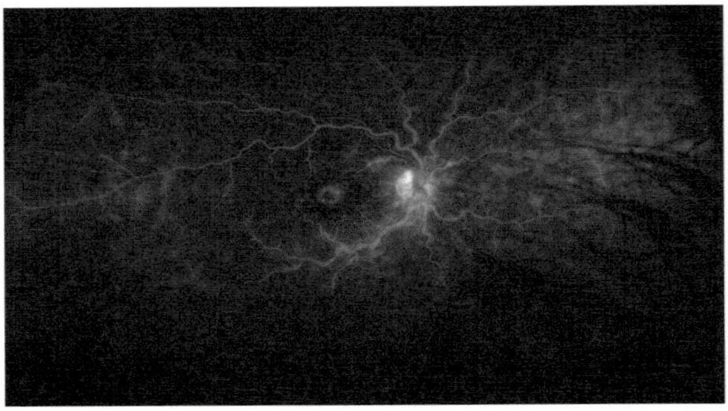

Fig. 2.1 Wide-field fluorescein angiogram of a male with Behçet's disease-associated retinal vasculitis. The photograph depicts tortuous vessels with diffuse leakage (veins and arteries) and angiographic cystoid macular edema. Courtesy: Bryn Burkholder, MD

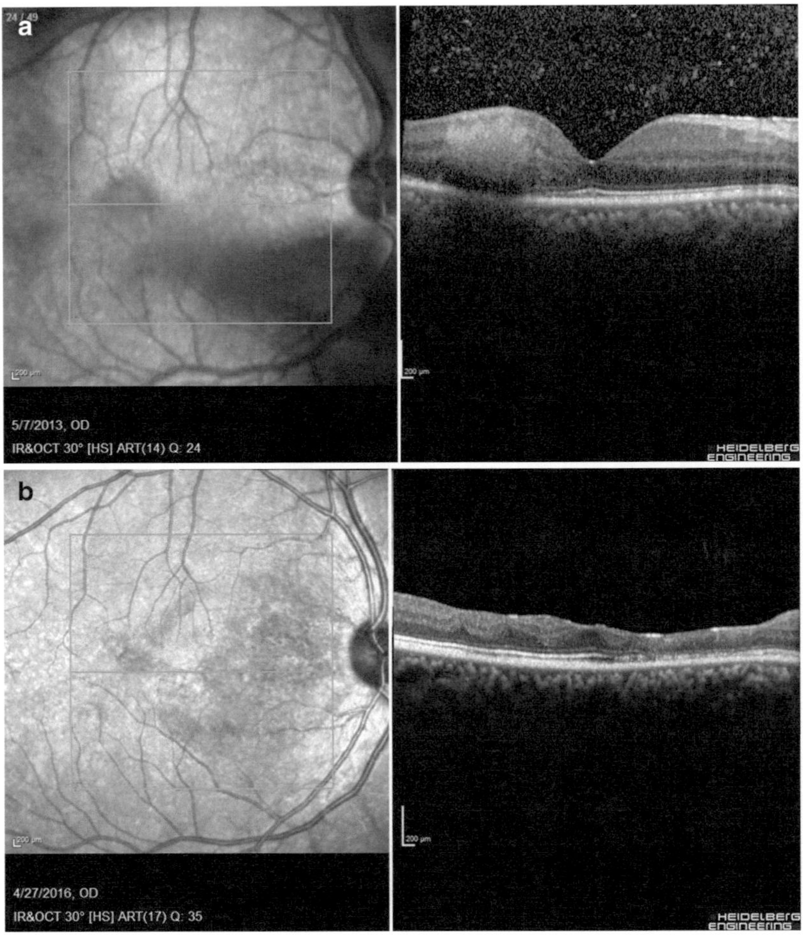

Fig. 2.2 Spectral domain OCT in a male with Behçet's disease-associated retinal vasculitis. Pictured above is a region of inner retinal edema corresponding to an acute arteriolar occlusion (**a**). Months later, after instituting therapy with infliximab, the residual inner retinal atrophic changes are noted (**b**). The patient maintained 20/35 visual acuity due to relative sparing of the fovea. Courtesy: Bryn Burkholder, MD

instituting early immunomodulatory therapy with azathioprine, alkylating agents, and, more recently, biologic mediators of inflammation such as infliximab. Given the expected chronic course, corticosteroid monotherapy is not considered to be an appropriate therapy given the side effects of long-term administration.

2.3 Systemic Lupus Erythematosus

Systemic lupus erythematosus (SLE) is an autoimmune disease characterized by the presence of circulating autoantibodies. The majority of these autoantibodies are targeted against cell nuclei, resulting in multisystem involvement.

In North America, the annual incidence of SLE ranges between 1.8 and 7.6 per 100,000 persons per year, with a reported prevalence of approximately 50 cases per 100,000 persons. The frequency of SLE varies by race and ethnicity, with higher rates reported in blacks, Asians, and Hispanics. Worldwide, the prevalence of SLE is variable, but the highest rates of prevalence have been reported in Italy, Spain, and the UK Afro-Caribbean population. More than 90% of cases of SLE occur in women of child-bearing age, suggesting a role for hormonal factors in the pathogenesis of the disease [2].

There are a variety of clinical manifestations of SLE ranging from the classic malar, or "butterfly" rash, to arthralgias (present in up to 85%) and nephropathy (present in 50%). The American College of Rheumatology has created and updated a list of clinical manifestations and serologic patterns that serve as diagnostic criteria for SLE (Table 2.3) [5].

Patients with SLE may also develop ocular involvement. The most common manifestations are surface disease, including episcleritis, scleritis, and keratoconjunctivitis sicca.

Table 2.3 American College of Rheumatology Diagnostic Criteria for SLE

1. Malar rash	Erythema over the malar eminences tending to spare the nasolabial folds
2. Discoid rash	Erythematous raised patches with adherent keratotic scaling and follicular plugging
3. Photosensitivity	Skin rash as a result of reaction to sunlight
4. Oral ulcers	Oral or nasopharyngeal ulceration, usually painless
5. Arthritis	Nonerosive arthritis involving two or more peripheral joints
6. Serositis	Pleuritis or pericarditis
7. Renal disorder	Persistent proteinuria greater than 0.5 g per day or cellular casts on urinalysis
8. Neurologic disorder	Seizures or psychosis in the absence of offending drugs or known metabolic derangements
9. Hematologic disorder	Hemolytic anemia, leukopenia, lymphopenia, or thrombocytopenia
10. Immunologic disorder	Anti-SM positivity or positive antiphospholipid antibodies
11. Anti-nuclear antibody	An abnormal titer of antinuclear antibody

A diagnosis is made if at least four of the listed features manifest simultaneously or serially over any length of time

The retinal and choroidal manifestations of SLE are potentially blinding and are considered to be important markers of systemic disease activity. Lupus retinopathy was initially described in 1929, by Bergmeister, and since then, numerous investigators have elaborated on its clinical signs and manifestations. The incidence of lupus retinopathy ranges from 3% in patients with mild disease to 29% in individuals with active disease affecting other organ systems. Additionally, a strong correlation between the presence of retinopathy and CNS disease has been described [2].

The most common signs of retinopathy are microangiopathic, mirroring the retinal vascular changes seen in diabetic and hypertensive retinopathy. Early on, retinal hemorrhages and cotton wool spots predominate. More advanced retinopathy includes the presence of inflammation of the retinal arterioles and/or venules. The most severe retinal lesion seen in lupus retinopathy is arterial occlusion, which can result in severe and permanent vision loss. Sudden vision loss from a central retinal vascular occlusion in a young individual without evident risk factors should prompt the clinician to consider an underlying diagnosis of SLE. Arterial occlusion in SLE can result in the same ischemic sequelae noted in other causes of retinal non-perfusion, such as neovascularization, vitreous hemorrhage, and tractional retinal detachment [6].

Individuals with retinal vasculopathy have a higher prevalence of concomitant antiphospholipid antibodies including anticardiolipin and lupus anticoagulant. In one study by Montehermoso et al., 77% of patients with SLE and retinal involvement had positive antiphospholipid antibody titers, whereas only 29% of SLE patients without retinal disease had positive titers [7].

The hemorrhages and vascular leakage noted in milder forms of lupus retinopathy are believed to be mediated by immune complex deposition and inflammation, while the histologic correlate of more severe occlusive disease is fibrinoid degeneration and necrosis without significant inflammation [8].

A rare ocular manifestation of SLE is lupus choroidopathy, presenting with exudative retinal detachment. Described in multiple case reports, choroidopathy is typically noted in patients with concurrent and highly active CNS and renal disease. Patients often have associated uncontrolled hypertension. The pathogenesis is suspected to be due to a combination of factors including the aforementioned uncontrolled blood pressure and immune complex deposition in the choriocapillaris. Anti-retinal pigment epithelium antibodies have also been implicated as a potential causative factor. Several series have indicated that choroidopathy may be a sensitive indicator of systemic lupus activity. The presence of SLE choroidopathy may be indicative of coexistent (although sometimes occult) nephropathy and CNS vasculitis [9].

The treatment for lupus retinopathy is immunosuppression, with corticosteroids used to rapidly control active inflammation, and steroid sparing immunomodulatory therapy used for long-term control. Retinal photocoagulation, intravitreal anti-vascular endothelial growth factor agents, and vitrectomy are used to treat the structural complications of advanced retinopathy and vaso-occlusive disease.

2.4 ANCA-Positive Vasculitis

The ANCA-associated vasculitides (AAV) include three clinical entities that are characterized by systemic vasculitis and a high prevalence of positive serologic testing for antineutrophil cytoplasmic antibodies. The three types of vasculitis are granulomatosis with polyangiitis (GPA), microscopic polyangiitis (MPA), and eosinophilic granulomatosis with polyangiitis (Churg–Strauss syndrome) (EGPA).

The worldwide annual incidence of ANCA-associated vasculitis is estimated to be 20 per million, with GPA accounting for about half in northern European populations, MPA a third, and the rest EGPA [10].

While ocular disease has been described in all of the ANCA-associated vasculitides, it has been best characterized and most frequent in GPA. The necrotizing vasculitis that characterizes GPA affects the upper and lower respiratory tracts and the kidneys. The antineutrophil cytoplasmic antibody (ANCA) occurs in 80% of patients with GPA. Ocular and orbital involvement can occur from 28% to 58% of patients with GPA. The typical inflammatory disease in individuals with GPA is scleritis, orbital inflammation, and peripheral ulcerative keratitis [2].

Posterior manifestations of ocular disease may include optic disk edema and subsequent atrophy from active orbital inflammation and serous retinal detachments from choroidal effusions in individuals with posterior scleritis.

Isolated retinal and choroidal disease is uncommon in most series, but reports of microangiopathy and occlusive retinal vasculitis have been described (Fig. 2.3). Microvascular changes such as cotton wool spots and retinal hemorrhages may be seen, as well as sequelae of retinal non-perfusion. Choroidal vascular occlusions and inflammatory masses have also been reported in individuals with GPA [11].

Similar to many autoimmune inflammatory diseases, the treatment of ANCA-associated vasculitis requires the use of corticosteroids and transition to immunomodulatory therapy including alkylating agents and biologics for long-term suppression of inflammation.

2.5 Susac's Syndrome

Susac's syndrome is an inflammatory microvasculopathy of undetermined etiology, affecting the brain, the cochlea, and the retina. This syndrome typically occurs in young women (20–40 years of age). Regarded as a rare disease, its true prevalence is unknown. At presentation, central nervous system signs and symptoms occur in 80% of patients, cochlear involvement (hearing loss) in 52%, and retinal findings in 46%. Only 20% of patients present with the complete triad, resulting in difficulty identifying the disorder. The diagnosis is based on clinical and radiographic findings, as there is no definitive laboratory test [2].

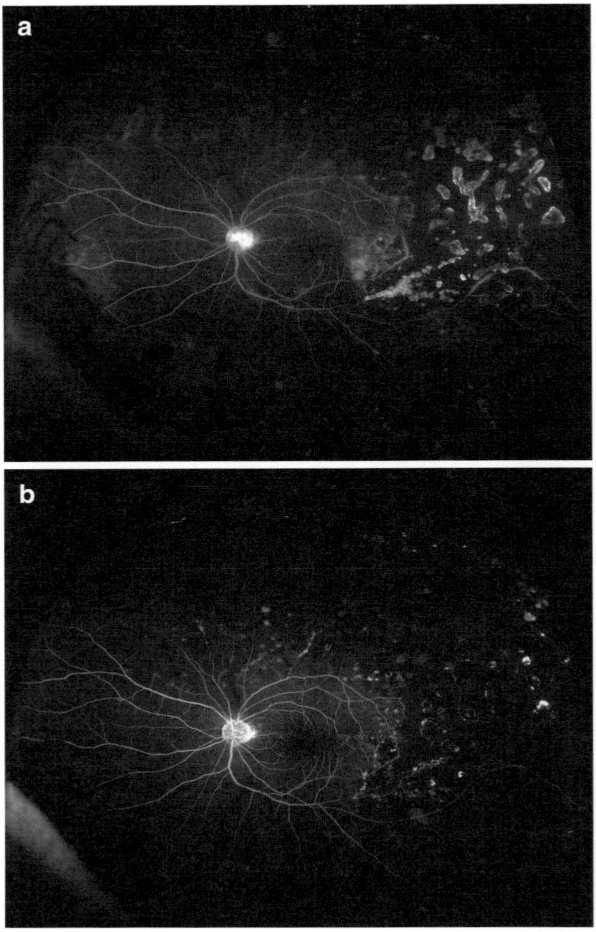

Fig. 2.3 Wide-field fluorescein angiography depicting occlusive vasculitis in an individual with GPA. There is a broad region of superior and temporal non-perfusion that was treated with laser photocoagulation (**a**). After instituting systemic anti-inflammatory therapy the patient's vasculitis stabilized with resolution of vascular leakage (**b**)

MRI findings include hyperintense foci on T2-weighted images. The lesions may occur in both gray and white matter, supratentorially or infratentorially. Lesions involving the central fibers of the corpus callosum are considered almost pathognomonic for Susac's syndrome in the appropriate clinical setting.

The ocular manifestations of this syndrome include focal arteriolar narrowing and occlusions (Fig. 2.4). Though the findings over time are usually bilateral, at the onset of disease, findings may predominate in one eye. Retinal hemorrhages and microaneurysms may be present. Over time, the occlusive retinal disease can lead to the formation of arteriolar collaterals. The vitreous and anterior chambers are usually quiet, or, at most, mildly inflamed.

The treatment of the microangiopathy generally involves immunosuppression with corticosteroids initially. Many types of steroid sparing immunosuppressive therapy have been employed with varying levels of success.

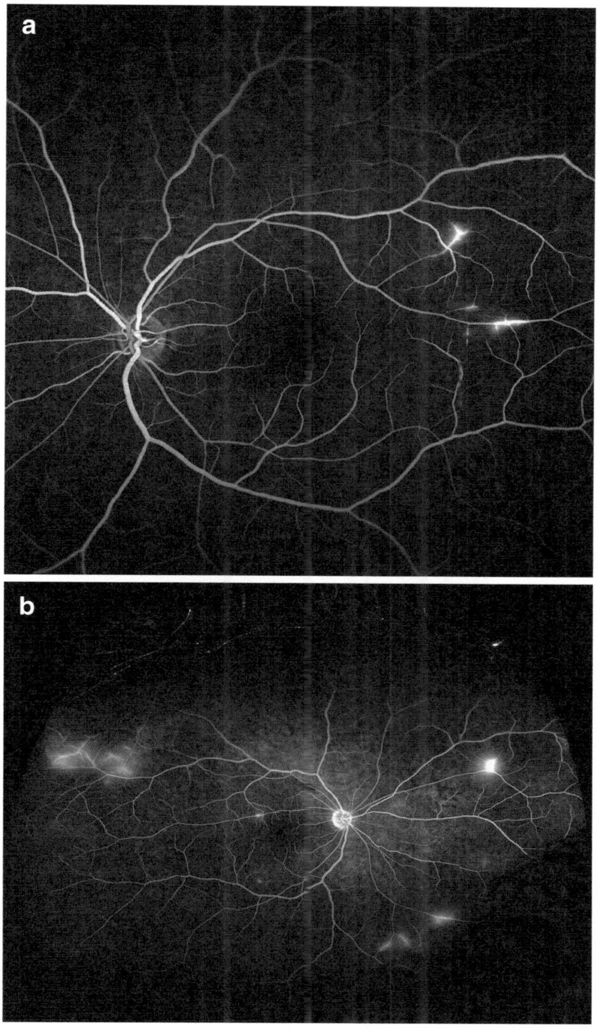

Fig. 2.4 Fluorescein angiography depicting segmental arteritis in a young female with Susac's syndrome

2.6 Other Systemic Vasculitides with Ophthalmic Manifestations

2.6.1 Polyarteritis Nodosa

Polyarteritis nodosa (PAN) is a systemic vasculitis affecting medium-sized and small muscular arteries, preferentially at bifurcations. The inflammation may result in aneurysmal dilatation which can be associated with rupture and thrombosis, yielding multisystem organ dysfunction. The skin, peripheral nerves, joints, intestines, and kidney may all be affected, in addition to the eye and orbit.

A variety of ocular manifestations have been described including scleritis, peripheral ulcerative keratitis, orbital inflammation, and retinal vasculitis. The descriptions of retinal vasculitis have included vitritis and both arterial and venous involvement (though arterial involvement has been more commonly described [12].

2.7 Kawasaki Disease

Kawasaki disease is a systemic vasculitis of children that typically affects the small- and medium-sized blood vessels of the body, in particular, the coronary arteries. It is most common in Asian children and the etiology is, as of yet, unknown.

Retinal vasculitis has not been described as a manifestation of this disease, though there is a case report demonstrating retinal ischemia suspected to be related to a thrombotic event from the systemic vasculitis [13]. The most common eye finding is bilateral conjunctival injection. Anterior uveitis, intermediate uveitis, and papilledema are less common findings. The anterior uveitis is usually bilateral and mild and responds to topical corticosteroids and systemic therapy for the vasculitis.

2.8 Takayasu's Arteritis

Takayasu's arteritis is a large-vessel granulomatous vasculitis that mostly commonly occurs in young or middle-aged Asian women. The vasculitis results in intimal fibrosis and narrowing of blood vessels, affecting pulmonary arteries and the aorta. As a result of the obstruction of the main branches from the aorta (subclavian artery, common carotid artery, brachiocephalic artery), the absence or weakening of the pulse in the upper extremities may be noted. The renal arteries may be markedly attenuated as well, leading to renovascular hypertension.

While Takayasu's arteritis is not associated with inflammation of the retinal vasculature, decreased blood flow to the retina and choroid as well as systemic hypertension may result in a variety of ocular manifestations including amaurosis fugax, hypertensive retinopathy (involvement of renal vasculature), and choroidal and retinal non-perfusion leading to ocular ischemic syndrome, retinal neovascularization, and its associated structural complications if left untreated, such as vitreous hemorrhage and neovascular glaucoma [8].

2.9 Retinal and Choroidal Imaging in Systemic Vasculitides

2.9.1 Fundus Photography

Fundus photography remains an important method for monitoring fundus changes over time and documenting findings such as hemorrhages, disk appearance, and retinal vascular caliber and branching patterns.

In addition, ultrawide-field (UWF) photography optical systems allow assessment of the retinal periphery in individuals with both media opacity and miotic pupils.

In individuals with retinal vasculitis, far peripheral vein sheathing and retinal infiltrates that denote disease activity can clearly be detected with pseudocolor imaging. Green laser and red laser separation images also provided additional informative value. Green laser light (red-free light) (532 nm) highlights the anterior retinal structures and retinal vasculature and has demonstrated utility in the visualization and quantification of lesions in the retina secondary to vasculitis. Even in patients with significant vitritis, high-definition images can be obtained to improve disease monitoring [14].

2.10 Fluorescein Angiography

The use of fluorescein angiography in ocular disease with a vasculitic component has been well established. This imaging modality allows for the direct observation of vascular hyperpermeability and capillary non-perfusion. As noted previously, the presence of predominant arteritis versus phlebitis can help narrow the differential in individuals with ocular inflammatory disease to an extent.

Behçet's disease shows a predominant phlebitis on FA, though severe arteritis and vascular occlusion may be noted rarely. Grading schema for the degree of retinal vascular leakage has been described by authors for assessing individuals with Behçet's disease and their response to treatment. Mean total vascular leakage scores based on fluorescein angiography have been shown to correlate with visual acuity over time [14].

Fluorescein angiography has been integral in diagnosing reported cases of Susac's syndrome. The pathognomonic lesions noted on FA in Susac's syndrome are multifocal, segmental areas of arteriolar narrowing with leakage of dye from the involved segments. The occlusions do not necessarily occur at the branches of the arterioles, in contrast to emboli or thrombi [12].

FA is also useful to follow treatment efficacy as steroids or other agents are tapered. The retinal and FA findings improve or resolve with treatment success and recur during flares of the syndrome. This information would allow the care team to intervene early, before further neurological or cochlear damage occurs.

The utility of ultrawide-field FA also allows for more accurate assessment of the extent of vasculitis in the retinal periphery, aiding in titration of medical therapy and also planning interventions such as laser photocoagulation.

In polyarteritis nodosa, the FA may reveal varying degrees of prolongation of the arm-to-retina circulation time given the narrowing of the proximal vessels branching from the aorta.

2.11 ICG Angiography

Angiographic evaluation with indocyanine green (ICG) can be used to study the choroidal circulation in systemic diseases.

ICG imaging has been used to visualize the choroidal circulation in lupus choroidopathy. Studies have revealed focal, transient early-phase hypofluorescence followed by late-phase diffuse hyperfluorescence, distortion of the large choroidal vessels, and also focal clusters of choroidal hyperfluorescence in the intermediate phase. It has been postulated that the focal areas of hyperfluorescence in the intermediate frames may actually represent ICG staining of immune complexes.

Baglio et al. used indocyanine green angiography to demonstrate that subtle changes in the choroidal circulation can be seen in patients with SLE-associated nephropathy, while similar findings are not seen in SLE patients without renal involvement [15].

2.12 Optical Coherence Tomography (OCT)

OCT is a noninvasive imaging modality that is now essential in assessing individuals with retinal vasculitis. Cystoid macular edema is a common occurrence in such patients and a primary cause of vision loss, which is easily and accurately measured by OCT. OCT can be used to monitor response to both local and systemic treatments.

Additionally, the presence of inner retinal edema noted on OCT can support a diagnosis of retinal vascular occlusion.

More recently, an OCT technique termed "enhanced depth imaging" (EDI) has been utilized to provide an enhanced view of the choroid and to measure choroidal thickness. Previous studies have indicated that choroid thickness is increased during the development of Vogt–Koyanagi–Harada (VKH) disease and is greater in the acute phase of the disease than in the convalescent phase. A recent study evaluating individuals with Behçet's disease has shown that subfoveal choroidal thickness is greater in the acute phase of uveitis than in the remission phase and correlates significantly with retinal vascular leakage by fluorescein angiography [16].

OCT has also been used to evaluate retinal nerve fiber layer and central macular thickness in individuals with a history of neuro-Behçet's disease and healthy control subjects. The average RNFL in patients with neuro-Behçet's disease was significantly lower than that of healthy controls, and average central macular thickness was significantly lower [17].

Retinal vasculitis may occur in the setting of a systemic vasculitic disorder. Recognizing the systemic context in which the ocular inflammation occurs may be of critical importance, both for limiting permanent ocular sequelae and also significant systemic morbidity and mortality. Therapeutic options include local ocular treatments (local steroid, laser), but systemic immunosuppressive therapy in conjunction with these measures is paramount. Retinal imaging may serve as an integral tool for gauging both the response to therapies and the need to escalate therapy.

References

1. Jennette JC, et al. Revised international Chapel Hill consensus conference nomenclature of vasculitides. Arthritis Rheum. 2012;65(1):1–11.
2. Foster CS, Vitale AT. Diagnosis and treatment of uveitis. New Delhi: Jaypee Brothers; 2013.

3. International Team for the Revision of the International Criteria for Behçet's Disease. The International Criteria for Behçet's Disease (ICBD): a collaborative study of 27 countries on the sensitivity and specificity of the new criteria. J Eur Acad Dermatol Venereol. 2014;28(3):338–47.
4. Davatchi F. Diagnosis/classification criteria for Behcet's disease. Pathol Res Int. 2012;2012: 607921.
5. American College of Rheumatology Ad Hoc Committee on Systemic Lupus Erythematosus Response Criteria. The American College of Rheumatology response criteria for systemic lupus erythematosus clinical trials: measures of overall disease activity. Arthritis Rheum. 2004;50:3418–26.
6. Au A, O'Day J. Review of severe vaso-occlusive retinopathy in systemic lupus erythematosus and the antiphospholipid syndrome: associations, visual outcomes, complications and treatment. Clin Exp Ophthalmol. 2004;32(1):87–100.
7. Montehermoso A, Cervera R, Font J, et al. Association of antiphospholipid antibodies with retinal vascular disease in systemic lupus erythematosus. Semin Arthritis Rheum. 1999;28(5): 326–32.
8. Nag TC, Wadhwa S. Histopathological changes in the eyes in systemic lupus erythematosus: an electron microscope and immunohistochemical study. Histol Histopathol. 2005;20(2):373–82.
9. Nguyen QD, Uy HS, Akpek EK, Harper SL, Zacks DN, Foster CS. Choroidopathy of systemic lupus erythematosus. Lupus. 2000;9(4):288–98.
10. Kallenberg CG. Pathogenesis and treatment of ANCA-associated vasculitides. Clin Exp Rheumatol. 2015;33(4 Suppl 92):S11–4.
11. Matlach J, Freiberg FJ, Gadeholt O, Göbel W. Vasculitis-like hemorrhagic retinal angiopathy in Wegener's granulomatosis. BMC Res Notes. 2013;6:364.
12. Morgan CM, Foster CS, D'Amico DJ, Gragoudas ES. Retinal vasculitis in polyarteritis nodosa. Retina. 1986;6(4):205–9.
13. Font RL, Mehta RS, Streusand SB, et al. Bilateral retinal ischemia in Kawasaki disease. Postmortem findings and electron microscopic observations. Ophthalmology. 1983;90(5): 569–77.
14. Mesquida M, Llorenç V, Fontenla JR, Navarro MJ, Adán A. Use of ultra-wide-field retinal imaging in the management of active Behçet retinal vasculitis. Retina. 2014;34(10):2121–7.
15. Baglio V, et al. Choroidopathy in patients with systemic lupus erythematosus with or without nephropathy. J Nephrol. 2011;24(4):522–9.
16. Kim M, Kim H, Kwon HJ, Kim SS, Koh HJ, Lee SC. Choroidal thickness in Behcet's uveitis: an enhanced depth imaging-optical coherence tomography and its association with angiographic changes. Invest Ophthalmol Vis Sci. 2013;54(9):6033–9.
17. Ucar D, Uygunoglu U, Dikkaya F, Yıldırım Y, Yuksel-Elgin C, Saip S, Siva A, Ozyazgan Y. Retinal nerve fiber layer structure abnormalities in patients with Neuro-Behcet's disease. Graefes Arch Clin Exp Ophthalmol. 2015;253(7):1181–5.

Multimodal Imaging in Drug-Related Retinal Toxicity

3

Remya Mareen Paulose, Jay Chhablani, and William F. Mieler

Abstract

The growth of various medical therapies has led to an increased frequency of medication induced side effects. The number of drugs that adversely affect the eye continues to rise, and their effects pose a great challenge to all ophthalmologists. Traditionally, most drug-induced side effects were diagnosed clinically according to the patient's presenting symptoms and signs and history of medication use. However, as imaging is used more and more commonly, many of these complications are initially diagnosed at imaging instead of at clinical presentation. Therefore, it is important for ophthalmologists to recognize the imaging appearance of common drug-induced complications and to include drug-induced toxicity in the differential diagnosis. Earlydetection of drug-induced retinal toxicity is important because many of theses changes can be reversed if the drug is discontinued promptly.

R.M. Paulose
Little Flower Hospital and Research Centre, Angamaly, Kerala, India

Smt.Kanuri Santhamma Retina Vitreous Centre, L.V. Prasad Eye Institute, Kallam Anji Reddy Campus, L.V. Prasad Marg, Banjara Hills, Hyderabad 500 034, Andhra Pradesh, India

J. Chhablani (✉)
Smt.Kanuri Santhamma Retina Vitreous Centre, L.V. Prasad Eye Institute, Kallam Anji Reddy Campus, L.V. Prasad Marg, Banjara Hills, Hyderabad 500 034, Andhra Pradesh, India
e-mail: jay.chhablani@gmail.com

W.F. Mieler
Department of Ophthalmology and Visual Sciences, University of Illinois at Chicago, 1200 W Harrison St, Chicago, IL 60607, USA

J. Chhablani et al. (eds.), *Retinal and Choroidal Imaging in Systemic Diseases*,
https://doi.org/10.1007/978-981-10-5461-7_3

Table 3.1 Classification of drugs based on the mechanism of retinal toxicity

Pigmentary retinopathy	Vascular damage	Crystalline retinopathy	CME
Quinolines	Talc	Tamoxifen	Latanoprost
Thioridazine	Cisplatin	Talc	Epinephrine
Clofazimine	Interferon	Canthaxanthin	Dipivefrin
Deferoxamine	Carmustine	Nitrofurantoin	Niacin
Phenothiazine	Quinine sulfate	Methoxyflurane	Taxols
Chlorpromazine	Aminoglycoside		
Cisplatin	Ergot derivatives		
Corticosteroid	Oral contraceptives		

The eye is a specialized organ in the body with high degree of sensitivity to the systemic use of toxic substances. The retina is privileged to have the blood retinal barrier, which limits the access of these toxic chemicals across it thus protecting this vital tissue. However, ocular side effects from systemic administration of drugs are well recognized, and more than 30 drugs have been associated with retinal toxicity.

Toxicity from these drugs is of serious ophthalmologic concern because even after cessation, many of these drugs continue to produce progressive visual loss. Hence, it is imperative to recognize the ocular involvement early. This review will focus on the use of multimodal imaging techniques which would aid the clinician with better understanding of the pattern of these toxicities which is important in the screening, diagnosis, and management of these adverse effects. Of all the investigations available to image the posterior segment, the ones which are crucial in the management of medication-related retinal toxicity will be described in detail.

With regard to the mechanism of toxicity, these drugs have been classified into different groups, as has been illustrated in Table 3.1. There are thousands of systemic medications, and it would be impractical to cover the retinal toxicity produced by each one of these medications. This chapter reviews the latest evidence on the imaging modalities in retinal toxicity caused by more commonly employed agents.

Broadly, drug-related retinal toxicity can be classified as shown below:

- Pigmentary retinopathy
- Crystalline retinopathy
- Retinal vasculopathy
- Retinal folds
- Cystoid macular edema (CME)

3.1 Drugs Causing Toxicity of the Retinal Pigment Epithelium (RPE)

These are the group of drugs that when administered systemically may lead to irreversible damage to the retina mainly to the retinal pigment epithelium. *Chloroquine and hydroxychloroquine* are the prototype drugs belonging to this category.

3.1.1 Chloroquine and Hydroxychloroquine

3.1.1.1 Mechanism of Retinal Damage

The mechanism of chloroquine (CQ) and hydroxychloroquine (HCQ) toxicity is not well understood. HCQ induces lysosomal dysfunction in photoreceptors and retinal pigment epithelium (RPE) cells which leads to accumulation of lipofuscin in RPE [1, 2]. Melanin binding increases the concentration of the drug in the retina and further contributes or prolongs the toxic effects. The macular localization of the disease suggests that light absorption or cone metabolism may play a role [1].

3.1.1.2 Clinical Features

In early stages, patients are usually asymptomatic, though rarely may note a paracentral scotoma that causes trouble with reading as well as diminished color vision. When allowed to advance, HCQ retinal toxicity leads to loss of up to three visual functions: visual acuity, peripheral vision, and night vision.

The characteristic finding in HCQ retinopathy is bull's eye maculopathy. It is caused by buildup of the systemic drug, and thus the findings are usually bilateral and symmetric. The early signs of hydroxychloroquine toxicity are macular edema and/or bilateral granular depigmentation of the RPE in the macula (Fig. 3.1a). With continued exposure to the drug, this can progress to an atrophic bull's eye maculopathy with concentric rings of hypopigmentation and hyperpigmentation surrounding the fovea (Figs. 3.1 and 3.2) [1, 3].

3.1.1.3 Imaging Modalities

Screening Tests

The risk of retinal toxicity is not precisely known, and the recent literature suggests that the true risk may be substantially higher [2]. A new study, comprising almost 4000 patients, reported that after 5–7 years of usage, the risk approaches 1% and continues to rise with prolonged exposure [4]. A greater overall risk of toxicity (above 1%) is believed to justify a more aggressive screening algorithm.

The various screening tests in this regard include:

- Spectral-domain OCT (SD-OCT)

SD-OCT empowered with high-speed high-resolution scanning has enabled us to detect significant structural alterations prior to development of clinically visible HCQ retinopathy. Earlier studies on optical coherence tomography in HCQ retinopathy have revealed findings such as loss of the external limiting membrane (ELM), disruption of the outer ellipsoid zone, parafoveal thinning of the outer nuclear layer, and RPE damage [5–8].

Relative foveal resistance has been noted in HCQ toxicity, which is observed as the preservation of the subfoveal outer retinal layers, accounting for the intact central visual acuity that can be seen even in advanced cases of retinopathy [9]. On the

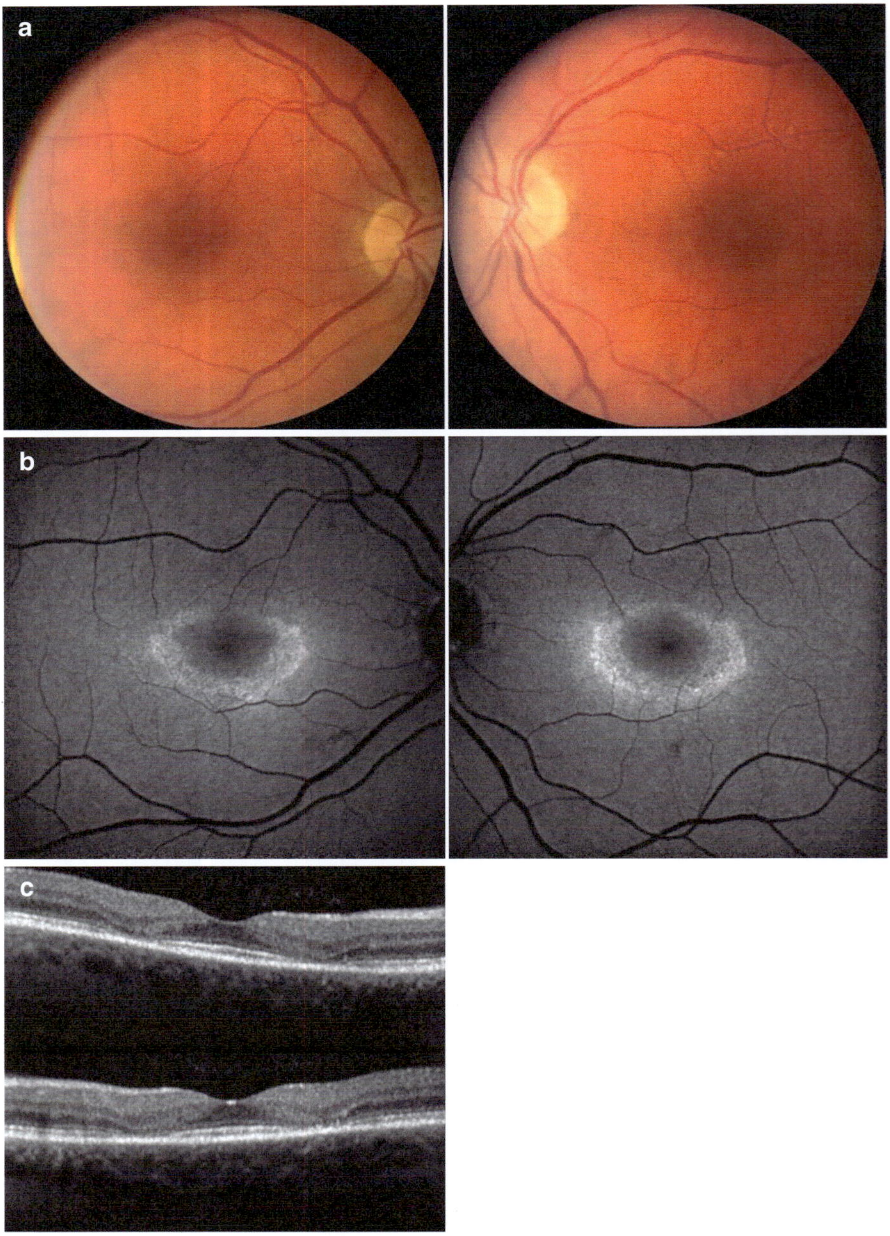

Fig. 3.1 (**a**) Color photographs of both eyes from a patient on hydroxychloroquine for the past 7 years, at 5.0 mg/kg/day, showing early bull's eye maculopathy. (**b**) On fundus autofluorescence, there is a ring of hypoautofluorescence. (**c**) Spectral-domain optical coherence tomography scans show slight thinning of the outer retina, with an early "flying saucer" sign. (**d**) A 10-2 Humphrey visual field documents mild diminution of function centrally. Visual acuity was 20/30 right eye and 20/40 left eye

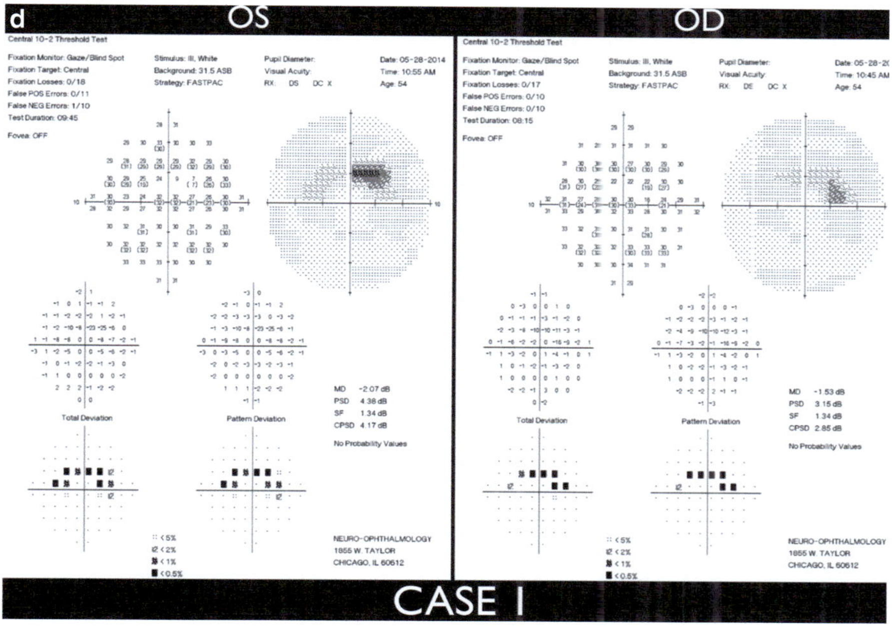

Fig. 3.1 (continued)

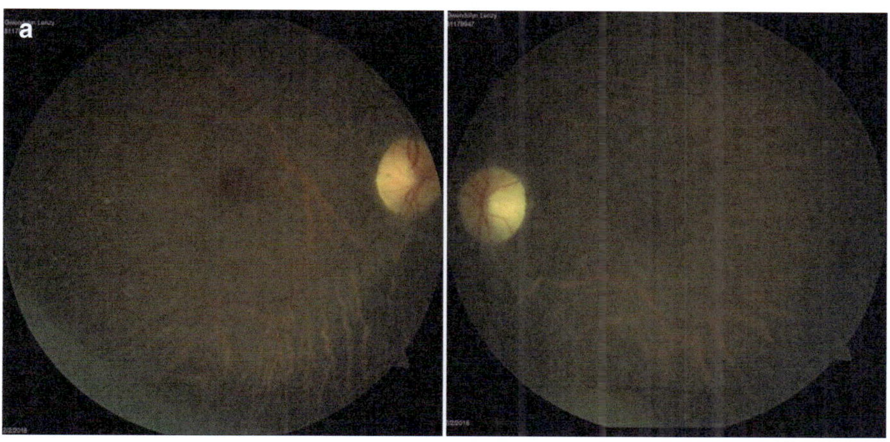

Fig. 3.2 (**a**) A patient on hydroxychloroquine for the past 25 years. In addition to a long duration of drug exposure, the patient had slowly developed renal dysfunction. The daily dosage exceeded 7.0 mg/kg/day. (**a**) Color photographs reveal widespread pigment thinning and mottling, while (**b**) the fundus autofluorescence highlights abnormalities well beyond a typical bull's eye lesion. (**c**) The fluorescein angiogram shows mottled hyperfluorescence throughout the entire posterior pole, and the (**d**) spectral-domain optical coherence tomography shows a very prominent "flying saucer" sign. Vision was 20/200 both eyes

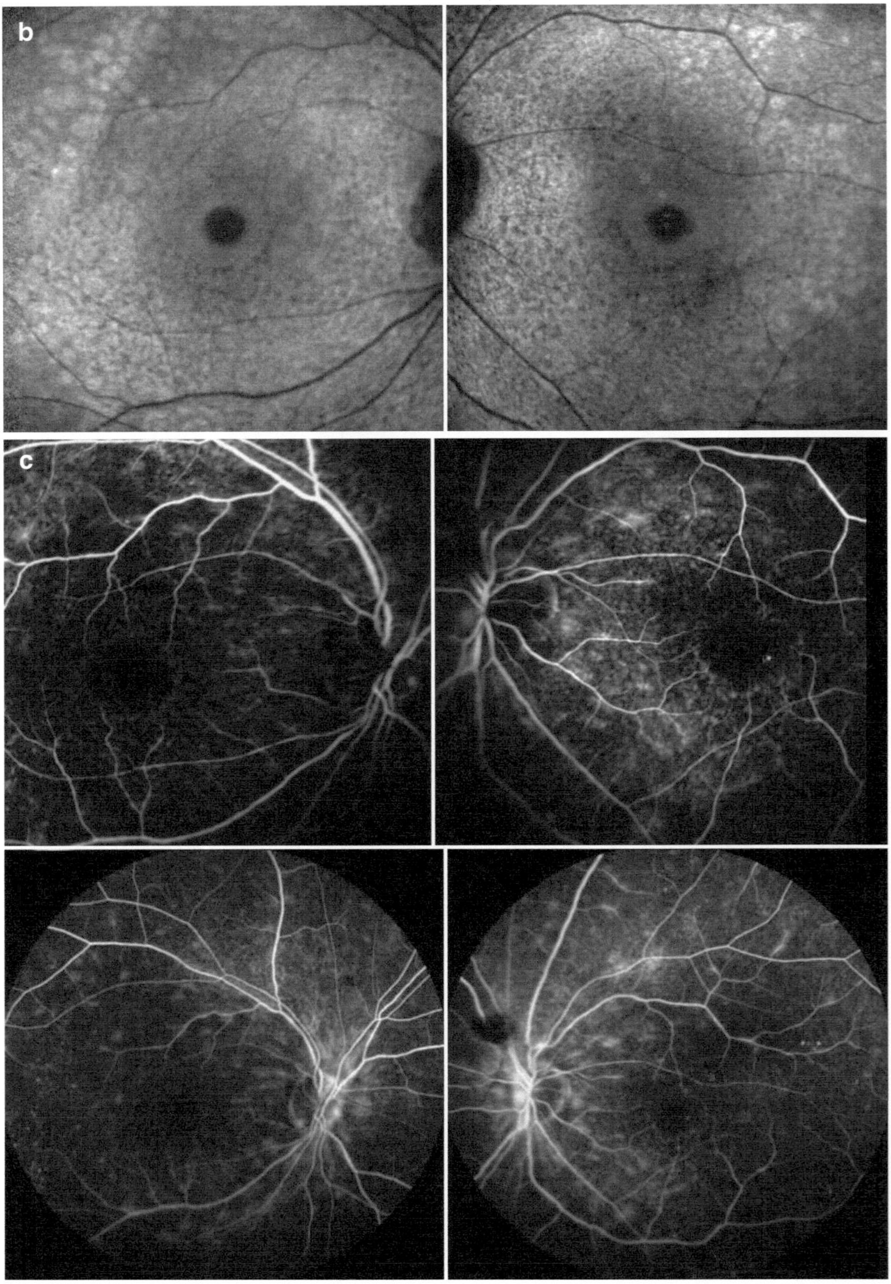

Fig. 3.2 (continued)

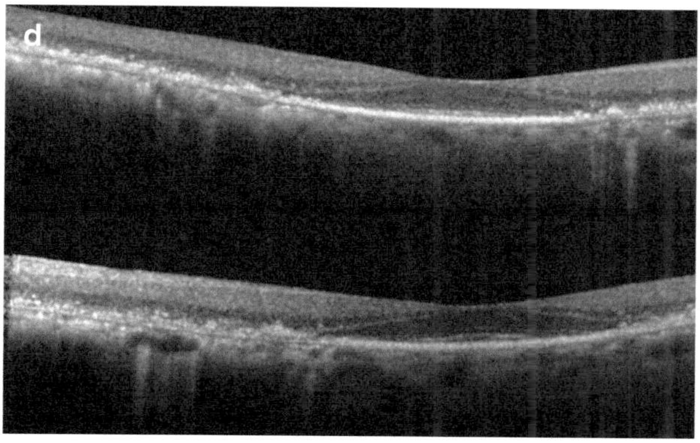

Fig. 3.2 (continued)

basis of this phenomenon, Eric Chen et al. have described *flying saucer* sign of HCQ retinopathy (Figs. 3.1 and 3.2). Here, an ovoid appearance is created by the intact central foveal outer retinal structures contrasting to the adjacent perifoveal loss of the photoreceptor ellipsoid band and outer nuclear layer atrophy [10].

While earlier researchers were focused on the outer retinal changes in HCQ retinopathy, the area of interest is slowly drifting toward the inner retinal alterations as well. Pasadhika et al. observed selective *thinning of the perifoveal inner retina* on SD-OCT, especially the inner plexiform and ganglion cell layers in the absence of structural changes to the outer retina [11, 12]. However, retinal nerve fiber layer thinning was not evident in these patients, which they proposed will happen eventually once significant retinal ganglion cell degeneration has occurred.

- Fundus autofluorescence (FAF)

FAF imaging is an effective noninvasive diagnostic method that can detect abnormalities of the RPE [13, 14]. Results of FAF imaging correspond to RPE lipofuscin characteristics which is a naturally occurring autofluorescent substance [13]. Absence of FAF indicates photoreceptor or pigment epithelial cell loss [14]. An increased FAF indicates accumulation of lipofuscin due to abnormal metabolism with increased phagocytosis of photoreceptor outer segments or an inherited or acquired defect of the phagocytic processes of the RPE cells [15, 16].

Early HCQ toxicity can also be detected on FAF as an *increased ring of signal within the parafoveal and perifoveal regions*, which is indicative of photoreceptor dysfunction and RPE abnormalities. More advanced disease will lead to *loss of autofluorescence* within these regions due to photoreceptor and RPE loss, often with surrounding hyperfluorescence (Figs. 3.2 and 3.3).

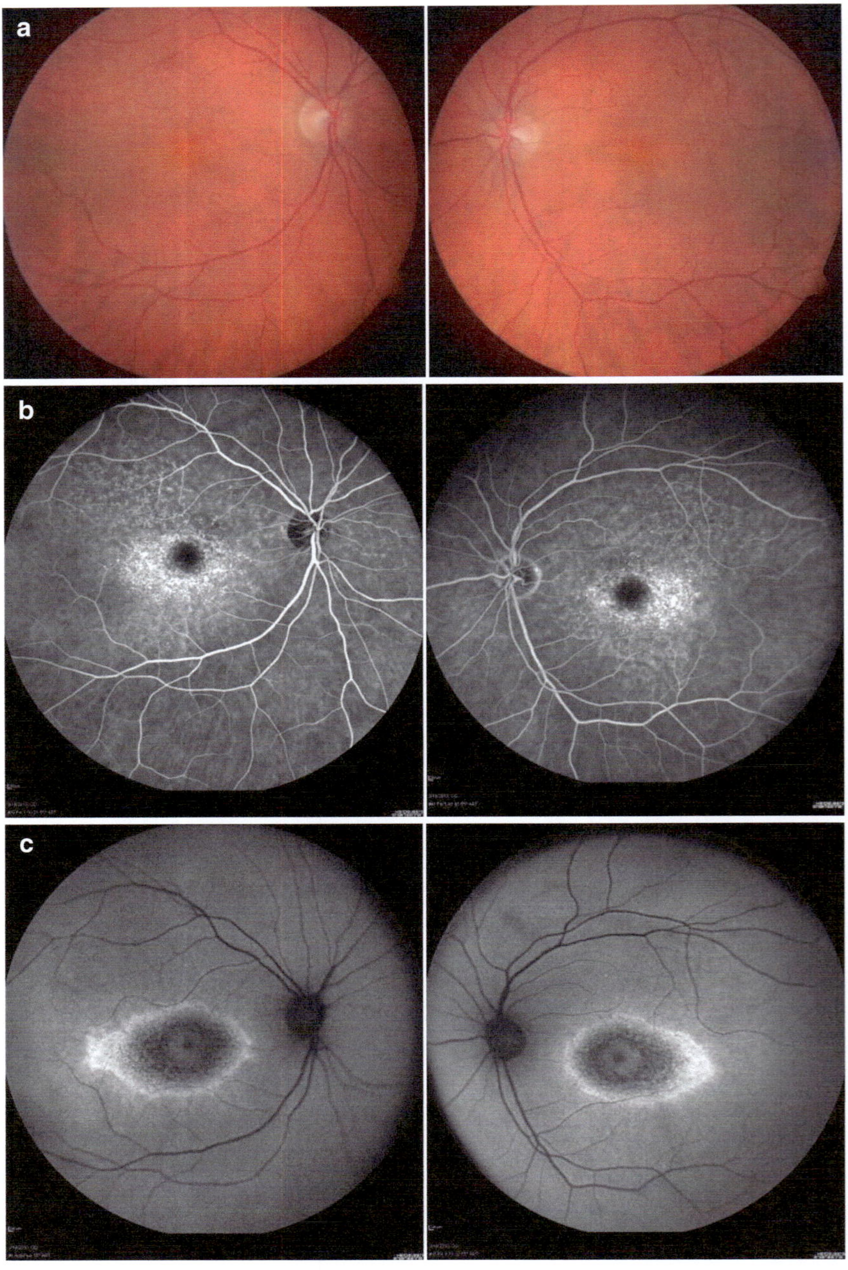

Fig. 3.3 (**a**) Color photographs from a patient of Asian descent on hydroxychloroquine showing signs of toxicity, with well-delineated bull's eye lesions, (**b**) mottled hyperfluorescence on fluorescein angiogram, and (**c**) a ring of hypoautofluorescence on fundus autofluorescence. (**d**) A spectral-domain optical coherence tomography shows pericentral retinal thinning with loss of the IS/OS junction, (**e**) the 10-2 HVF shows prominent loss of visual field, and the (**f**) mf-ERG documents marked suppression of function surrounding an annual pattern around the fovea (courtesy of David Sarraf, MD, Los Angeles, CA)

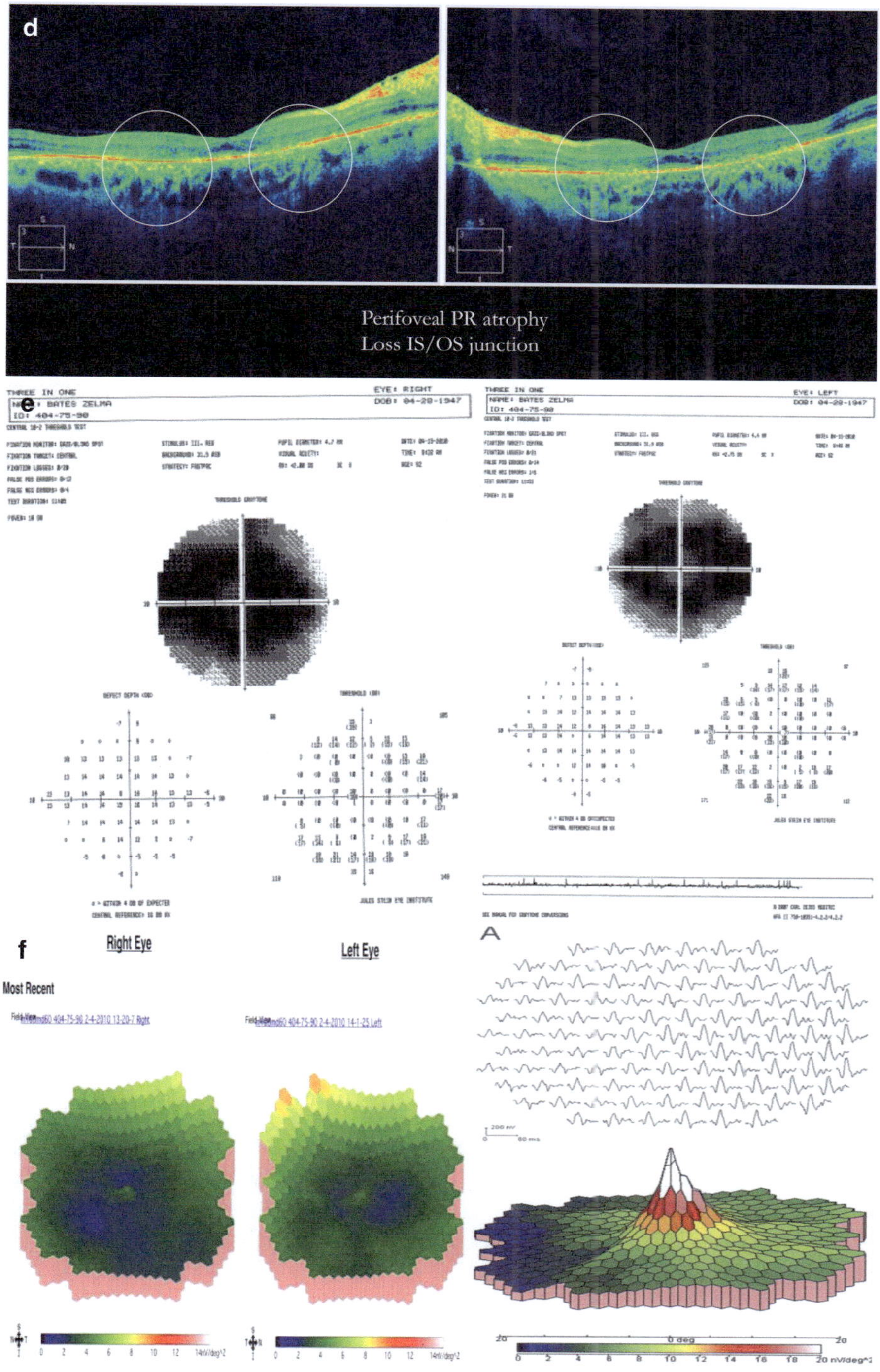

Fig. 3.3 (continued)

FAF is a good tool to monitor progression in known cases of HCQ retinopathy even after stopping the therapy. FAF intensity depends on the degree of RPE damage. Early changes include mottled or speckled appearance in the pericentral macula which eventually coalesces into dark areas of absent FAF signal once the cells have died. These dark regions may be bordered by a rim of increased autofluorescence, indicating which RPE cells will undergo degeneration next [14].

- Multifocal electroretinogram (mf-ERG)

Identifying retinal toxicity due to CQ or HCQ is a pertinent application of mf-ERG. HCQ toxicity that first affects small areas of the retina between *5° and 15° from the fovea* shows a color display of normal mf-ERGs. The amplitude of the mathematically derived b-wave of the mf-ERG is displayed in a color scale. White represents maximum b-wave amplitude, and black indicates no measureable b-wave. Clinically, areas that map black usually represent blind spots to the patient, and dark blue reflects areas of blurry vision (Fig. 3.3).

The mf-ERG may show "a moat around a small hill" appearance. The most common waveform pattern seen in patients with HCQ toxicity is paracentral amplitude loss, indicative of decreased perifoveal retinal function. Latest reports suggest that serial mf-ERGs may detect decreased retinal function even earlier than other modalities in patients with otherwise normal clinical examinations, though this has not been fully proven.

Maturi et al. in their study on the use of mf-ERG in long-term HCQ users suggested that prolonged implicit time in addition to the reduction in parafoveal amplitude may be a more specific feature [17]. Furthermore, they demonstrated three additional configurations of mf-ERG amplitudes in HCQ users:

1. Central foveal loss
2. Peripheral loss
3. Generalized loss

Overall mf-ERG testing has emerged as a promising objective measure for detecting early HCQ toxicity. It is generally employed after a patient has been on HCQ for five or more years.

- Humphrey visual field (HVF 10-2)

HCQ toxicity is characterized by subtle paracentral visual field defects. 10-2 white pattern deviation plots or red 10-2 fields can be done which often times shows a loss of sensitivity 2–6° off center and is very significant (Fig. 3.1). Even the most subtle change should be thoroughly evaluated with additional objective testing. In progressive disease, patients usually will have paracentral and central or foveal defects, whereas in late-stage or advanced disease, there is paracentral scotoma. Please also note that patients of Asian descent more typically exhibit perifoveal patterns of toxicity, rather than central changes.

- Adaptive optics (AO)

Adaptive optics is a technology used to improve the performance of optical systems by reducing the effect of wavefront distortions. The advent of AO has enabled in vivo visualization of cone mosaic to resolutions of ≤2 μm [18–20]. Thus, using adaptive optics, photoreceptor abnormalities have been revealed in various retinal diseases that were otherwise not discernible with other imaging modalities [19, 21].

The data regarding the use of AO in HCQ remain in its early stages. Few anecdotal reports demonstrate the disruption of cone photoreceptor mosaic in areas corresponding to HVF 10-2 defects and SD-OCT ellipsoid zone abnormalities [21]. Although AO serves as a noninvasive and high-resolution imaging modality, the findings are yet to be validated in HCQ retinopathy.

Other investigative modalities for drug-induced pigment epithelial and retinal toxicity include microperimetry, full-field ERG, and fluorescein angiography (FA). Microperimetry can be a useful tool to study the impact of macular RPE changes on visual function in this disease. The latest models of microperimeters incorporate a color fundus camera for image registration and an auto-tracking system to facilitate the accurate measurement of retinal sensitivity within the central visual field, even in patients with unstable or extrafoveal fixation. This allows detection of absolute scotomata, relative scotomata, or abnormally reduced retinal sensitivity in patients with macular pathologies.

Clinical pearls—HCQ retinopathy
• *Hall mark*—pigmentary retinopathy
• *Bull's eye maculopathy*
• *SD-OCT*—relative foveal resistance *"Flying saucer sign"*
• *FAF-increased AF signal in the parafoveal and perifoveal regions* Late stages—loss of AF
• *Mf-ERG-reduced b-wave amplitude in 5–15°*
• *HVF 10-2—loss of sensitivity 2—6° off center*
• *Adaptive optics—cone photoreceptor mosaic disruption*

3.1.2 Deferoxamine (DFO)

Deferoxamine is a widely used chelating agent in treating transfusional hemochromatosis. It is indicated in patients who require long-term blood transfusions. DFO prevents iron overload due to these repeated transfusions and thus protects from systemic iron toxicity. However, retinal toxicity due to DFO has been recognized widely, and there are different estimates of the incidence of retinal toxicity due to DFO ranging from 1 to 9% [22–27].

Although a clear relationship between drug dosage and development of DFO retinopathy could not be identified in most studies, it has been found that older age and longer duration of DFO treatment may be associated with more advanced forms of retinopathy.

3.1.2.1 Mechanism of Toxicity

The mechanism of DFO toxicity has been extensively studied; however, it is still not well understood. But recent studies have identified DFO-mediated direct toxic effect on the RPE cells, thus leading to acceleration of the programmed cell death of these cells [27].

3.1.3 Clinical Features

The acute stage of DFO retinopathy is characterized by retinal opacification or loss of transparency, as well as EOG and ERG attenuation. This stage is followed by macular and/or equatorial RPE pigmentary mottling, which persists even after functional recovery. Multiple case reports have described characteristic fundus lesions of DFO retinopathy seen by ophthalmoscopy and fundus photography; these lesions included pigmentary retinopathy, Bull's eye maculopathy, and possible vitelliform maculopathy (Fig. 3.4) [28, 29].

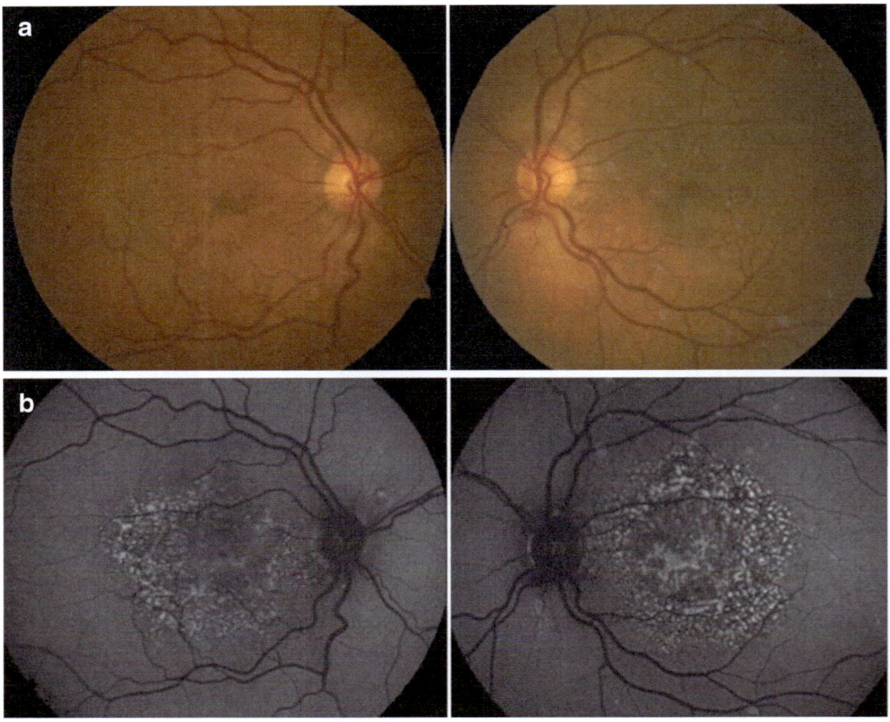

Fig. 3.4 (**a**) Color photographs of both eyes documenting diffuse pigment mottling in a patient on long-term deferoxamine. (**b**) The fundus autofluorescence highlights the areas of pigment mottling

3.1.4 Investigations

3.1.4.1 Fundus Autofluorescence on Confocal Scanning Laser Ophthalmoscopy

To date, FAF imaging using cSLO seems to be the most effective clinical adjunct for the diagnosis and evaluation of patients with DFO retinopathy [25]. Viola et al. in 2012 described four phenotypic patterns of abnormal FAF in thalassemic patients who needed long-term DFO treatment with the use of a cSLO device [26]. The characteristics of each pattern are described below.

- *Minimal change pattern*—Eyes with only minimal variations from the normal FAF appearance, with irregularly increased or decreased background FAF, are included in this group.
- *Focal pattern*—This pattern is defined by the presence of at least one medium-sized spot (diameter, 101–199 μm), of markedly increased FAF that is much brighter than the surrounding background autofluorescence. On color fundus photographs, these spots may correspond to visible alterations, such as focal hyperpigmented areas.
- Patchy pattern—This pattern is characterized by the presence of at least one large area (>200 μm) of markedly increased FAF. These areas are brighter than the surrounding background FAF, usually with well-defined borders.
- Speckled pattern—The speckled pattern is defined by the presence of multiple small areas of irregularly increased and decreased FAF that extend beyond the macula (Fig. 3.4).

3.1.4.2 Spectral-Domain OCT

In the early stage of the disease, SD-OCT usually shows only focal thickenings or bumps of the RPE, resembling basal laminar drusen. With further advancement of the disease, these RPE bumps coalesce to form hyperreflective dome-shaped lesions that disrupt the architecture of the overlying outer retinal layers. Later stages show progressive atrophy of RPE and photoreceptors. End stage shows migration of hyperreflective subretinal deposits toward the outer plexiform layer interrupting the overlying external limiting membrane.

3.1.4.3 Visual Field

The deterioration of visual fields with long-term DFO treatment has been well documented in the literature. The most common alterations were generalized constriction of the visual field [26, 30] or central-paracentral scotomata [31]. However, it was noticed that these abnormalities resolved after withdrawal of high-dose therapy.

3.1.4.4 Electrophysiology

Electroretinogram (ERG) or also electrooculogram (EOG) is essential for analyzing the location, extent, and degree of functional loss due to DFO retinopathy. Electrophysiology performed in rats given intravenous DFO showed early dose-related suppression of b-wave amplitude [32, 33].

Fortunately, these changes were found to normalize after splenectomy and cessation of DFO therapy.

3.1.5 Drugs Causing Crystalline Retinopathy

3.1.5.1 Tamoxifen Toxicity

The prototype of this group of drugs is tamoxifen which is quite commonly employed for cancer chemotherapy in the setting of metastatic breast carcinoma and advanced glioblastoma. Perifoveal crystalline maculopathy (Fig. 3.5) is the hallmark of tamoxifen toxicity, though it was observed that this correlation was mainly

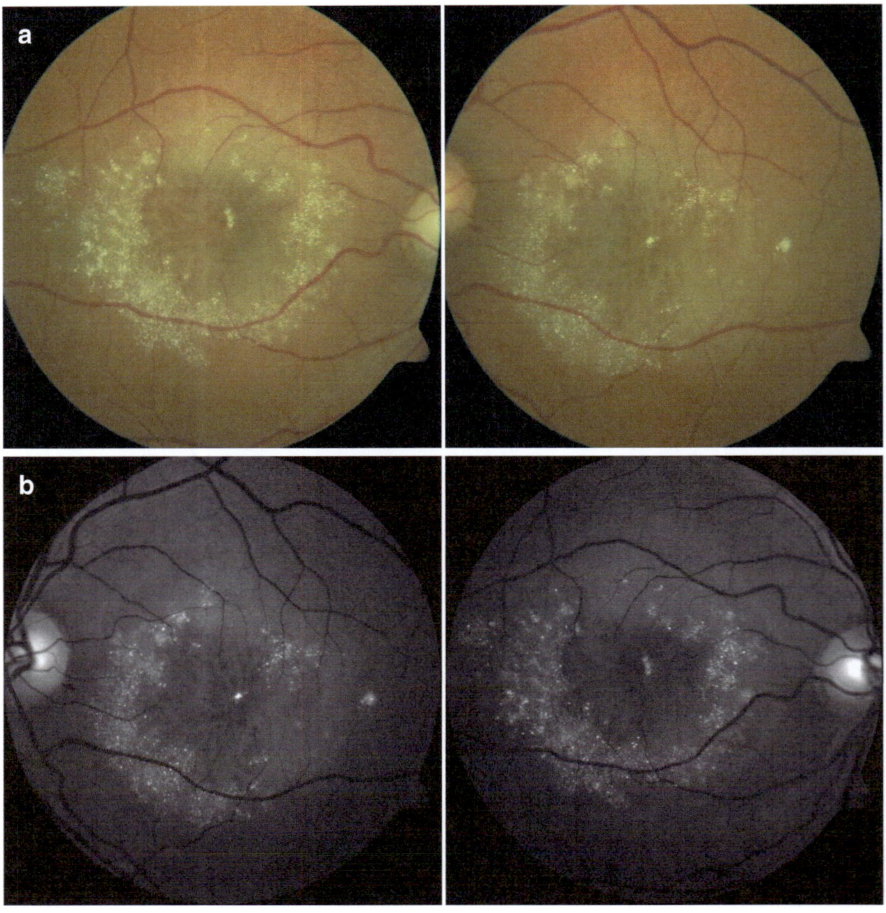

Fig. 3.5 (**a**) Color photographs of both eyes showing a ring of intraretinal perifoveal crystals in a patient on high-dose tamoxifen (200 mg/day), for treatment of glioblastoma. (**b**) A red free image highlights the crystals (images courtesy of Dave Sarraf, MD, Los Angeles, CA)

dose related and was seen in patients with daily dose more than 60–100 mg. Ever since the reduction of the dose to 20 mg/day, there have been only fewer reports of documented toxicity (approximately 3% of patients). Interestingly, with the advent of newer investigative modalities, a higher percentage of drug users have been noted to have subtle evidence of toxicity [34–38].

3.1.6 SD-OCT

Without the benefit of SD-OCT imaging, many cases of tamoxifen maculopathy would have been overlooked just by the clinical examination alone. SD-OCT picks up pseudocystic cavitary spaces in the central macula (Fig. 3.6) [39–41]. Most of these cases are diagnosed much before other signs and symptoms appeared in the patient. Foveal cavitation may predispose to full-thickness macular holes, which have been reported to develop five times more often in tamoxifen users than in women of similar age [42].

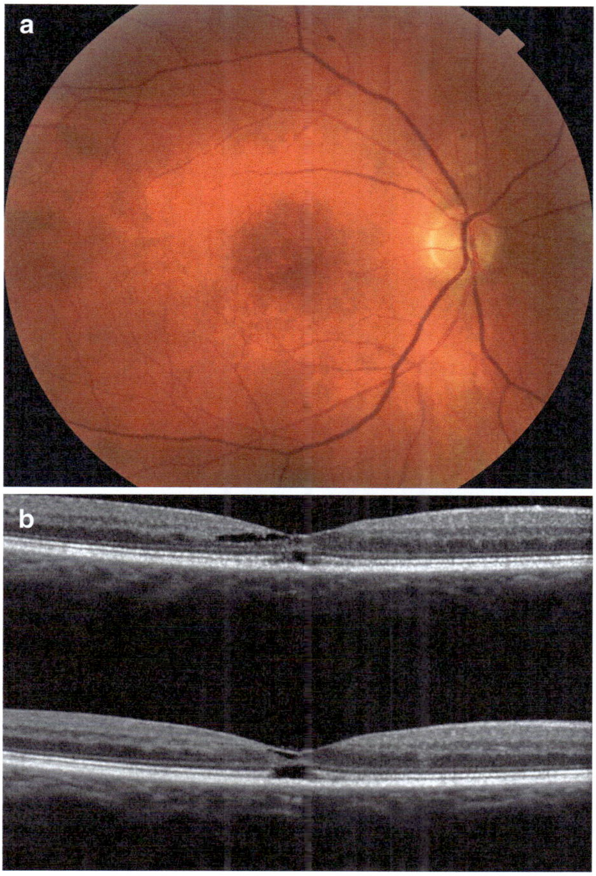

Fig. 3.6 (**a**) Color photograph of the right eye from a patient on tamoxifen, showing only minimal evidence of intraretinal crystals in a perifoveal pattern. (**b**) The spectral-domain optical coherence tomography documents a cavitary pattern seen in the setting of tamoxifen (images courtesy of Richard F Spaide, MD, New York, New York)

Both the cavitations and the crystalline retinopathy of tamoxifen toxicity are strikingly similar to those produced by idiopathic macular telangiectasia type 2. In MacTel 2, there is disturbance in the Muller cell functioning and structural integrity, ultimately leading to a loss of macular pigment and pseudocystic atrophy [42]. Crystals are found superficially in areas of altered Muller cell morphology and are hypothesized to be located within Muller cell footplates and adjacent processes surrounding retinal neurons [34].

The highest incidence of retinopathy was reported by Chung and associates, who screened breast cancer patients on 20 mg of daily tamoxifen with both time-domain OCT and SD-OCT and found that 6 of 49 patients (12.2%) had retinal cavitations, visualized reliably only with high-resolution scans [38].

3.1.7 Fundus Autofluorescence

Autofluorescence imaging shows punctate hyperautofluorescent foci corresponding to the yellow spots seen clinically, as well as absence of the normal foveal hypoautofluorescence.

3.1.8 Fluorescein Angiography (FA)

Unlike the angiographic macular edema seen in various other drug toxicities, FA reveals mild hyperfluorescence in the central macula corresponding to the area of pseudocystic atrophy of the retina but with no leakage. This proves that it is not a true macular edema (yet typical leaking cystoid macular edema has been seen in select cases).

The recent consensus is that patients on tamoxifen therapy may benefit from baseline and yearly screening with fundus examination and SD-OCT imaging. Isolated crystalline retinopathy without SD-OCT findings does not warrant stoppage of the drug. However, the presence of cavitary spaces on SD-OCT should prompt reconsideration of tamoxifen treatment. In such cases, the patient's oncologist should be consulted, and consideration should be given to modifying the dose or discontinuing the drug.

Clinical pearls in crystalline retinopathy
• Prototype—tamoxifen
• Underdiagnosed in early stages
• SD-OCT—pseudocystic cavitation at the fovea, early sign
• FAF—hyper-AF at the area of crystalline deposits and altered foveal hypoautofluorescence
• FA—mild hyperfluorescence in the central macula without active leak
• Recent consensus—baseline and yearly screening with fundus examination and SD-OCT

3.1.9 Vascular Toxicity

3.1.9.1 Talc Retinopathy

An important drug in this group is talc, which is an insoluble inert particulate filler material used in the preparation of certain oral, inhalational, and intravenous drugs. When injected systemically, these fine particles enter into the systemic circulation which further embolize and get lodged in the retinal vessels, thus causing ischemia.

Talc retinopathy is characterized by the appearance of these crystals, which are found inside the small retinal arteries throughout the fundus (Fig. 3.7). Talc crystals should be differentiated from other conditions causing crystalline retinopathy and from other causes of retinal embolism.

3.1.10 Adaptive Optics and SD-OCT

The advent of adaptive optics has made it possible to detect the deposits of talc in the blood vessels in the retina. As reported by Soliman et al., AO imaging revealed multiple shiny refractile dots distributed both intravascularly and extravascularly corresponding to those seen in the fundus. The high resolution of AO allowed detection of some tiny particles that were not detectable clinically [41].

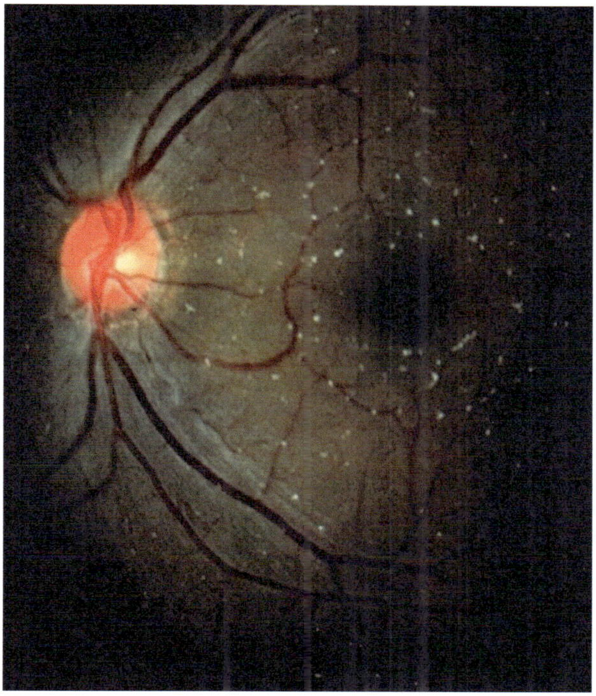

Fig. 3.7 Color photograph of the left eye from a drug abuser, showing numerous intra-arterial talc particles

With SD-OCT, the locations of these crystals with respect to retinal layers have been demonstrated. They were found distributed among the inner retinal layers where retinal blood vessels reside [43]. SD-OCT demonstrated multiple hyperreflective dots of varying sizes scattered among the nerve fiber layer, ganglion cell layer, inner plexiform, and inner nuclear layer. Thinning of the inner retinal layers in temporal part of the macula was noted in the same patient [43].

3.1.11 Aminoglycoside Toxicity

Another important drug which causes vascular damage is aminoglycoside antibiotics, presenting as macular or retinal infarction. In such cases, FA reveals the areas of non-perfusion, but more interestingly SD-OCT shows inner retinal layer hyperreflectivity suggestive of ischemia.

3.1.11.1 Drugs Causing Macular Edema

Several medicines have been associated with the development of CME, and these include agents such as prostaglandin analogues like latanoprost, nicotinic acid, epinephrine, and taxols (Fig. 3.8).

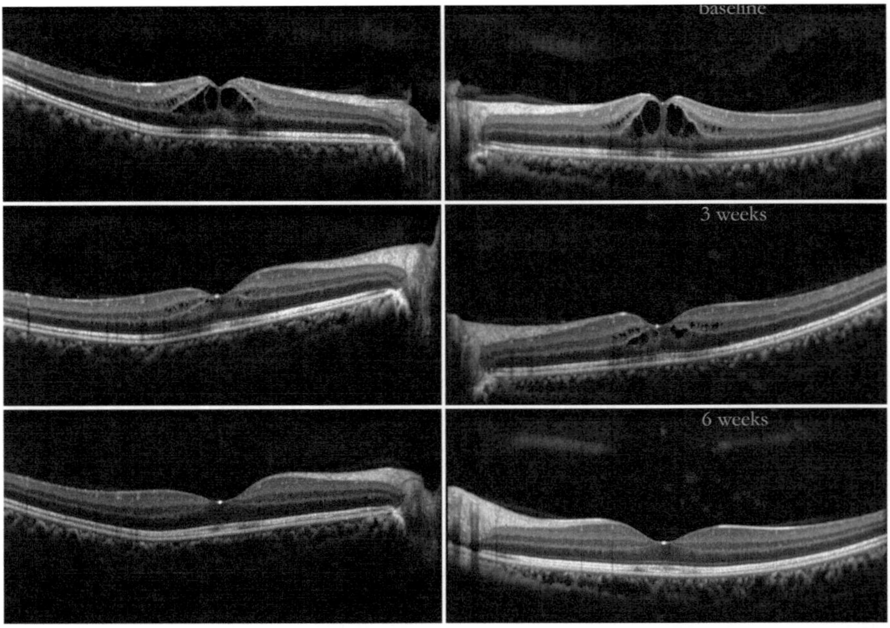

Fig. 3.8 Fluorescein angiogram showing macular cystic spaces from a patient on paclitaxel. Upon discontinuation of the medication, the cystic spaces resolved. A fluorescein angiogram (not shown) did not reveal any late leakage even when the cystic spaces were present

3.1.11.2 Mechanism of Action

The macular edema caused by these drugs cannot be called true macular edema, as this "pseudo-macular edema" is probably caused by intracellular fluid accumulation, as opposed to true edema, which is in the extracellular space [44].

3.1.11.3 Investigations

Fluorescein angiography and OCT are useful to confirm the diagnosis.

FA—Fluorescein angiogram shows absence of fluorescein leakage or vascular alteration contrary to that expected in a case of typical cystoid macular edema. The petaloid appearance caused by fluorescein dye leakage typical of CME is absent [45].

OCT—Optical coherence tomography shows fluid accumulation in the form of intraretinal cystoid spaces that appear more numerous and larger in the outer plexiform layer than that in the inner nuclear zone [46, 47] (Fig. 3.8).

3.1.11.4 Treatment

Treatment is discontinuation of the medication, which generally allows for rapid resolution of the pseudo-CME and restoration of visual function (Fig. 3.8).

3.1.11.5 Miscellaneous Agents

Sildenafil

Mechanism of Action

Sildenafil improves erectile function in men with ED (erectile dysfunction) by selectively inhibiting cyclic guanosine monophosphate (cGMP)-specific phosphodiesterase type 5 (PDE-5), which is present in all vascular tissues and enhances the smooth muscle relaxant effects of nitric oxide [48].

The choroid being analogous in many respect to the corpus cavernosum has been described as an erectile tissue in the literature [49]. The fenestrated choroidal vasculature is highly responsive to both local and neurogenic stimuli, and the uveal system may hold up to 97% of the intraocular blood volume. Sildenafil, thus inducing smooth muscle relaxation, causes increased choroidal perfusion. This can secondarily affect retinal and retinal pigment epithelial function and could predispose users to serous retinal detachment or retinal edema [50].

Imaging in sildenafil toxicity.

Enhanced depth imaging—Enhanced depth imaging (EDI) OCT moves the imaging focal point of spectral-domain OCT (the zero-delay line) more posteriorly, allowing for a stronger returning reflection from the choroid, resulting in better definition of details [51]. A study by Kim et al. on the measurement of choroidal perfusion and thickness following systemic sildenafil showed statistically significant increase in choroidal thickness as measured by EDI-OCT 2 h after 50 mg of sildenafil [52].

Neurosensory detachment on OCT—The increase in choroidal thickness following sildenafil ingestion [51] favors the prior reports on the development of the central serous retinopathy following the pharmacological use of sildenafil [53, 54]. This has led to greater global concern for the need to limit the prescription and usage of these agents.

Swept-scan ultrasound—The study conducted by Kim et al. also demonstrated that 2 h after ingestion of 50 mg of sildenafil, there was an increase in choroidal perfusion as measured by 20 MHz swept-scan ultrasound which was found to be statistically significant [52].

Conclusion

Retinal toxicity from systemic medications is of serious ophthalmologic and medicolegal concern because even after cessation of therapy, many of these drugs continue to produce progressive visual loss. In the majority of cases, the damage remains permanent. With the newer enhanced imaging modalities, it is possible for the ophthalmologist to identify the retinal toxicities at a very early stage before the clinical signs appear. But the standardization of the results with these sophisticated methods needs to be better assessed via randomized controlled trials in the future, or at least further observatory studies.

References

1. Mahon GJ, Anderson HR, Gardiner TA, et al. Chloroquine causes lysosomal dysfunction in neural retina and RPE: implications for retinopathy. Curr Eye Res. 2004;28:277–84.
2. Marmor MF, Carr RE, Easterbrook M, Farjo AA, Mieler WF. Recommendations on screening for chloroquine and hydroxychloroquine retinopathy: a report by the American Academy of Ophthalmology. Ophthalmology. 2002;109:1377–82.
3. Bernstein HN, Ginsberg J. The pathology of chloroquine retinopathy. Arch Ophthalmol. 1964;71:238–45.
4. Yam JC, Kwok AK. Ocular toxicity of hydroxychloroquine. Hong Kong Med J. 2006;12(4): 294–304.
5. Lai TY, Ngai JW, Chan WM, et al. Visual field and multifocal electroretinography and their correlations in patients on hydroxychloroquine therapy. Doc Ophthalmol. 2006;112:177–87.
6. Mititelu M, Wong BJ, Brenner M, Bryar PJ, Jampol LM, Fawzi AA. Progression of hydroxychloroquine toxic effects after drug therapy cessation: new evidence from multimodal imaging. JAMA Ophthalmol. 2013;131:1187–97.
7. Marmor MF. Comparison of screening procedures in hydroxychloroquine toxicity. Arch Ophthalmol. 2012;130:461–9.
8. Elder M, Rahman AM, Mc LJ. Early paracentral visual field loss in patients taking hydroxychloroquine. Arch Ophthalmol. 2006;124:1729–33.
9. Kellner S, Weinitz S, Kellner U. Spectral domain optical coherence tomography detects early stages of chloroquine retinopathy similar to multifocal electroretinography, fundus autofluorescence and near-infrared autofluorescence. Br J Ophthalmol. 2009;93(11):1444–7.
10. Chen E, Brown DM, Benz MS, et al. Spectral domain optical coherence tomography as an effective screening test for hydroxychloroquine retinopathy (the "flying saucer" sign). Clin Ophthalmol. 2010;4:1151–8.

11. Pasadhika S, Fishman GA, Choi D, Shahidi M. Selective thinning of the perifoveal inner retina as an early sign of hydroxychloroquine retinal toxicity. Eye (Lond). 2010;24(5):756–62. quiz 763
12. Pasadhika S, Fishman GA. Effects of chronic exposure to hydroxychloroquine or chloroquine on inner retinal structures. Eye (Lond). 2010;24(2):340–6.
13. Delori FC, Dorey CK, Staurenghi G, et al. In vivo fluorescence of the ocular fundus exhibits retinal pigment epithelium lipofuscin characteristics. Invest Ophthalmol Vis Sci. 1995;36:718–29.
14. Holz FG, Bellmann C, Staudt S, Schutt F, Volcker HE. Fundus autofluorescence and development of geographic atrophy in age-related macular degeneration. Invest Ophthalmol Vis Sci. 2001;42:1051–6.
15. Kennedy CJ, Rakoczy PE, ConstableI J. Lipofuscin of the retinal pigment epithelium: a review. Eye. 1995;9:763–71.
16. Okubo A, Rosa BH, Bunce CV, et al. The relationship of age changes in retinal pigment epithelium and Bruch's membrane. Invest Ophthalmol Vis Sci. 1999;40:443–9.
17. Maturi RK, Yu M, Weleber RG. Multifocal electroretinographic evaluation of long-term hydroxychloroquine users. Arch Ophthalmol. 2004;122:973–81.
18. Roorda A, Romero-Borja F, Donnelly Iii W, Queener H, Hebert T, Campbell M. Adaptive optics scanning laser ophthalmoscopy. Opt Express. 2002;10(9):405–12.
19. Park SP, Chung JK, Greenstein V, Tsang SH, Chang S. A study of factors affecting the human cone photoreceptor density measured by adaptive optics scanning laser ophthalmoscope. Exp Eye Res. 2013;108:1–9.
20. Kim JE, Chung M. Adaptive optics for retinal imaging: current status. Retina. 2013;33:1483–6.
21. Stepien KE, Han DP, Schell J, Godara P, Rha J, Carroll J. Spectral-domain optical coherence tomography and adaptive optics may detect hydroxychloroquine retinal toxicity before symptomatic vision loss. Trans Am Ophthalmol Soc. 2009;107:28–33.
22. Brittenham GM. Iron-chelating therapy for transfusional iron overload. N Engl J Med. 2011;364:146–56.
23. Stummvoll HK, Graf H, Meisinger V. Effect of desferrioxamine on aluminum kinetics during hemodialysis. Miner Electrolyte Metab. 1984;10:263–6.
24. Chen H, et al. Auditory and visual toxicity during deferoxamine therapy in transfusion-dependent patients. J Pediatr Hematol Oncol. 2005;27:651–3.
25. Martin CM, Mizanin J, Konkle DF, Schwartz E. Vision and hearing during deferoxamine therapy. J Pediatr. 1990;117:326–30.
26. Baath JS, Lam WC, Kirby M, Chun A. Deferoxamine-related ocular toxicity: Incidence and outcome in a pediatric population. Retina. 2008;28:894–9.
27. Viola F, Barteselli G, Dell'Arti L, et al. Abnormal fundus autofluorescence results of patients in long-term treatment with deferoxamine. Ophthalmology. 2012;119:1693–700.
28. Blake DR, Winyard P, Lunec J, et al. Cerebral and ocular toxicity induced by desferrioxamine. Q J Med. 1985;56:345–55.
29. Bansal V, Elgarbly I, Ghanchi FD, Atkinson PL. Bull's eye maculopathy with deferoxamine. Eur J Haematol. 2003;70:420–1.
30. Arden GB, Wonke B, Kennedy C, Huehns ER. Ocular changes in patients undergoing long-term desferrioxamine treatment. Br J Ophthalmol. 1984;68(12):873–7.
31. Ravelli M, Scaroni P, Mombelloni S, et al. Acute visual disorders in patients on regular dialysis given desferrioxamine as a test. Nephrol Dial Transplant. 1990;5:945–9.
32. Gehlbach PL, Purple RL, Hallaway PE, Hedlund BE. Polymer conjugation reduces deferoxamine induced retinopathy in an albino rat model. Invest Ophthalmol Vis Sci. 1993;34:2871–7.
33. Good PA, Claxson A, Morris CJ, Blake DR. A model for desferrioxamine-induced retinopathy using the albino rat. Ophthalmologica. 1990;201:32–6.
34. Kaiser-Kupfer MI, Kupfer C, Rodrigues MM. Tamoxifen retinopathy. A clinicopathologic report. Ophthalmology. 1981;88(1):89–93.
35. Nair AG, Das D, Goyal A, Gandhi RA. The eyes have it! Tamoxifen maculopathy revisited: a case report. J Ocul Pharmacol Ther. 2012;28(6):640–2.

36. Chung SE, Kim SW, Chung HW, Kang SW. Estrogen antagonist and development of macular hole. Korean J Ophthalmol. 2010;24(5):306–9.
37. Gualino V, Cohen SY, Delyfer MN, Sahel JA, Gaudric A. Optical coherence tomography findings in tamoxifen retinopathy. Am J Ophthalmol. 2005;140(4):757–8.
38. Mauget-Faysse M, Gambrelle J, Quaranta-El MM. Optical coherence tomography in tamoxifen retinopathy. Breast Cancer Res Treat. 2006;99(1):117–8.
39. Park SS, Zawadzki RJ, Truong SN, Choi SS, Werner JS. Microcystoid maculopathy associated with tamoxifen use diagnosed by high-resolution Fourier-domain optical coherence tomography. Retin Cases Brief Rep. 2009;3(1):33–5.
40. Chung H, Kim D, Ahn SH, et al. Early detection of tamoxifen-induced maculopathy in patients with low cumulative doses of tamoxifen. Ophthalmic Surg Lasers Imaging. 2010;42:1–5.
41. Soliman MK, Sarwar S, Hanout M, Sadiq MA, Agarwal A, Gulati V, Dong Q. High-resolution adaptive optics findings in talc retinopathy. Int J Retina Vitreo. 2015;1:10.
42. Cronin BG, Lekich CK, Bourke RD. Tamoxifen therapy conveys increased risk of developing a macular hole. Int Ophthalmol. 2005;26(3):101–5.
43. Shah VA, Cassell M, Poulose A, Sabates NR. Talc retinopathy. Ophthalmology. 2008; DOI: 10.1016/j.ophtha.2007.10.043.
44. Jampol LM. Niacin maculopathy. Ophthalmology. 1988;95:1704–5.
45. Bressler NM. Cystoid macular edema from niacin typically is not accompanied by fluorescein leakage on angiography. Am J Ophthalmol. 2005;139(5):951.
46. Spirn MJ, Warren FA, Guyer DR, Klancnik JM, Spaide RF. Optical coherence tomography findings in nicotinic acid maculopathy. Am J Ophthalmol. 2003;135(6):913–4.
47. Dajani HM, Lauer AK. Optical coherence tomography findings in niacin maculopathy. Can J Ophthalmol. 2006;41(2):197–200.
48. Ballard SA, Gingell CJ, Tang K, Turner LA, Price ME, Naylor AM. Effects of sildenafil on the relaxation of human corpus cavernosum tissue in vitro and on the activities of cyclic nucleotide phosphodiesterase isozymes. J Urol. 1998;159:2164–71.
49. Duke-Elder S, Wybar K. Anatomy of the visual systems. In: Duke-Elder S, editor. System of ophthalmology, vol. 2. St. Louis: CV Mosby Co; 1961. p. 132.
50. Paris G, Sponsel WE, Sandoval SS, Elliott WR, Trigo Y, Sanford DK, Harison JM. Sildenafil increases ocular perfusion. Int Ophthalmol. 2001;23(4–6):355–8.
51. Mrejen S, Spaide RF. Optical coherence tomography: imaging of the choroid and beyond. Surv Ophthalmol. 2013;58:387–429.
52. David Y. Kim et al Measurement of Choroidal Perfusion and Thickness Following Systemic Sildenafil (Viagra®). Acta Ophthalmol. 2013 Mar;91(2):183–8.
53. Allibhai ZA, Gale JS, Sheidow TS. Central serous chorioretinopathy in a patient taking sildenafil citrate. Ophthalmic Surg Lasers Imaging. 2004;35:165–7.
54. Fraunfelder FW, Fraunfelder FT. Central serous chorioretinopathy associated with sildenafil. Retina. 2008;28:606–9.

Retinal Manifestations in Hematological Disorders

4

Giulio Barteselli, Maura Di Nicola, and Laura Dell'Arti

Abstract

Red blood cell, white blood cell, and platelet disorders often lead to a large variety of hematologic effects in ocular tissues, and especially in the retina. Although retinal findings may not be pathognomonic of a specific blood disorder, ophthalmologists can directly visualize characteristic retinal changes and be the first to diagnose a blood dyscrasia. Typical findings on indirect ophthalmoscopy are retinal hemorrhages, microaneurysms, hard exudates, cotton wool spots, macular edema, retinal vascular edema, pallor of the disc, edema of the disc, retinal and optic disc neovascularization, vitreous hemorrhage and inflammation, retinal and retinal pigment epithelium detachment, and retinal and choroidal infiltrates. Other retinal findings may be more indicative of a specific blood disorder, such as thalassemia or sickle cell disease. High-resolution imaging can help ophthalmologists in the detection of early retinal changes or more peculiar findings and can guide physicians in an early diagnosis of a specific blood dyscrasia.

G. Barteselli (✉)
Genentech Inc., South San Francisco, CA, USA

Department of Ophthalmology, Shiley Eye Institute, University of California San Diego, La Jolla, CA 92093, USA
e-mail: giuliobart@gmail.com

M. Di Nicola • L. Dell'Arti
Ophthalmological Unit, Department of Clinical Sciences and Community Health, Ca' Granda Foundation-Ospedale Maggiore Policlinico, University of Milan, Milan, Italy
e-mail: mauradinicola@gmail.com; ldellarti@gmail.com

J. Chhablani et al. (eds.), *Retinal and Choroidal Imaging in Systemic Diseases*,
https://doi.org/10.1007/978-981-10-5461-7_4

4.1 Introduction

The term "dyscrasia" is used in medical context to indicate a disease of the blood, usually referring to disorders of the cellular elements including red blood cells, white blood cells, and platelets, which represent 45% of the total blood volume. About 55% of the blood is an aqueous solution called *plasma*, containing 92% water. The remaining 8% of the plasma consists of proteins (albumin, globulin, fibrinogen, and enzymes), lipids, carbohydrates, hormones, vitamins, and salts. The term *serum* refers to plasma from which the clotting proteins have been removed.

Disorders of the red blood cells are associated with mutations in the globing genes determining abnormal synthesis of hemoglobin. These are the most frequent monogenic disorders worldwide and affect approximately 7% of the global population [1]. Adult hemoglobin (HbA) is formed by the combination of two α-globin and β-globin proteins with a central heme molecule [2]. Hemoglobin abnormalities might be a result of synthesis of abnormal molecules or reduced synthesis of normal α- or β-globin chains (thalassemias)..

- α-Thalassemia is more common in the far east, and the clinical severity of the disease varies according to the number of missing/inactive genes.
- β-Thalassemia is more frequent in the Mediterranean region, presumably due to the selective pressure from *Plasmodium falciparum* malaria in this area. In β-thalassemia major either small amounts or no β-chains are synthetized. As a result, both erythroblasts and mature red cells are deformed and precipitate, resulting in ineffective erythropoiesis and hemolysis. Blood transfusions are necessary for patient's sustainment, along with chelation therapy in order to avoid iron overload. β-Thalassemia trait (minor) is a common and usually symptomless condition with mild anemia, while cases of thalassemia of moderate severity not requiring regular transfusion are usually referred to as β-thalassemia intermedia.
- Sickle cell disease includes a group of disorders in which the sickle β-globin gene is inherited. Inheritance of the disease is autosomal recessive, so either two copies of sickle hemoglobin (HbS) or one copy of HbS plus another variant (such as HbC) is required for disease expression [2]. Several combinations are possible: HbSS (homozygous) is the most common, but HbSC and HbSβ-thal might also cause sickling disease. HbS is insoluble and forms crystals with low oxygen tension: as a result, red cells sickle and might block microvessels or larger vessels causing infarcts of various organs. Clinical features include severe hemolytic anemia punctuated by different types of crises: vaso-occlusive, visceral, aplastic, or hemolytic. Prophylaxis aiming at preventing crisis is mandatory in the management of sickle cell disease, along with the use of different combinations of folic acid and hydroxyurea. Sickle cell trait is a benign condition with no anemia and normal appearance of red blood cells.

Disorders of the white cells are secondary to either an increase or decrease of white blood cells, which are classified into myeloid leukocytes and the lymphocytes [3–5]. The myeloid lineage includes neutrophils, monocytes, eosinophils, and basophils. Lymphocytes include T cells, B cells, and natural killer cells. White blood cell diseases may involve only one of the five types of white blood cells, or a few or all five types together. Disorders of neutrophils and lymphocytes are the most common, while abnormalities of monocytes, eosinophils, and basophils are less common.

- Leukocytosis refers to a higher than normal number of the total white blood cells due to any cause. It may be caused by an increase of neutrophils (neutrophilia), lymphocytes (lymphocytosis), monocytes (monocytosis), eosinophils (eosinophilia), basophils (basophilia), or immature cells (blasts). Leukocytosis can be caused by infection, inflammation, allergic reaction, malignancy, hereditary disorders, physiologic processes (stress, exercise), or other miscellaneous causes. This condition causes vascular occlusions, often resulting in organs' ischemia, hemorrhage, and edema.
- Leukemias are heterogeneous neoplastic disorders of white blood cells. They can be divided into myeloid or lymphoid, depending on their origin, and into acute or chronic. A clone of leukemic cells may arise at any stage of maturation, in the lymphoid, myeloid, or pluripotential stage. Rearrangement of the DNA due to both external factors (chemicals, alkylating agents, ionizing radiation) and internal factors (such as chromosomal abnormalities) seems to represent the cause of the clonal expansion. Acute leukemias, acute lymphocytic leukemia (ALL), and acute myelogenous leukemia (AML) usually present with progressive weakness and fatigue secondary to anemia, infection secondary to leukopenia, and bleeding secondary to thrombocytopenia. Many patients with chronic leukemias, chronic myelogenous leukemia (CML), and chronic lymphocytic leukemia (CLL) are asymptomatic. In other patients, clinical manifestations include splenomegaly, lymphadenopathy, hepatomegaly, fever, weight loss, malaise, frequent infections, bleeding, and thrombosis.
- Leukopenia is an abnormally low number of the white blood cells found in the blood; the clinical sequelae of leucopenia usually manifest as infections. Neutropenia refers to a decrease in the number of circulating neutrophil granulocytes, the most abundant white blood cells. Low white cell count may be due to acute viral infections, chemotherapy, radiation therapy, myelofibrosis, aplastic anemia, other systemic diseases and other medications. Lymphocytopenia is due to a decreased number of lymphocytes in the blood. The most common causes are AIDS and undernutrition.
- Plasma cell dyscrasias form a heterogeneous group of diseases characterized by the expansion of the number of monoclonal bone marrow plasma cells that produce monoclonal immunoglobulins. Plasma cell dyscrasias include multiple myeloma, Waldenström's macroglobulinemia, heavy chain diseases, amyloidosis, and benign monoclonal hypergammaglobulinemia (or monoclonal gammopathies of undetermined significance).

Inherited or acquired disorders of platelet count or function might be responsible for abnormal bleeding. In case of thrombocytopenia or abnormal platelet function, spontaneous skin purpura, mucosal hemorrhage, and prolonged bleeding after trauma represent the characteristic manifestations. Main causes of thrombocytopenia include failure of platelet production, increased consumption of platelets, and abnormal distribution of platelets. Management varies according to the underlying condition [3–5].

Inherited or acquired diseases of clotting factors determine an abnormal coagulation cascade; this can affect hemostasis and finally lead to thrombosis and/or hemorrhage [3–5].

- The most common and most severe disorder is factor VIII deficiency (hemophilia A). Typical manifestations of this X-linked disease include severe and protracted bleeding, after even minor trauma, and spontaneous bleeding into joints, the central nervous system, and the abdominal cavity.
- Other coagulation-impeding conditions include anticoagulant afibrinogenemia/dysfibrinogenemia, factor V deficiency, factor VII deficiency, factor X deficiency, factor XI deficiency, factor XII deficiency, factor XIII deficiency, hemophilia B, and hypoprothrombinemias.
- The thrombotic disorders (thrombophilia) include primary hypercoagulable states that are caused by abnormalities of specific coagulation proteins (such as procoagulant afibrinogenemia/dysfibrinogenemia, protein C deficiency, protein S deficiency, antithrombin III deficiency, factor V Leiden deficiency, activated protein C resistance, disseminated intravascular coagulation) and secondary hypercoagulable states that cause a thrombotic tendency by complex and often multifactorial mechanisms (i.e., malignancies, myeloproliferative disorders).

The clinical exam of the fundus oculi provides a direct view of the hematologic effects of blood dyscrasias in ocular tissues. By observing the characteristic changes in the retina, the ophthalmologist may actually be the first to diagnose a blood dyscrasia. Ocular findings of blood dyscrasias aren't pathognomonic signs and may be observed in many local and systemic diseases. Typical findings are retinal hemorrhages, microaneurysms, hard exudates, cotton wool spots, macular edema, retinal vascular edema, pallor of the disc, edema of the disc, retinal and optic disc neovascularization, vitreous hemorrhage and inflammation, retinal and retinal pigment epithelium detachment, and retinal and choroidal infiltrates. In this chapter, we will focus on hematologic diseases of interest for the ophthalmologist.

4.2 Retinal Manifestations in β-Thalassemia Syndromes

A variety of retinal findings have been reported in patients with β-thalassemia syndromes; these may occur as a result of the disease itself or of the iron chelation therapy [6]. Because patients affected by the most severe form need regular blood transfusions to survive, subsequent iron overload may potentially occur in several organs (i.e., the liver, spleen, myocardium, endocrine organs) including the eye. Several iron-chelating agents, such as desferrioxamine (DFO), deferiprone (DFP), and deferasirox, are currently approved to address this problem. Retinal manifestations of β-thalassemia include retinal pigment epithelium (RPE) degeneration and mottling, retinal edema, retinal hemorrhages, angioid streaks, papillitis, and macular scarring [7–9].

Recent advancement in multimodal retinal imaging using confocal laser scanning ophthalmoscopy (cSLO) has better characterized these retinal abnormalities in β-thalassemia. Specifically, abnormalities can be separated in two groups: (1) pseudoxanthoma elasticum (PXE)-like and (2) non-PXE-like abnormalities. This is likely due to a pathological mechanism that these two disorders seem to share and that is associated with the ABCC6 gene, which results in mutated PXE, and diminished expression in βhis is likely [11, 12]. PXE-like retinal abnormalities include peau d'orange (which was previously described as "salt-and-pepper" appearance in the macula or pigmentation in the periphery) [9] which appear as confluent dark yellowish lesions at the level of RPE which occur posteriorly and then spread centrifugally, often preceding angioid streaks; angioid streaks (Fig. 4.1), which result from dehiscence in Bruch's membrane and atrophy of the overlying RPE, that might develop vision-threatening complications such as macular choroidal neovascularization; and finally optic nerve head drusen (Fig. 4.2) [10]. On the other hand,

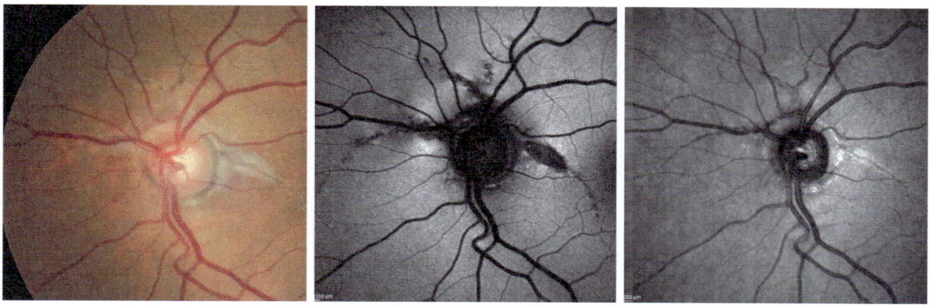

Fig. 4.1 Angioid streaks. Color fundus image (*left*), fundus autofluorescence (*middle*), and near-infrared imaging (*right*) showing peripapillary angioid streaks in a patient affected by β-thalassemia

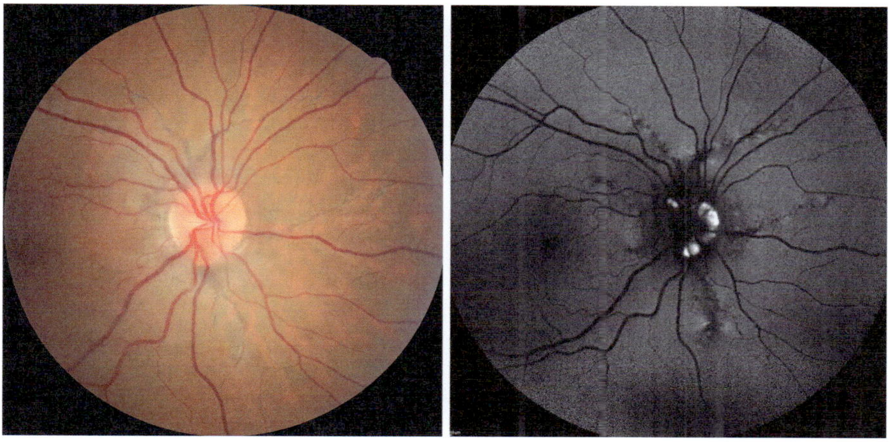

Fig. 4.2 Optic disc drusen associated with angioid streaks. Color fundus image (*left*) and fundus autofluorescence (*right*) showing peripapillary optic disc drusen and angioid streaks in a patient affected by β-thalassemia

non-PXE-like abnormalities include retinal venous tortuosity, which increases with age and in case of splenectomy, while it has an inverse relationship with hematocrit [8, 10].

DFO-induced ocular toxicity includes symptoms such as impaired color vision, night blindness, reduced visual acuity, and loss of visual field. Ocular findings include cataract, optic neuropathy, optic atrophy, and macular or equatorial pigmentary degeneration. Characteristic fundus lesions of DFO retinopathy include pigmentary retinopathy, bull's eye maculopathy, and vitelliform maculopathy [6, 12]. These alterations might affect functional tests (such as electrophysiological studies, visual field, and microperimetry) but can be efficiently assessed with the support of multimodal imaging [13]. More specifically, fundus autofluorescence (FAF) has been established as a superior noninvasive prognostic tool that can detect early RPE changes, with the characterization of four abnormal patterns: minimal change, focal, patchy, and speckled [14]. Because the type of FAF pattern may affect the visual outcome of patients with DFO toxicity, this test is a prerequisite for identifying specific high-risk characteristics that may be helpful in the decision to discontinue or switch therapy for patients to prevent disease progression. Optical coherence tomography (OCT) has also been proven to be extremely useful in detecting early sign of DFO retinopathy and in following up patients who need regular transfusions [13].

4.3 Retinal Manifestations in Sickle Cell Disease

A variety of manifestations may occur in patients with sickle cell disease (SCD). Vascular tortuosity is likely due to arteriovenous anastomoses in the retinal periphery and appears to be more frequent in SS patients [15]. Vascular occlusion is usually peripheral, where the retinal vessels may terminate as *hairpin loops*. Only arterioles and capillaries are occluded in children, whereas both arteries and veins can occlude in adults, along with occlusions at the posterior pole (such as branch retinal artery occlusion and submacular choroidal infarction) [2]. Peripheral arteriolar occlusion and capillary loss are two of the most typical signs of ocular involvement in SCD. It progresses with age and might lead to massive remodeling of the peripheral vasculature, with final clear distinction between vascular and avascular retina [16]. The macula might be affected by abnormal perfusion, with small vessel obstructions causing remodeling of the arcades around the foveal avascular zone (FAZ). Macular infarcts can easily be confirmed by OCT [17], which has enabled the capture of detailed in vivo images of morphologic macular features. Recently, spectral-domain OCT has also revealed temporal and/or macular thinning (macular splaying) in some patients with SCR (Fig. 4.3) [18]. Functional consequences are variable, and they do not relate to the extent of macular change and range from decreased visual acuity to abnormal color vision and central scotomas. However, retinal sensitivity is decreased in areas of macular thinning [19], and macular thinning is correlated with the presence of proliferative SCR [18]. Other manifestations in the macular area include epiretinal membranes, schisis, holes, and posterior pole

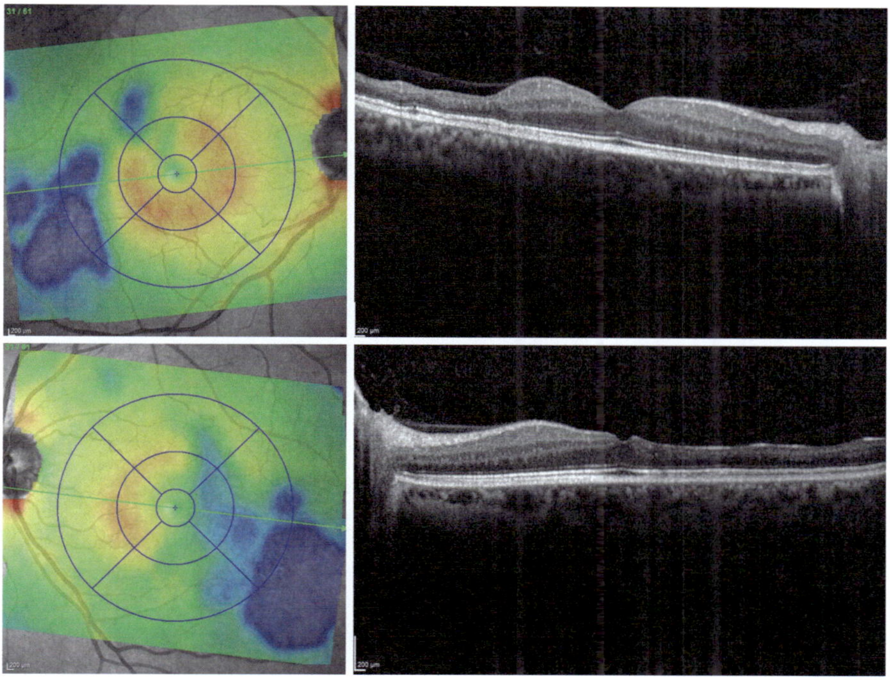

Fig. 4.3 Bilateral temporal retinal thinning. Optical coherence tomography color-coded retinal map (*left column*) and B-scan through the fovea (*right column*) demonstrating temporal retinal thinning in both eyes of a patient affected by sickle cell disease

neovascularization, but these occur more rarely [2]. Hemorrhages in the peripheral retina are common: preretinal hemorrhages appear as circumscribed red lesions in front of the retinal vasculature (*salmon-patch hemorrhages*) and leave mottled brown areas and refractile iridescent deposits when they resolve [20]. Intraretinal hemorrhages may track into the subretinal space, eliciting a RPE reaction with stellate and speculate hyperpigmentation (*black sunburst sign*) and may resolve to a schisis cavity with iridescent deposits [2]. Angioid streaks are rare and most commonly found in SS patients, have a relatively benign course, and might present either as narrow dark lines radiating from the disc or with surrounding atrophic areas [2].

Proliferative sickle cell retinopathy (PSR) is the major sight-threatening complication of sickle eye disease. It is associated with visual loss, which most commonly results from vitreous hemorrhage and traction retinal detachment. It is most frequent in SC disease (frequencies up to 70%) and Sβ-Thal disease, although these variants have a milder systemic course. On the other hand, patients with SS disease have frequent vaso-occlusive crises and severe systemic course but less frequently display PSR [2]. Incidence of PSR increases with age. Recent recommendations suggest to initiate screening for retinopathy at 9 years for SC patients and at 13 years

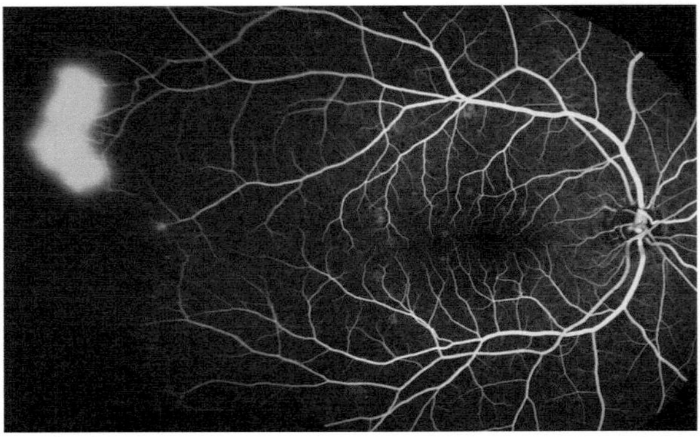

Fig. 4.4 Sea fan. Fluorescein angiography showing sea fan proliferation at the temporal avascular retina in a patient affected by sickle cell disease

for SS and Sβ-Thal patients, since SC patients show earlier onset (neither sex nor presence of systemic manifestations seems to be predictive for prevalence or age of onset of retinopathy) [21]. In addition to the effects of genotype and age, PSR is affected by hematological risk factors, such as low fetal hemoglobin in both sexes. In PSR, neovascular lesions develop at the border between the vascular and avascular retina, usually in the temporal periphery (superotemporal quadrant is considered the most common location for early neovascularization). These lesions display a typical *sea fan* appearance and might be unilateral or bilateral (Fig. 4.4). Large fibrovascular lesions may exert traction on the retina, thus leading to retinal detachment in advanced cases [2].

Classification of PSR includes five stages [22]:

- Stage I: peripheral arterial occlusion
- Stage II: peripheral arteriovenous anastomoses (*hairpin loop*)
- Stage III: neovascular and fibrous proliferation (*sea fan*)
- Stage IV: vitreous hemorrhage
- Stage V: retinal detachment

Spontaneous regression of the lesions can occur in up to 30% of cases [23], through the development of autoinfarcted or atrophic lesions, and is more common in SS disease. Management of PSR includes either observation or scatter photocoagulation, which destroys the ischemic retina that is responsible for neovascularization [24]. Complications such as vitreous hemorrhage or retinal detachment require a surgical approach.

Sickle cell trait (HbAS) has traditionally been considered a benign condition. Systemic and ocular complications are rarely seen in these patients. Nevertheless, in case of concomitant systemic diseases or trauma, retinopathy can occur, thus requiring a comprehensive medical workup [25]. Previously described ocular findings include retinal hemorrhage and exudates, angioid streaks, chorioretinal infarction, chorioretinitis, vitreous hemorrhage, central retinal artery occlusion, and PSR, some of which might also be coincidental given the large number of patients with sickle cell trait [26].

Finally, other ocular manifestations include orbit involvement and anterior segment changes. Patients affected by SCD are predisposed to both orbital wall infarction and orbital cellulitis, which might present as orbital compression syndrome with inflammation (facial pain, lid edema, proptosis, and fever). Transient saccular dilatations of conjunctival vessels packed with red cells, described as comma-shaped capillaries in the bulbar conjunctiva, are considered pathognomonic of SCD [27]. They are more common in SS disease and diminish under the heat from a slit lamp beam. Sectoral iris atrophy with pupillary irregularity may result from iris infarcts. Anterior segment ischemia is a rare but potentially devastating complication of treatment of retinal detachment and vitreous hemorrhage in PSR by scleral buckling and pars plana vitrectomy [2].

4.4 Retinal Manifestations in Leukemias

The ocular fundus manifestations of leukemia are secondary to the clinical picture of pancytopenia. The retinal findings include vitreous inflammation and/or hemorrhage, papilledema, optic disc infiltration (Fig. 4.5), intraretinal hemorrhages (flame-shaped, dot blot Roth spots), microaneurysms, cotton wool spots, hard exudates, retinal edema or infiltrates, retinal artery occlusion (Fig. 4.6), venous stasis retinopathy or vein occlusion (Fig. 4.7), perivascular sheathing, retinal and optic disc neovascularization, perifoveal ischemia (retinal ischemia and leukemia are more common in the peripheral fundus but rarely will present in the macula itself), retinal serous detachment, and choroidal infiltrates [28, 29]. Treatment of the underlying cause of the ocular fundus manifestations (i.e., anemia, thrombocytopenia, retinal or choroidal leukemic infiltrate, hyperviscosity syndrome, circulating neoplastic white blood cells, and/or bone marrow infiltration) will often result in improvement or complete resolution of the ocular fundus findings [30]. Leukemia may involve ocular tissues by toxicity due to chemotherapeutic agents. Furthermore, retinal findings may also be seen in graft-versus-host reactions in patients undergoing allogeneic bone marrow transplantation or as a sign of secondary infections following immunosuppressive therapy. Infections can lead to severe ocular involvement such as endophthalmitis [31].

Central nervous system involvement occurs most commonly in children and is becoming more frequent because of the increased survival rate associated with more effective treatment [32]. The optic nerve is one of the disease-relapse sites in a patient with systemic or meningeal leukemia, and early diagnosis is fundamental for prolonging survival. Leukemic infiltration of the optic nerve represents an emergency because vision might rapidly decline as a consequence of either the leukemic infiltration itself or a retinal vascular occlusion (due to the direct invasion of the neoplastic cells and the higher blood viscosity). According to the literature, orbital and/or ocular involvement is associated with a significantly lower survival rate than those who lack ophthalmic manifestations. Thus, the optic nerve is considered a pharmacologic sanctuary, relatively unaffected by systemic chemotherapy. A separate treatment modality, often radiotherapy, is required for both visual recovery and possibly for prolonging survival [33].

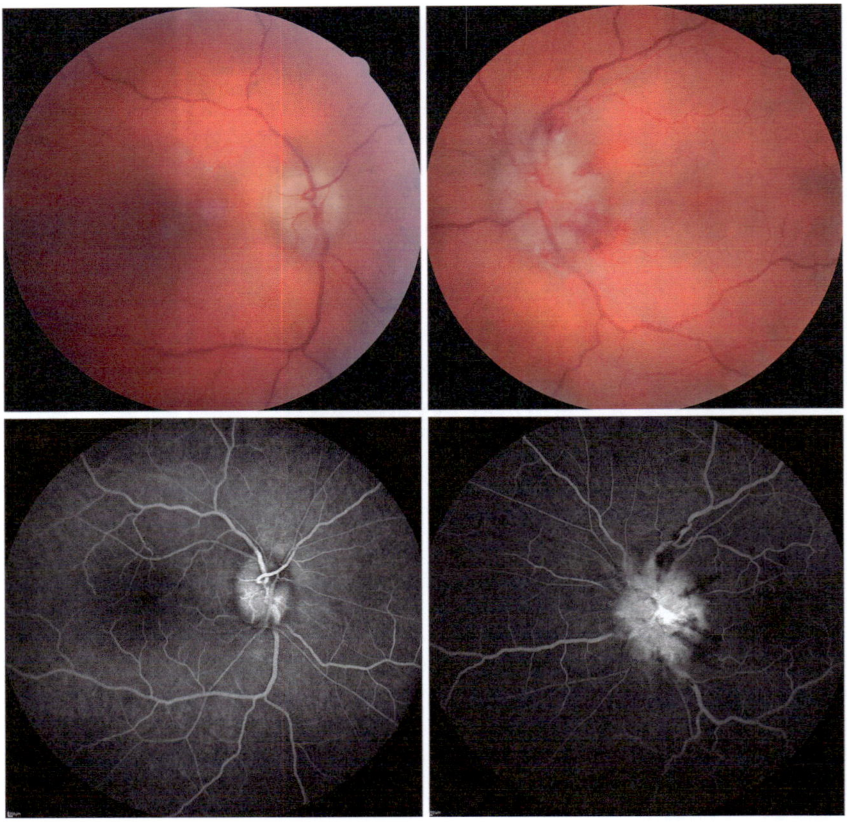

Fig. 4.5 Optic disc infiltration. Color fundus images (*top row*) and fluorescein angiography (*bottom row*) showing bilateral optic disc infiltration in a leukemic patient

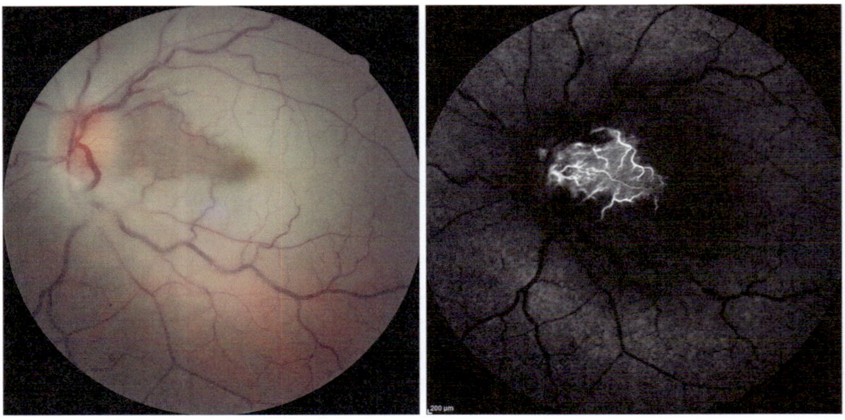

Fig. 4.6 Central retinal artery occlusion. Color fundus image (*left*) and fluorescein angiography (*right*) showing central retinal artery occlusion with cilioretinal artery sparing in a leukemic patient

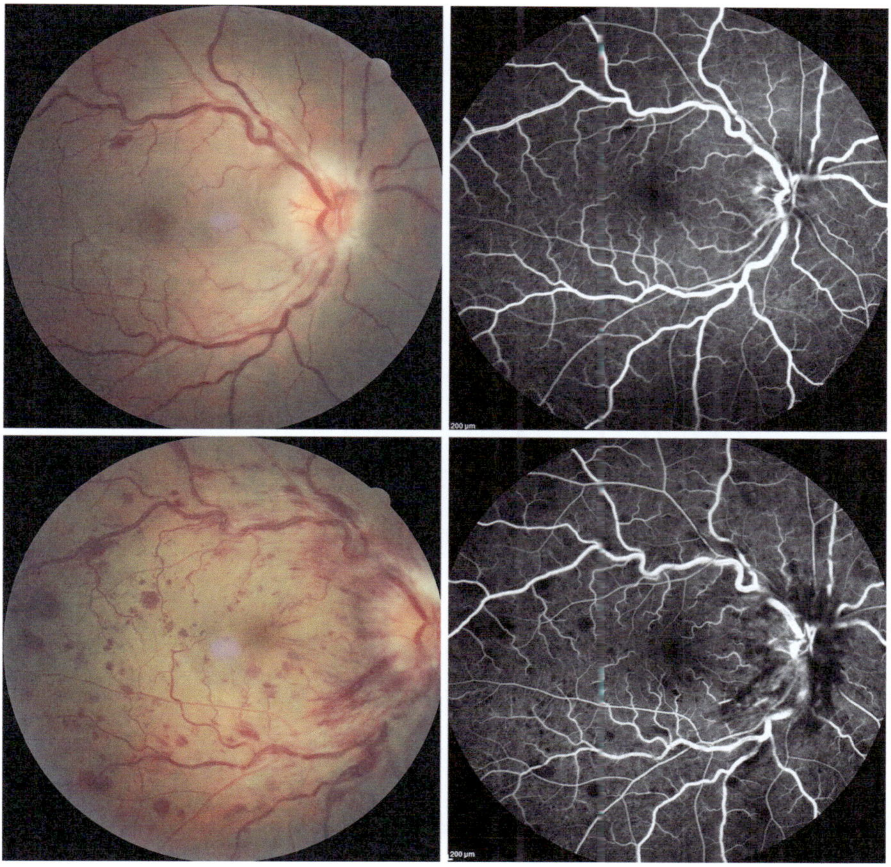

Fig. 4.7 Venous stasis retinopathy followed by central retinal venous occlusion. Color fundus image (*upper left*) and fluorescein angiography (*upper right*) showing venous stasis retinopathy associated with optic disc swelling in a leukemic patient. One month later, the same patient developed a central retinal venous occlusion (*bottom row*)

Reddy and Menon recommended routine ophthalmologic examination as part of a complete evaluation at the time of diagnosis in childhood acute leukemia because of the high prevalence of asymptomatic ocular lesions [34].

4.5 Retinal Manifestation in Plasma Dyscrasia

The most common cause of hyperviscosity syndrome due to a paraproteinemia is Waldenström's macroglobulinemia (WM). Hypersecretion of clonal IgM in WM increases the blood viscosity promoting erythrocyte aggregation [35]. The most common ocular manifestation is venous stasis retinopathy secondary to the hyperviscous state. Venous stasis may progress to retinal vein occlusion, with associated

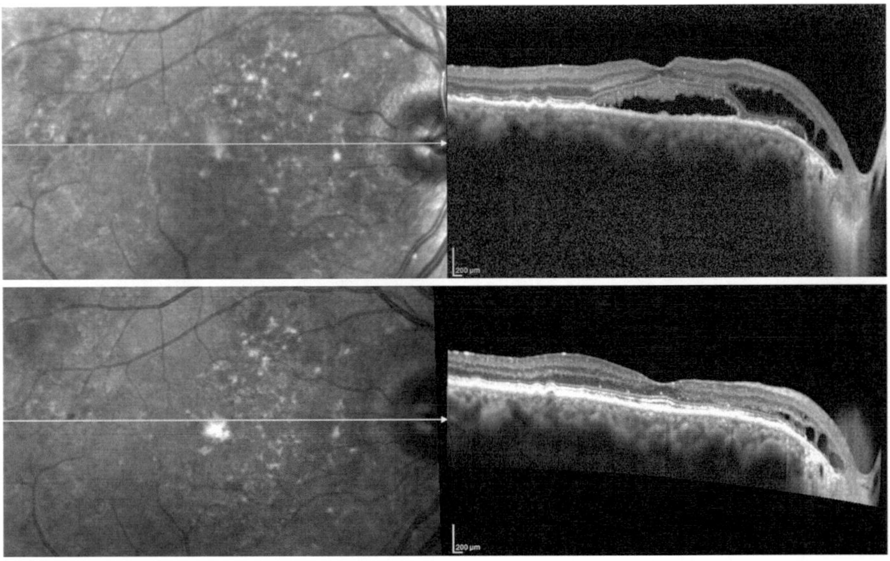

Fig. 4.8 Resolution of serous detachment of the neurosensory retina. Near-infrared image (*upper left*) and corresponding optical coherence tomography B-scan through the fovea (*upper right*) demonstrating serous detachment of the neurosensory retina associated with intraretinal edema and choroidal thickening in a patient with Waldenström's macroglobulinemia. After plasmapheresis, significant reduction of intraretinal fluid and resolution of subretinal fluid were detected (*bottom row*)

hemorrhagic and exudative findings [36]. Serous macular detachments and cystoid macular edema in these disorders have been recently termed paraproteinemic maculopathy (Fig. 4.8) [37]. These findings may easily be mistaken for central serous chorioretinopathy; however, leakage patterns on fluorescein angiography indicative of central serous chorioretinopathy are not observed in paraproteinemic maculopathy. Optic nerve edema may be observed [38]. A paraneoplastic phenomenon involving an autoimmune reaction against retinal photoreceptors may occur [39]. Systemic treatment of WM with plasmapheresis and cytotoxic agents improves retinal findings [40]. Ocular manifestations of amyloid syndromes may include perivascular sheathing, vitreous veils, cotton wool spots, retinal hemorrhages, retinal and choroidal infiltrates in a perivascular distribution, RPE mottling, and choroidal hypofluorescence on fluorescein and indocyanine green angiography [41].

4.6 Retinal Manifestations in Thrombophilic and Hyperviscosity Syndromes

Although not frequently, retinal vascular disease may result from inherited or acquired defects in blood components that may either alter blood viscosity or disrupt the coagulation cascade. Several cases of retinal vascular disease linked to mutations of the clotting factors have been reported. Despite this, prospective clinical trials often failed to show a significant association with the gene mutation [42]. A prospective study demonstrated Leiden mutation in 17% of young patients affected by retinal venous occlusion [43]. Other prospective clinical trials have shown an association of elevated homocysteine levels [44], MTHFR gene mutation [45], and protein C and S deficiencies [46, 47] with retinal vascular diseases. A definite link between the antiphospholipid syndrome and retinal vascular disease remains elusive [42]. The most common ophthalmic finding is retinal vein occlusion; however, abnormalities of the arterial system, the choroid, and the macula are also possible. A systemic investigation is warranted in cases with lack of typical predispositions. Visual symptoms may be the only manifestation of the disease, making ophthalmologist's diagnosis critical for both treatment and thrombotic prophylaxis [42].

4.7 Retinal Manifestations in Platelet Disorders and Coagulopathies

With consumption or lack of the platelets and clotting factors, the blood becomes hypocoagulable, leading to hemorrhage, tissue hypoxia, and further release of thromboplastin [48]. The major ocular fundus manifestations of disseminated intravascular coagulation include serous detachments of the retina (particularly in the macular and peripapillary regions), retinal and choroidal hemorrhages, and vitreous hemorrhage [49].

Key Learning Points

- A large variety of hematologic effects can be directly visualized in the retina by ophthalmologists, which may be the first to diagnose a blood dyscrasia.
- Although many retinal findings may not be pathognomonic, other may be more indicative of a specific blood disorder.
- High-resolution retinal imaging has important clinical relevance in the diagnosis and follow-up of retinopathies secondary to blood dyscrasias because it contributes to the detection of early macula changes that may be missed during ophthalmoscopy.

References

1. Hoffbrand AV, Moss PAH, Pettit JE. Essential hematology. 5th ed. Hoboken, NJ: Blackwell Publishing; 2006.
2. Elagouz M, Jyothi S, Gupta B, et al. Sickle cell disease and the eye: old and new concepts. Surv Ophthalmol. 2010;55:359–77.
3. Jameson JN, Kasper DL, Harrison TR, et al. Harrison's principles of internal medicine. NewYork: McGraw-Hill Medical Publishing Division; 2005.

4. Robbins SL, Vinay K, Abul KA, et al. Robbins and cotran pathologic basis of disease. 8th ed. Philadelphia: WB Saunders Company; 2010.
5. Porter RS. The Merck manual. 19th ed. Kenilworth, NJ: Merk & Co.; 2011.
6. Bhoiwala DL, Dunaief JL. Retinal abnormalities in β-thalassemia major. Surv Ophthalmol. 2016;61:33–50.
7. Gartaganis S, Ismiridis K, Papageorgiou O, et al. Ocular abnormalities in patients with beta thalassemia. Am J Ophthalmol. 1989;108:699–703.
8. Sorcinelli R, Sitzia A, Figus A, et al. Ocular findings in beta-thalassemia. Metab Pediatr Syst Ophthalmol. 1990;13:23–5.
9. Taher A, Bashshur Z, Shamseddeen WA, et al. Ocular findings among thalassemia patients. Am J Ophthalmol. 2006;142:704–5.
10. Barteselli G, Dell'Arti L, Finger RP, et al. The spectrum of ocular alterations in patients with beta-thalassemia syndromes suggests a pathology similar to pseudoxanthoma elasticum. Ophthalmology. 2014;121:709–18.
11. Martin L, Douet V, VanWart CM, et al. A mouse model of beta-thalassemia shows a liver-specific down-regulation of Abcc6 expression. Am J Pathol. 2011;178:774–83.
12. Di Nicola M, Barteselli G, Dell'Arti L, et al. Functional and structural abnormalities in Deferoxamine retinopathy: a review of the literature. Biomed Res Int. 2015;2015:249617.
13. Viola F, Barteselli G, Dell'Arti L, et al. Multimodal imaging in deferoxamine retinopathy. Retina. 2014;34:1428–38.
14. Viola F, Barteselli G, Dell'Arti L, et al. Abnormal fundus autofluorescence results of patients in long-term treatment with deferoxamine. Ophthalmology. 2012;119:1693–700.
15. Welch RB, Goldberg MF. Sickle-cell hemoglobin and its relation to fundus abnormality. Arch Ophthalmol. 1966;75:353–62.
16. Galinos SO, Asdourian GK, Woolf MB, et al. Spontaneous remodelling of the peripheral retinal vasculature in sickling disorders. Am J Ophthalmol. 1975;79:853–70.
17. Witkin AJ, Rogers AH, Ko TH, et al. Optical coherence tomography demonstration of macular infarction in sickle cell retinopathy. Arch Ophthalmol. 2006;124:746–7.
18. Mathew R, Bafiq R, Ramu J, et al. Spectral domain optical coherence tomography in patients with sickle cell disease. Br J Ophthalmol. 2015;99:967–72.
19. Chow CC, Genead MA, Anastasakis A, Chau FY, Fishman GA, Lim JI. Structural and functional correlation in sickle cell retinopathy using spectral-domain optical coherence tomography and scanning laser ophthalmoscope microperimetry. Am J Ophthalmol. 2011;152:704–11.
20. Gagliano DA, Goldberg MF. The evolution of salmon-patch hemorrhages in sickle cell retinopathy. Arch Ophthalmol. 1989;107:1814–5.
21. Gill HS, Lam WC. A screening strategy for the detection of sickle cell retinopathy in pediatric patients. Can J Ophthalmol. 2008;43:188–91.
22. Goldberg MF. Natural history of untreated proliferative sickle retinopathy. Arch Ophthalmol. 1971;85:428–37.
23. Downes SM, Hambleton IR, Chuang EL, et al. Incidence and natural history of proliferative sickle cell retinopathy: observations from a cohort study. Ophthalmology. 2005;112:1869–75.
24. Myint KT, Sahoo S, Thein AW, et al. Laser therapy for retinopathy in sickle cell disease. Cochrane Database Syst Rev. 2015:9–10. DOI: 10.1002/14651858.CD010790.pub2.
25. Reynolds SA, Besada E, Winter-Corella C. Retinopathy in patients with sickle cell trait. Optometry. 2007;78:582–7.
26. Nagpal KC, Asdourian GK, Patrianakos D, et al. Proliferative retinopathy in sickle cell trait. Arch Intern Med. 1977;137:325–8.
27. Paton D. The conjunctival sign of sickle cell disease. Arch Ophthalmol. 1961;66:90–4.
28. Rosenthal AR. Ocular manifestations of leukemia. A review. Ophthalmology. 1983;90:899–905.
29. Awh CC, Miller JB, Wu DM, et al. Leukostasis retinopathy: a new clinical manifestation of chronic myeloid leukemia with severe hyperleukocytosis. Ophthal Surg Lasers Imaging Retina. 2015;46:768–70.
30. Mehta AB, Goldman JM, Kohner E. Hyperleucocytic retinopathy in chronic granulocytic leukaemia: the role of intensive leucapheresis. Br J Haematol. 1984;56:661.

31. Sharma T, Grewal J, Gupta S, Murray PI. Ophthalmic manifestations of acute leukaemias: the ophthalmologist's role. Eye (Lond). 2004;18:663–72.
32. Nikaido H, Mishima H, Ono H, et al. Leukemic involvement of the optic nerve. Am J Ophthalmol. 1988;105:294–8.
33. Lin YC, Wang AG, Yen MY. Leukaemic infiltration of the optic nerve as the initial manifestation of leukaemic relapse. Eye. 2004;18:546–50.
34. Reddy SC, Menon BS. A prospective study of ocular manifestations in childhood acute leukaemia. Acta Ophthalmol Scand. 1998;76:700.
35. Gertz MA, Kyle RA. Hyperviscosity syndrome. J Intensive Care Med. 1995;10:128–41.
36. Feman SS, Stein RS. Waldenstrom's macroglobulinemia, a hyperviscosity manifestation of venous stasis retinopathy. Int Ophthalmol. 1981;4:107–12.
37. Mansour AM, Arevalo JF, Badal J, et al. Paraproteinemic maculopathy. Ophthalmology. 2014;121:1925–32.
38. Chong DY, Comer GM, Trobe JD. Optic disc edema, cystoid macular edema, and elevated vascular endothelial growth factor in a patient with POEMS syndrome. J Neuroophthalmol. 2007;27:180–3.
39. Sen HN, Chan CC, Caruso RC, et al. Waldenstrom's macroglobulinemia-associated retinopathy. Ophthalmology. 2004;111:535–9.
40. Gertz MA. Waldenstrom macroglobulinemia: 2011 update on diagnosis, risk stratification, and management. Am J Hematol. 2011;86:411–6.
41. Pece A, Yannuzzi L, Sannace C, et al. Chorioretinal involvement in primary systemic nonfamilial amyloidosis. Am J Ophthalmol. 2000;130:250.
42. Rajagopal R, Apte RS. Retinal manifestations of thrombophilic and hyperviscosity syndromes. Surv Ophthalmol. 2016;61:236–47.
43. Kuhli C, Hattenbach LO, Scharrer I, et al. High prevalence of resistance to APC in young patients with retinal vein occlusion. Graefes Arch Clin Exp Ophthalmol. 2002;240:163–8.
44. Martin SC, Rauz S, Marr JE, et al. Plasma total homocysteine and retinal vascular disease. Eye (Lond). 2000;14:590–3.
45. Loewenstein A, Goldstein M, Winder A, et al. Retinal vein occlusion associated with methylenetetrahydrofolate reductase mutation. Ophthalmology. 1999;106:1817–20.
46. Bertram B, Remky A, Arend O, et al. Protein C, protein S, and antithrombin III in acute ocular occlusive diseases. Ger J Ophthalmol. 1995;4:332–5.
47. Greiner K, Hafner G, Dick B, et al. Retinal vascular occlusion and deficiencies in the protein C pathway. Am J Ophthalmol. 1999;128:69–74.
48. Meyer CH, Callizo J, Mennel S, Schmidt JC. Complete resorption of retinal hemorrhages in idiopathic thrombocytopenic purpura. Eur J Ophthalmol. 2007;17:128–9.
49. Cogan DG. Ocular involvement in disseminated intravascular coagulopathy. Arch Ophthalmol. 1975;93:1.

5 Retinal Manifestations of Renal Diseases

Aniruddha Agarwal and Alessandro Invernizzi

Abstract

Various diseases affecting the renal excretory system can be associated by or secondary cause of pathological changes in the retina and choroid. Some of these entities such as tubulointerstitial nephritis and uveitis (TINU) are well recognized for their characteristic clinical manifestations. Similarly, patients with systemic lupus erythematosus may present with protean clinical manifestations. Recently, it has been recognized that fundus examination among patients with renal diseases may provide insights into the disease pathogenesis, severity, and progression. Thus, careful correlation between renal and retinal diseases may enable the clinician scientist to understand the pathophysiology of the disease and its natural history. In the index chapter, retinal findings of various diseases affecting the renal system have been elucidated. In addition, the features on imaging evaluation have also been provided. A brief note on their management has been discussed.

A. Agarwal (✉)
Department of Ophthalmology, Advanced Eye Center, Post Graduate Institute of Medical Education and Research (PGIMER), Sector 12, Chandigarh 160012, India

Ocular Imaging Research and Reading Center (OIRRC), Menlo Park, CA 94025, USA
e-mail: aniruddha9@gmail.com

A. Invernizzi
Eye Clinic, Department of Biomedical and Clinical Science "Luigi Sacco", Luigi Sacco Hospital, University of Milan, Milan, Italy

J. Chhablani et al. (eds.), *Retinal and Choroidal Imaging in Systemic Diseases*,
https://doi.org/10.1007/978-981-10-5461-7_5

5.1 Introduction

Patients with renal diseases especially autoimmune conditions may present with various pathological alterations involving the ocular tissues. Although several ocular tissues may be involved, the most commonly affected tissue is the retinochoroid. A host of autoimmune, metabolic, and biochemical processes affect the chorioretinal milieu resulting in characteristic tissue abnormalities and/or ocular inflammation. If the ocular symptoms precede diagnosis of systemic involvement, there may be a clinical challenge in determining the exact etiology and planning appropriate treatment. Thus, recognition of the disease phenotype and comprehensive systemic evaluation form the cornerstone of the management.

With numerous advances in the techniques of noninvasive imaging and recognition of disease patterns, our understanding of renal disease pathogenesis has been greatly enhanced. A number of asymptomatic and symptomatic changes have been described among patients with renal conditions such as tubulointerstitial nephritis and uveitis (TINU), systemic lupus erythematosus (SLE), and end-stage renal disease, among others. A thorough review of these ocular associations may aid in our knowledge of the complex mechanisms involved in the pathogenesis of these diseases. Establishing correlation between ocular signs and systemic disease severity may help in clinical decision-making and altering the line of management.

In the subsequent sections, clinically relevant and common renal diseases with chorioretinal involvement have been described. A brief summary of SLE has also been provided (described in details in a separate chapter). The relevance of retinal imaging in these conditions has been highlighted.

5.2 Glomerulonephritides

5.2.1 Membranoproliferative Glomerulonephritis

5.2.1.1 Introduction and Types

Membranoproliferative glomerulonephritis (MPGN) is characterized by proliferation of cellular elements in the glomerular tissue and basement membrane changes [1]. Histological studies show increased mesangial matrix deposition (electron dense material) and hypercellularity [2]. MPGN is associated with features of chronic glomerulonephritis, secondary hypertension, and systemic features due to immune complex deposition. The most common age of diagnosis is 5–15 years, and within a period of 10 years, approximately 50% of patients may progress to end-stage renal disease (ESRD) [3].

Type 1 MPGN is characterized by subendothelial glomerular electron dense deposits; type 2 MPGN is characterized by deposition of electron dense material of unknown origin in the lamina densa of the glomerular basement membrane; and type 3 MPGN is characterized by the presence of both type I and type II lesions [4]. Recently, a consensus conference on MPGN has reclassified the disease into two types: immune complex mediated and complement mediated [5].

5.2.1.2 Ocular Manifestations

Classically, pathological manifestations of the posterior segment of the eye have been observed in patients with type 2 MPGN (dense deposit disease). These pathological alterations commonly affect the outer retina and retinal pigment epithelium (RPE)-Bruch's membrane complex [4]. Due to RPE and outer retinal involvement, these patients may have altered visual fields and color perception, prolonged dark adaptation, and electroretinogram changes. The pathogenesis of these RPE changes has been attributed to the dense deposits at the RPE-Bruch's membrane complex. In a study by Michielsen et al., 11 out of 12 patients with type 2 MPGN were diagnosed with diffuse RPE alterations [6]. Various manifestations of the condition include RPE-Bruch's deposits similar to basal laminar deposits, exudative drusen, and pigment epithelial detachments [7]. This condition may also be complicated by development of subretinal/choroidal neovascularization (CNV) [6, 8, 9]. Development of CNV may be higher among patients with bilateral widespread RPE alterations and outer retinal changes. Fluorescein angiography (FA) and spectral-domain optical coherence tomography (SD-OCT) greatly aid in the detection of subretinal fluid, pigment epithelial detachments, and atypical central serous retinopathy [10].

Due to the decompensation of the RPE, patients may also develop central serous retinopathy-like picture with subretinal fluid and drusen-like deposits (DLDs) at the RPE-Bruch's membrane complex (Fig. 5.1) [7, 11]. DLDs may be common finding among patients with type 2 MPGN [12]. Presence of DLDs in patients of type 2 MPGN was first reported in 1989. Usually, the DLDs are located in the posterior pole and the mid-periphery. However, the presence of peripheral drusen has also been described in the literature [13]. SD-OCT imaging of DLDs in type 2 MPGN gives an appearance of subretinal RPE-Bruch's membrane elevations and hyper-reflectivity due to the deposition of matrix material [14]. Using high-speed ultra-high-resolution OCT, irregular thickening of the Bruch's membrane has been observed in patients with MPGN [15].

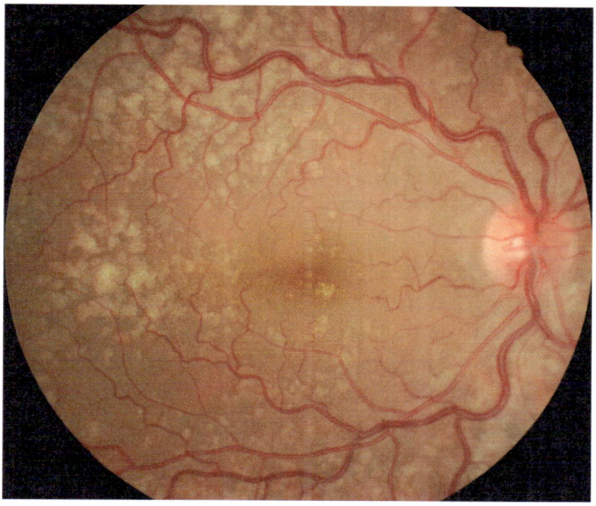

Fig. 5.1 Fundus photograph of a patient with biopsy-proven membranoproliferative glomerulonephritis with subretinal drusen-like deposits

Fundus autofluorescence (FAF) imaging shows multifocal hyper-autofluorescence in the areas with DLDs. Similarly, FA and indocyanine green angiography show multifocal hyperfluorescence associated with the subretinal deposits [16].

In the past, presence of DLDs and other outer retinal/RPE abnormalities were noted only in patients with type 2 MPGN. However, recent literature has shown that such changes may be observed even in patients with type 1 and 3 MPGN. Recently, Han et al. have described presence of extensive DLDs in a patient with type 1 MPGN [17]. These recent investigations have shed the light on the importance of the newer classification of MPGN which is based on molecular methods rather than anatomical location of the dense deposits. In a report by Dalvin et al., DLDs were observed in two patients with type 1 and 3 MPGN (based on anatomical classification). Thus, the authors proposed that ophthalmologists must recognize the importance of recognizing the newer classification of MPGN based on complement activation or immune complex-mediated disease [18]. Such an approach may aid in the better understanding of the pathophysiological mechanisms behind these complex diseases.

5.2.2 IgA Nephropathy

5.2.2.1 Introduction and Pathogenesis

IgA nephropathy (also known as Berger's disease) is a complement-mediated condition characterized by glomerulonephritis and progression to ESRD in approximately 40% individuals [19]. This condition was first described by Berger and Hingais in 1968 [20]. The disease is characterized by complement activation and deposition of IgA (as well as IgG) immune complexes in the mesangium of the glomeruli leading to a chronic disease. The deposition of polymeric IgA1, IgG, and complement C3 occurs in a diffuse granular manner. Recent progress in the diagnostic techniques has improved our understanding of the glycosylation pathways of IgA1 glycans and binding galactose-deficient IgA1 complexes to mesangial cells responsible for development of IgA nephropathy. While the trigger of inflammation is suggested to be autoimmune in nature, various antigenic stimuli due to bacteria, viruses, and fungi have been implicated in the pathogenesis [21]. The diagnosis of IgA Nephropathy requires renal biopsy and examination of mesangial matrices with periodic acid-Schiff staining.

5.2.2.2 Ocular Manifestations

The major clinical findings of IgA nephropathy include secondary hypertension (more than 40% patients at presentation) and chronic kidney disease [22]. Thus patients with IgA nephropathy may develop features of hypertensive retinopathy including arteriolar narrowing, changes in the arteriovenous crossings, and ischemia of retinal nerve fiber layer (cotton-wool spots) [23]. Patients may also develop serous retinal detachments which may be bilateral. These can be confirmed on SD-OCT. [23, 24] The findings of cotton-wool spots and serous retinal detachments are reversible on therapy with hemodialysis, peritoneal dialysis, or plasmapheresis.

In a case report by Taban et al., imaging evaluation using FA demonstrated presence of choroidal infarction secondary to possible immune complex deposition [23]. Other manifestations of IgA nephropathy include presence of bilateral subretinal drusenoid deposits (SDDs). In a case report by Lally et al., a 42-year-old Asian woman with renal biopsy-proven IgA nephropathy showed presence of well-defined yellow clusters of SDDs in the macula. These were well appreciated using SD-OCT imaging. On SD-OCT, SDDs appeared as perifoveal hyper-reflective convex deposits internal to the retinal pigment epithelium (RPE)-Bruch's membrane complex. There was elevation of the ellipsoid zone and granular reflectivity between the ellipsoid and interdigitation bands adjacent to the deposits. In the report, the authors postulate that SDDs are histopathological correlate of reticular pseudodrusen and occur due to deposition of circulating serum IgA1 complexes [25].

Figure 5.2 shows a patient with subretinal hyper-reflective deposits at the fovea due to possible subretinal complement deposition.

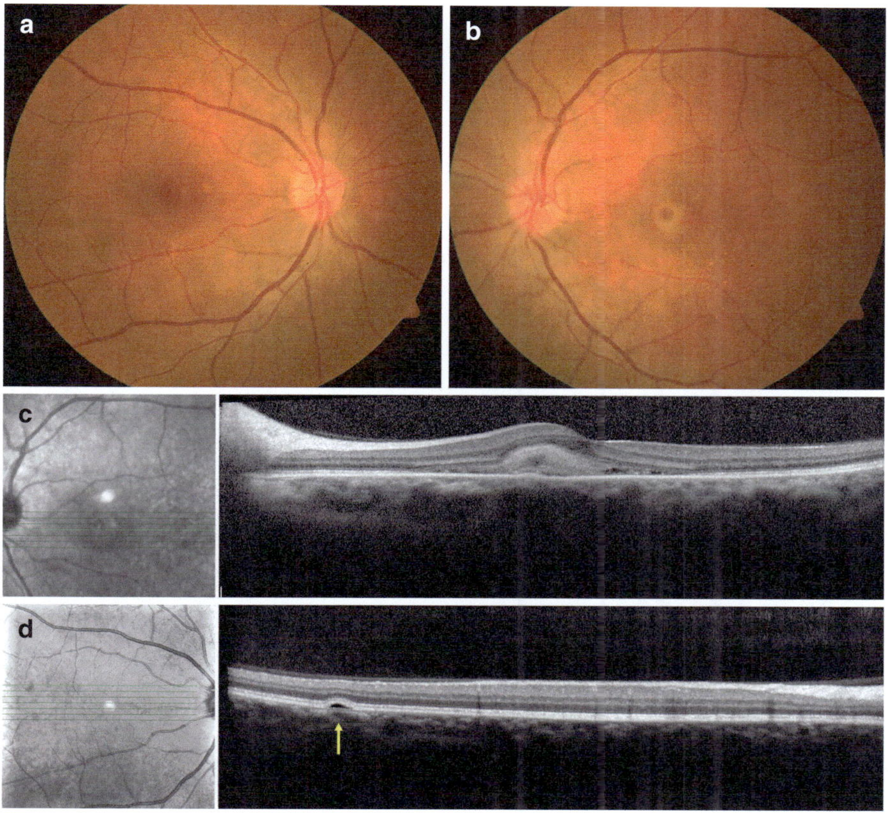

Fig. 5.2 A 33-year-old male with proteinuria was diagnosed with stage III renal disease associated with biopsy-proven IgA nephropathy. Fundus examination revealed the presence of yellow-white ring-shaped deposit in the macula of OS and discrete, small, subretinal deposits in the macula OU (**a** and **b**). Spectral-domain optical coherence tomography (OCT) showed the presence of subretinal hyper-reflective deposits at the fovea of OS suggestive of complement and/or IgA complex deposition (**c**). OCT scan through the small discrete lesions (**d**) revealed hyper-reflective drusenoid deposits at the level of the retinal pigment epithelial (RPE)-Bruch's membrane complex and elevation of the RPE

5.3 Tubulointerstitial Nephritis and Uveitis (TINU)

5.3.1 Introduction and Etiopathogenesis

Tubulointerstitial nephritis and uveitis (TINU) is an autoimmune oculorenal syndrome common in younger aged population (mean age 15 years) with female predominance (3:1). TINU is characterized by the acute interstitial nephritis (AIN) and uveitis with no known etiology [26]. TINU was first described in 1975 by Dobrin et al. and has a reported prevalence of 1–2%. Although the exact pathogenesis of TINU is unknown, it is thought to have an autoimmune basis triggered by infections, antibiotics, or NSAIDs. TINU has an established association with HLA-DRB1*01 and HLADQA1*01 and a particularly strong association (RR = 167) with HLA-DRB1*0102 [27]. Clinically the patients with TINU present nonspecific systemic symptoms of fever, malaise, myalgia, and fatigue. About one third of patients present with signs and symptoms of AIN characterized by flank pain, hematuria, sterile pyuria (eosinophiluria), and mild proteinuria [28, 29].

5.3.2 Ocular Manifestations

Approximately 21% cases of TINU present with ocular manifestations preceding systemic symptoms. Ocular symptoms in TINU predominantly present as bilateral, non-granulomatous anterior uveitis (80% cases) [29–31]. The anterior uveitis is sudden in onset and is characterized by pain, redness, and photophobia. On slit-lamp examination, fine keratic precipitates, anterior chamber cells, occasionally a high flare, and rarely a hypopyon can be seen. Posterior synechiae can also be visualized in certain cases. Figure 5.3 illustrates anterior segment inflammation in a patient with TINU.

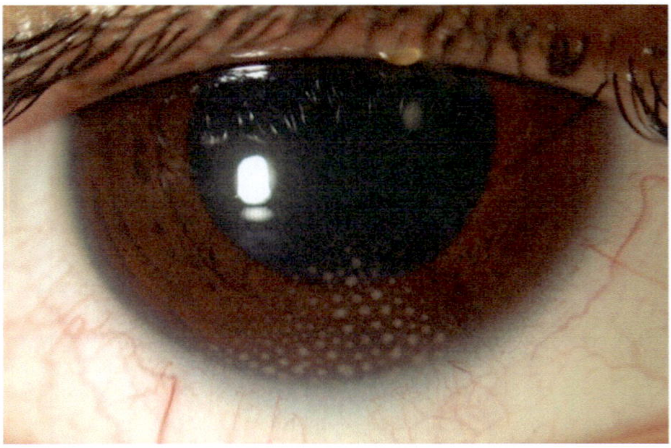

Fig. 5.3 Figure shows anterior segment photograph of a patient with tubulointerstitial nephritis and uveitis (TINU). There is presence of anterior chamber cells and flare and granulomatous keratic precipitates *(Image courtesy: Peter McCluskey, MD, Australia)*

Posterior segment involvement in TINU is usually limited to occasional mild vitreous cells and rare complications of disk and macular edema. Other associations include development of cataract and glaucoma. It is imperative to note that while diagnosing TINU may be challenging especially in cases with unexplained chronic or recurrent uveitis, the prognosis is generally good. Timely diagnosis and management with corticosteroids and/or immunosuppression improve the long-term outcomes in these patients [28, 32].

5.4 Metabolic Renal Diseases: Hyperoxaluria

5.4.1 Incidence and Pathogenesis

Although rare, primary hyperoxaluria is a clinical entity of considerable importance due to its association with nephrolithiasis, nephrocalcinosis, and renal failure [33]. Primary hyperoxaluria is inherited in an autosomal recessive manner and is caused by a deficiency of a liver enzyme alanine-glyoxylate aminotransferase (AGT). AGT catalyzes the conversion of glyoxylate to glycine. Absence of AGT results in formation of oxalate crystals which deposit in the kidneys and other organ systems [34].

5.4.2 Ocular Manifestations

Retinal involvement in patients with hyperoxaluria has been recognized as early as 1974 [35]. Hyperoxaluria manifests as deposition of crystals in the macula (*crystalline retinopathy*) [36, 37]. Ocular involvement in hyperoxaluria may be bilateral and symmetrical. The pathological changes are usually confined to the posterior pole and mid-periphery. Fundus lesions are usually small (100–200 microns) and appear dark due to deposition of calcium oxalate crystals. Sometimes, the fundus lesions may be large (*retinal oxalosis*) and appear geographic in nature [38]. Hyperoxaluria may also be associated with retinal flecks [39]. *Oxalate maculopathy* may also be associated with diffuse optic disk pallor [36].

The subretinal deposits in hyperoxaluria may also be visualized using SD-OCT imaging [40]. Due to outer retinal/RPE damage, there may be development of secondary choroidal neovascular membranes [41]. These can be confirmed using FA. Choroidal neovascularization usually occurs adjacent to the site of macular scarring. Recently, Derveaux et al. proposed phenotypic classification of oxalate maculopathy in type 1 primary hyperoxaluria. The authors described four distinct retinal phenotypes: bilateral perifoveal retinal pigment epithelium hyperplasia, subretinal crystals, confluent macular RPE hyperplasia, and subretinal fibrosis. Thus, retinopathy in hyperoxaluria may show considerable phenotypic variations [42]. A thorough understanding of this phenotypic manifestation may aid the clinician in predicting visual outcome in these patients.

5.5 Systemic Lupus Erythematosus

5.5.1 Introduction and Pathogenesis

Systemic lupus erythematosus (SLE) is a multi-organ disease with a characteristic relapsing/remitting course due to activation of autoimmune mechanisms leading to production of polyclonal antibodies, development of immune tolerance against nuclear antigens, and deposition of immune complexes in tissues [43–45]. Due to widespread organ-tissue damage, SLE has protean clinical manifestations. Diagnosis of SLE is based on the presence of clinical criteria defined by the American Rheumatology Association (ARA). These criteria include the presence of nephritis, skin rash, arthritis, and other organ dysfunction due to serositis. The presence of 4 out of 11 criteria is necessary for establishing a diagnosis of SLE [46].

SLE is most commonly seen in women of child-bearing age. In pregnancy, SLE may result in severe comorbidities and complicate the course of the pregnancy. In the following section, ocular findings of SLE have been highlighted. Details of ocular involvement in SLE have also been listed elsewhere in this book.

5.5.2 Ocular Findings

Approximately 2–30% patients with SLE present with ocular manifestations [47]. Retinal manifestations of SLE may be asymptomatic, such as the presence of isolated cotton-wool spots, DLDs, or few retinal hemorrhages, or may be severe sight threatening such as near-complete vaso-occlusion [47–50]. While various ocular tissues may be involved in SLE, retinal vessels are predominantly affected in SLE. Involvement of retinal vasculature in SLE is termed as *lupus vasculitis*. Lupus vasculitis is typically a *vasculopathy* due to fibrinoid necrosis rather than true vessel wall inflammation [51]. On FA, lupus vasculopathy may present with mild late perivascular hyperfluorescence unlike typical inflammatory retinal vasculitis. The spectrum of findings in lupus vasculitis include cotton-wool spots, intra-retinal hemorrhages, vascular occlusion (especially arteriolar in severe cases), and secondary neovascularization that may lead to vitreous hemorrhage or tractional retinal detachment [50].

Patients with SLE may present with *Purtscher-like retinopathy* due to widespread complement activation leading to large cotton-wool spots, optic disk edema, retinal hemorrhages and edema, and arteriolar occlusion on FA [52]. Due to the hypercoagulable state in patients with SLE and the presence of antiphospholipid antibodies (APLA) that predispose to a prothrombotic state [53], patients with SLE may present with a *central retinal vein occlusion (CRVO)-like picture*. This condition may mimic typical CRVO with widespread hemorrhages, cotton-wool spots, and optic disk edema.

Lupus choroidopathy is characterized by multifocal serous retinal elevations and RPE detachments [54, 55]. This condition is relatively rare and occurs in severe conditions. On the other hand, DLDs may be a more common outer retinal/RPE/

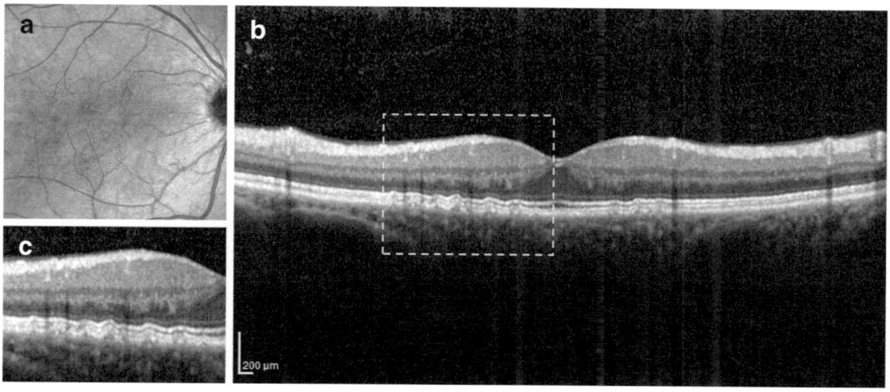

Fig. 5.4 Optical coherence tomography (OCT) using the enhanced depth imaging (EDI) mode shows the presence of drusen-like deposits (DLDs) temporal to the fovea. These DLDs can be well appreciated on the reflectance image (**a**). The vertical line scan through the fovea shows presence of DLDs as irregular elevations of the retinal pigment epithelium (**b**). Magnified view (**c**) shows the detailed structure of these drusen

inner choroidal manifestation of SLE [56]. Classically, DLDs were thought to be present in retinae of patients with SLE-associated nephritis but not in those with SLE and no renal involvement. However, it has been recently recognized that DLDs may be present in patients with SLE without kidney involvement. Recognition of DLDs in patients with SLE may therefore have prognostic significance and may serve as a useful biomarker in assessing the natural history of the disease.

Figure 5.4 shows a patient with typical DLDs as observed on EDI-OCT.

5.6 Conclusions and Summary

A number of pathologies involving renal system result from complex autoimmune pathological processes that may be associated with ocular findings. *Investigations into these processes demonstrate the anatomical similarities between the renal glomeruli and the choriocapillaris/RPE-Bruch's membrane complex.* Certain ocular findings may not be sight threatening, such as presence of few cotton-wool spots or DLDs away from the fovea. However, recognition of these pathological changes especially sight-threatening conditions that sometimes precede the development of renal manifestations may lead to diagnostic challenges. Clinicians may face difficulty in deciphering the etiology of the ocular manifestations and determine its clinical relevance. In addition, due to the wealth of information in the recent literature on certain manifestations such as DLDs may lead to confusion on the prognostic significance of these lesions.

Advanced imaging modalities such as SD-OCT and EDI-OCT and improved fluorescein angiography techniques have improved our understanding of the distinct and remarkable changes that occur in various chorioretinal layers in diseases of the kidney. For instance, due to newer technologies such as near-infrared reflectance imaging, autofluorescence, and EDI-OCT, the morphology and significance of DLDs in conditions such as MPGN and SLE have been recently recognized. Updated and newer classification of entities such as MPGN have changed our understanding and highlighted the importance of ocular examination in type 1 and 3 MPGN. Similarly, modalities such as laser flare photometry have advanced our abilities of monitoring patients with inflammatory conditions such as TINU.

In summary, comprehensive analyses of various ocular conditions and their clinical presentations using advanced retinal imaging techniques are relevant in a number of diseases affecting the kidneys. As the wealth of information in literature continues to expand, it is likely that the pathogenetic mechanisms of these conditions will be more clearly elucidated in the near future.

Financial Support The authors have no financial disclosure/proprietary interest. No conflicting relationship exists for any author.

Supported in part by an unrestricted grant from Research to Prevent Blindness (RPB) to the Truhlsen Eye Institute at the University of Nebraska Medical Center.

References

1. Floege J, Amann K. Primary glomerulonephritides. Lancet. 2016;387(10,032):2036–48.
2. Cook HT, Pickering MC. Histopathology of MPGN and C3 glomerulopathies. Nature reviews. Nephrology. 2015;11(1):14–22.
3. Appel GB, Cook HT, Hageman G, et al. Membranoproliferative glomerulonephritis type II (dense deposit disease): an update. J Am Soc Nephrol. May 2005;16(5):1392–403.
4. Kim DD, Mieler WF, Wolf MD. Posterior segment changes in membranoproliferative glomerulonephritis. Am J Ophthalmol. 1992;114(5):593–9.
5. Salvadori M, Rosso G. Reclassification of membranoproliferative glomerulonephritis: identification of a new GN: C3GN. World J Nephrol. 2016;5(4):308–20.
6. Michielsen B, Leys A, Van Damme B, Missotten L. Fundus changes in chronic membranoproliferative glomerulonephritis type II. Adv Ophthalmol. 1990;76(3):219–29.
7. Ulbig MR, Riordan-Eva P, Holz FG, Rees HC, Hamilton PA. Membranoproliferative glomerulonephritis type II associated with central serous retinopathy. Am J Ophthalmol. 1993; 116(4):410–3.
8. Leys A, Michielsen B, Leys M, Vanrenterghem Y, Missotten L, Van Damme B. Subretinal neovascular membranes associated with chronic membranoproliferative glomerulonephritis type II. Graefes Arch Clin Exp Ophthalmol. 1990;228(6):499–504.
9. Hassenstein A, Richard G. Choroidal neovascularisation in type II membranoproliferative glomerulonephritis, photodynamic therapy as a treatment option--a case report. Klin Monbl Augenheilkd. 2003;220(7):492–5.
10. Awan MA, Grierson DJ, Walker S. Bilateral macular sub-retinal fluid and retinal pigment epithelial detachment associated with type 2 membrano-proliferative glomerulonephritis. Clin Exp Optom. 2008;91(5):476–9.
11. Polk TD, Kimura AE, Park D, Gass JD. Subretinal fluid associated with membranoproliferative glomerulonephritis type 2. Arch Ophthalmol. 1997;115(7):927–8.
12. Kim RY, Faktorovich EG, Kuo CY, Olson JL. Retinal function abnormalities in membranoproliferative glomerulonephritis type II. Am J Ophthalmol. 1997;123(5):619–28.
13. Huang SJ, Costa DL, Gross NE, Yannuzzi LA. Peripheral drusen in membranoproliferative glomerulonephritis type II. Retina. 2003;23(3):429–31.

14. Venkatesh P, Sony P, Garg SP. Optical coherence tomography of fundus findings in type II mesangiocapillary glomerulonephritis. Eye. 2006;20(4):497–9.
15. Adhi M, Read SP, Liu JJ, Fujimoto JG, Duker JS. High-speed ultrahigh-resolution OCT of Bruch's membrane in membranoproliferative glomerulonephritis type 2. Ophthal Surg Lasers Imag Retina. 2014;45(6):614–7.
16. Cebeci Z, Bayraktar S, Oray M, Kir N. Multimodal imaging of membranoproliferative glomerulonephritis type II. Saudi J Ophthalmol. 2016;30(4):260–3.
17. Han DP, Sievers S. Extensive drusen in type I membranoproliferative glomerulonephritis. Arch Ophthalmol. 2009;127(4):577–9.
18. Dalvin LA, Fervenza FC, Sethi S, Pulido JS. Shedding light on fundus drusen associated with membranoproliferative glomerulonephritis: breaking stereotypes of types I, II, AND III. Retinal Cases Brief Rep. 2016;10(1):72–8.
19. Tomino Y. Diagnosis and treatment of patients with IgA nephropathy in Japan. Kidney Res Clin Pract. 2016;35(4):197–203.
20. Berger J, Hinglais N. Intercapillary deposits of IgA-IgG. J Urol Nephrol (Paris). 1968;74(9):694–5.
21. Julian BA, Novak J. IgA nephropathy: an update. Curr Opin Nephrol Hypertens. 2004;13(2):171–9.
22. Payton CD, McLay A, Jones JM. Progressive IgA nephropathy: the role of hypertension. Nephrol Dial Transplant. 1988;3(2):138–42.
23. Taban M, Chand D, Sears JE. Ocular findings in IgA nephropathy with renal failure and hypertension. J Pediatr Ophthalmol Strabismus. 2006;43(6):378–80.
24. Andion-Fernandez M, Dorado-Fernandez T, Juarez-Casado MA, Santamarina-Pernas R. Bilateral serous retinal detachments associated with IgA nephropathy. Arch Soc Esp Oftalmol. 2015;90(11):531–5.
25. Lally DR, Baumal C. Subretinal drusenoid deposits associated with complement-mediated IgA nephropathy. JAMA Ophthalmol. 2014;132(6):775–7.
26. Mackensen F, Billing H. Tubulointerstitial nephritis and uveitis syndrome. Curr Opin Ophthalmol. 2009;20(6):525–31.
27. Mackensen F, David F, Schwenger V, et al. HLA-DRB1*0102 is associated with TINU syndrome and bilateral, sudden-onset anterior uveitis but not with interstitial nephritis alone. Br J Ophthalmol. 2011;95(7):971–5.
28. Mandeville JT, Levinson RD, Holland GN. The tubulointerstitial nephritis and uveitis syndrome. Surv Ophthalmol. 2001;46(3):195–208.
29. Levinson RD. Tubulointerstitial nephritis and uveitis syndrome. Int Ophthalmol Clin. 2008;48(3):51–9.
30. Biester S, Muller C, Deuter CM, Doycheva D, Altpeter E, Zierhut M. Tubulointerstitial nephritis and uveitis in siblings. Ocul Immunol Inflamm. 2010;18(5):370–2.
31. Ramakrishnan S, Dilip R. Syndrome of tubulointerstitial nephritis and uveitis. J Assoc Physicians India. 2009;57:177–9.
32. Johnson BS, Austin JK, Pizio HF. Tubulointerstitial nephritis and uveitis syndrome. Optometry. 2003;74(4):240–4.
33. Hulton SA. The primary hyperoxalurias: a practical approach to diagnosis and treatment. Int J Surg. 2016;36(Pt D):649–54.
34. Coulter-Mackie MB, White CT, Lange D, Chew BH. Primary hyperoxaluria type 1. In: Pagon RA, Adam MP, Ardinger HH, et al., editors. GeneReviews(R). Seattle WA: University of Washington. GeneReviews is a registered trademark of the University of Washington, Seattle; 1993.
35. Morgan JM, Hartley MW, Miller AC Jr, Diethelm AG. Successful renal transplantation in hyperoxaluria. Arch Surg. 1974;109(3):430–3.
36. Small KW, Letson R, Scheinman J. Ocular findings in primary hyperoxaluria. Arch Ophthalmol. 1990;108(1):89–93.
37. Yuan A, Ehlers JP. Crystalline retinopathy from primary hyperoxaluria. Retina. 2012;32(9):1994–5.

38. Munir WM, Sharma MC, Li T, Dealba F, Goldstein DA. Retinal oxalosis in primary hyperoxaluria type 1. Retina. 2004;24(6):974–6.
39. Besirli CG. Retinal flecks in primary hyperoxaluria. JAMA Ophthalmol. 2015;133(10):e151532.
40. Querques G, Bouzitou-Mfoumou R, Soubrane G, Souied EH. Spectral-domain optical coherence tomography visualisation of retinal oxalosis in primary hyperoxaluria. Eye. 2010;24(5): 941–3.
41. Theodossiadis PG, Friberg TR, Panagiotidis DN, Gogas PS, Pantelia EM, Moschos MN. Choroidal neovascularization in primary hyperoxaluria. Am J Ophthalmol. 2002;134(1): 134–7.
42. Derveaux T, Delbeke P, Walraedt S, et al. Detailed clinical phenotyping of oxalate maculopathy in primary hyperoxaluria type 1 and review of the literature. Retina. 2016;36(11):2227–35.
43. Thong B, Olsen NJ. Systemic lupus erythematosus diagnosis and management. Rheumatology. 2016;56(suppl_1):i3–i13.
44. Yap DY, Chan TM. Lupus nephritis in Asia: clinical features and management. Kidney Dis. 2015;1(2):100–9.
45. Adinolfi A, Valentini E, Calabresi E, et al. One year in review 2016: systemic lupus erythematosus. Clin Exp Rheumatol. 2016;34(4):569–74.
46. Tan EM, Cohen AS, Fries JF, et al. The 1982 revised criteria for the classification of systemic lupus erythematosus. Arthritis Rheum. 1982;25(11):1271–7.
47. Read RW. Clinical mini-review: systemic lupus erythematosus and the eye. Ocul Immunol Inflamm. 2004;12(2):87–99.
48. Lally L, Sammaritano LR. Vasculitis in antiphospholipid syndrome. Rheum Dis Clin N Am. 2015;41(1):109–23. ix
49. Preble JM, Silpa-archa S, Foster CS. Ocular involvement in systemic lupus erythematosus. Curr Opin Ophthalmol. 2015;26(6):540–5.
50. Silpa-archa S, Lee JJ, Foster CS. Ocular manifestations in systemic lupus erythematosus. Br J Ophthalmol. 2016;100(1):135–41.
51. Stanford MR, Graham EM. Systemic associations of retinal vasculitis. Int Ophthalmol Clin. 1991;31(3):23–33.
52. Wu C, Dai R, Dong F, Wang Q. Purtscher-like retinopathy in systemic lupus erythematosus. Am J Ophthalmol. 2014;158(6):1335–41. e1331
53. Unlu O, Zuily S, Erkan D. The clinical significance of antiphospholipid antibodies in systemic lupus erythematosus. Eur J Rheumatol. 2016;3(2):75–84.
54. Nguyen QD, Uy HS, Akpek EK, Harper SL, Zacks DN, Foster CS. Choroidopathy of systemic lupus erythematosus. Lupus. 2000;9(4):288–98.
55. Altinkaynak H, Duru N, Uysal BS, et al. Choroidal thickness in patients with systemic lupus erythematosus analyzed by spectral-domain optical coherence tomography. Ocul Immunol Inflamm. 2016;24(3):254–60.
56. Invernizzi A, Dell'Arti L, Leone G, et al. Drusen-like deposits in young adults diagnosed with systemic lupus erythematosus. Am J Ophthalmol. 2016;175:68–76.

Imaging of Retinal and Choroidal Manifestations of Gastrointestinal Disease

6

Francisco J. Rodríguez, Catalina Becerra, and María Cristina Gabela

Abstract

Ocular manifestations of gastrointestinal diseases are uncommon. This chapter describes multimodal imaging of the most frequent gastrointestinal disorders, and associated retinal and choroidal findings. Inflammatory bowel disease, Whipple's disease, and Behçet's disease may have vaso-occlusive manifestations, as well as vasculitis, retinitis, and changes in the choroid, due to inflammation.

Purtscher's like retinopathy associated with pancreatitis presents with changes associated to vaso-occlusive disease. Avitaminosis A has degenerative flecks in the retina that may be reversible with adequate supplementation.

Familial adenomatous polyposis syndrome, also considered in this chapter, has typical clinical characteristic changes in the retinal pigment epithelium that help in the diagnosis.

F.J. Rodríguez, M.D. (✉)
Fundación Oftalmológica Nacional, Escuela de Medicina y Ciencias de la Salud, Universidad del Rosario, Bogotá, DC, Colombia

Fundación Oftalmológica Nacional, Bogotá, DC, Colombia
e-mail: fjrodriguez@fon.org.co

C. Becerra, M.D.
Fundación Oftalmológica Nacional, Bogota, DC, Colombia

M.C. Gabela, M.D.
Fundación Oftalmológica Nacional, Escuela de Medicina y Ciencias de la Salud, Universidad del Rosario, Bogotá, DC, Colombia

J. Chhablani et al. (eds.), *Retinal and Choroidal Imaging in Systemic Diseases*, https://doi.org/10.1007/978-981-10-5461-7_6

6.1 Inflammatory Bowel Disease

6.1.1 Introduction

Inflammatory bowel disease (IBD) is a chronic inflammatory disorder of unknown etiology, and it is used to describe two entities: Crohn's disease (CD) and ulcerative colitis (UC). The annual incidence of CD is about 3.1–14.6 per 100,000 people and for UC 2.2–14.3 per 100,000 people. In recent years the incidence of CD has increased. CD is more frequent in females, while UC is more common in males, and it appears to be higher in urban areas [1].

This multisystemic disorder usually presents with gastrointestinal symptoms (i.e., abdominal pain, diarrhea, and rectal bleeding), and it is associated with a wide spectrum of extraintestinal manifestations, between 21% and 36% of patients, that include ocular, pulmonary, cardiovascular, neurological, and renal, among others [1, 2]. The risk factors for extraintestinal manifestations in Crohn's disease are active disease, family history of IBD, and smoking. And for ulcerative colitis, undergoing gastrointestinal surgery and steroid dependency [3].

These manifestations are due to active systemic vasculitis, vessel wall inflammation, and coagulation abnormalities that lead to an occlusive effect on arteries and veins and structural changes in vessels walls [1]. Angiogenesis has emerged as an additional pathophysiological mechanism [4].

6.1.2 Ocular Manifestations

Ocular involvement is considered as a marker of active bowel disease. However, there is no definite data of the prevalence of ophthalmological manifestations. It has been reported to be between 4% and 30%, being less than 1–10% the posterior segment complications [2, 4, 5]. Around 50% of the patients will have more than one ocular manifestation and at least one other extraintestinal complication [6, 7].

The anterior segment is more commonly involved, and it manifests as dry eye, conjunctivitis, keratitis, episcleritis, self-limited scleritis, and recurrent nongranulomatous iridocyclitis [2, 6, 8].

Posterior segment findings described in IBD are variable, nonspecific, and sometimes occur concurrently [7]. These include panuveitis, vitritis, optic neuritis (retrobulbar optic neuritis and papillitis), neuroretinitis, serous retinal detachment, vasculitis, retinal vascular occlusion, retinal edema, macular edema, central serous retinopathy, macular hemorrhage, and retinal neovascularization [5, 9, 10] (Fig. 6.1a, b, e, f and Fig. 6.2a, b).

Choroidal findings include steroid-responsive choroidal infiltrates, choroidal folds, chorioretinitis, choroiditis, choroidal neovascularization (CNV), and acute posterior multifocal placoid pigment epitheliopathy (APMPPE) [2, 8, 10, 11]. Although CNV is not common, it is another complication that can be related or not to ocular inflammation in IBD patients [12, 13].

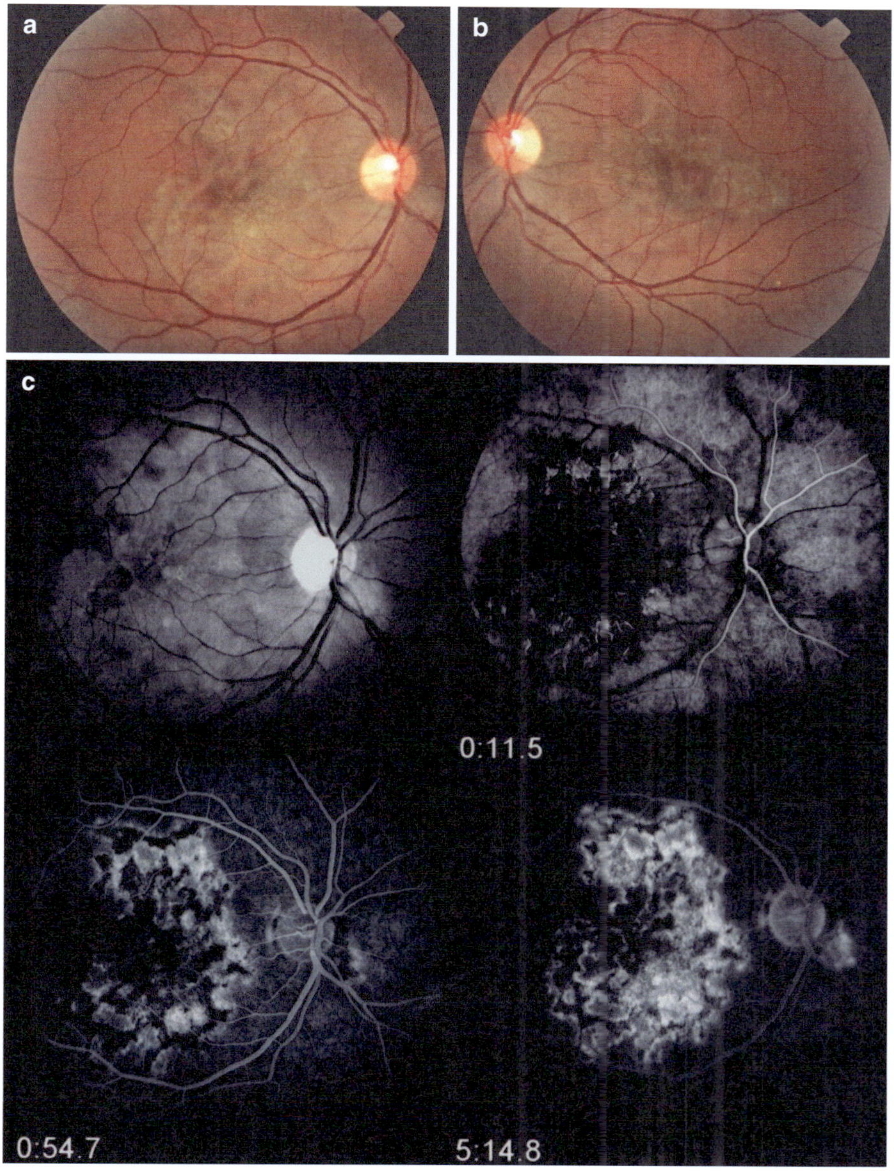

Fig. 6.1 (**a**, **b**) Right and left eye of a 25 years old women, with plaque-like, confluent, inactive lesions in the posterior pole. (**c**, **d**) Fluorescein angiogram showing early hypofluorescent macular lesions with late hyperfluorescence and staining. (**e**, **f**) Five years later the patient returned with a diagnosis of Crohn's disease. Visual acuity was 20/25 in both eyes. Fundus examination showed non-active lesions in both eyes. (**g**, **h**) Fluorescein angiography shows hypofluorescent non-active lesions in the macular area in both eyes

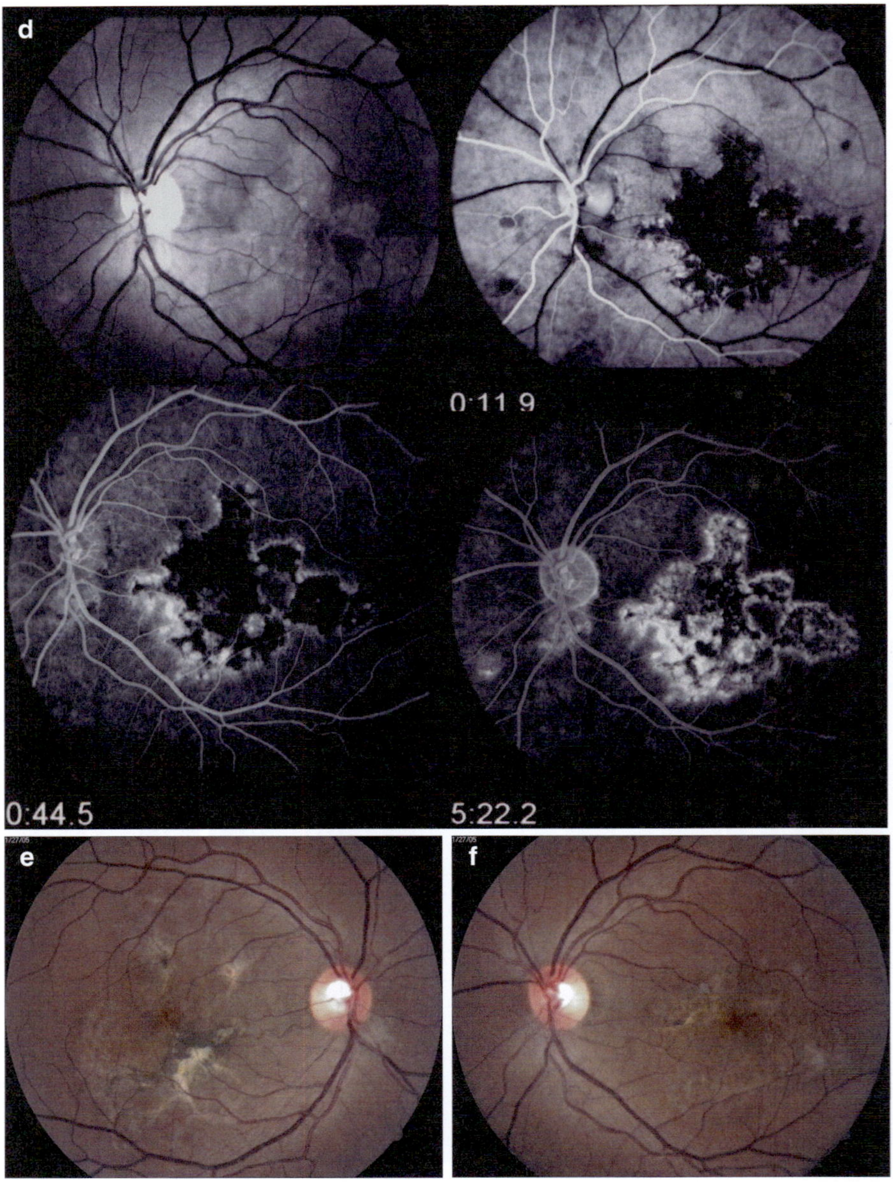

Fig. 6.1 (continued)

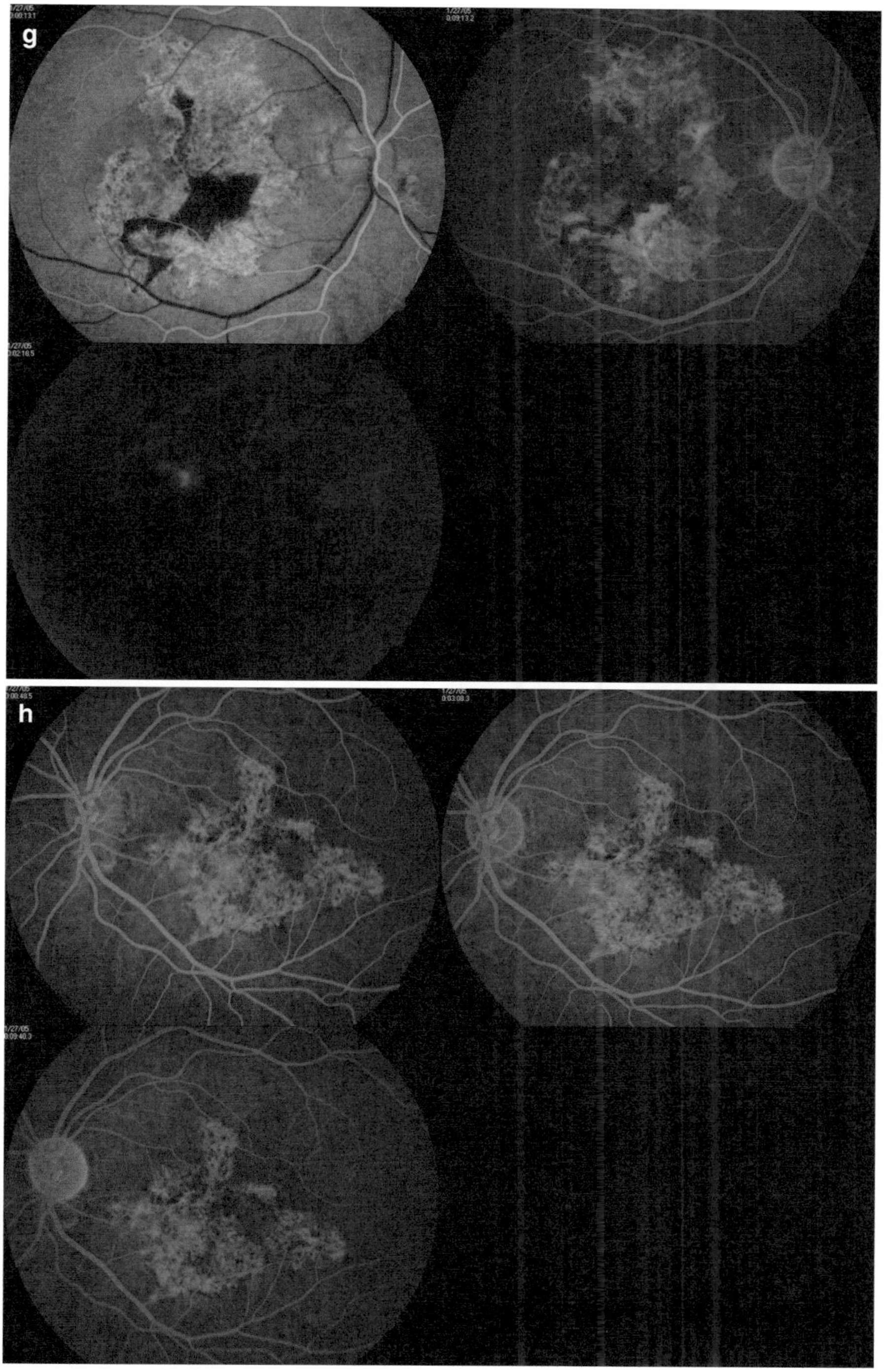

Fig. 6.1 (continued)

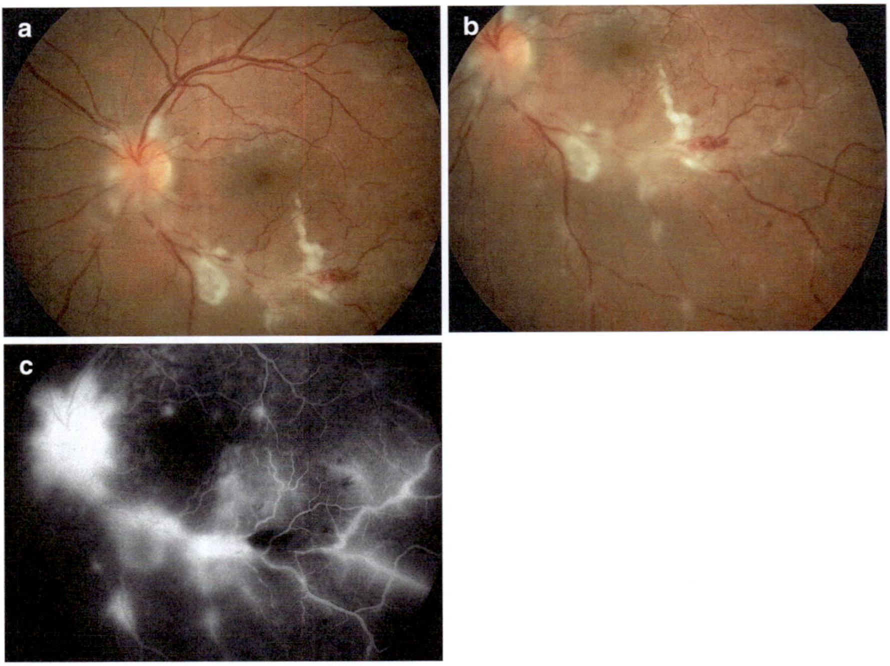

Fig. 6.2 (**a**, **b**) Retinal vasculitis and ischemia in a patient with Crohn's disease. Observe cotton wool spots and intraretinal hemorrhages. (**c**) Late phase of fluorescein angiography shows staining of the retina vessels, areas of ischemia also observed in the color photographs and optic disc staining

6.1.3 Imaging

6.1.3.1 Fundus Fluorescein Angiography and Indocyanine Green Angiography

FFA is useful in cases with retinal vasculopathy, choroidopathy, and optic neuropathy [2]. Capillary dropout is a common finding in vascular occlusions, vasculitis, and retinal neovascularization [5]. Patients with retinal vein occlusions can present with or without associated vasculitis [11] (Fig. 6.1c, d, g, h and Fig. 6.2c).

ICG angiography can show normal choroidal appearance [6], areas of hypoperfusion, and variable focal hypofluorescent spots, as found in choroiditis [12].

6.1.3.2 Optical Coherence Tomography

EDI-OCT choroidal thickness measurement in patients with IBD does not show increase or correlation to the degree of disease activity, except for patients with ileal involvement [4].

6.2 Whipple's Disease

6.2.1 Introduction

Whipple's disease was first reported in 1907 by Georges H. Whipple [14]. It is caused by *Tropheryma whipplei*, a bacterium found ubiquitously in the environment [15, 16]. Most of the cases have been reported in the United States and Europe. *T. whipplei* can be found in stool, and fecal-oral transmission is considered to be the cause of infection [17].

It is a rare disease, with an incidence less than 1 per 1,000,000 people per year [18]. It is more common in men (3:1 ratio), and the age of diagnosis ranges between 48 and 54 years [19].

It is a multisystemic disorder characterized by arthralgia, weight loss, diarrhea, and abdominal pain [18, 20]. Fever, lymphadenopathy steatorrhea, anemia, skin darkening, and ocular symptoms may be present. Neurologic manifestations are the most serious and include progressive supranuclear ophthalmoplegia, oculomasticatory myorhythmia, or oculofacial-skeletal myorhythmia that is pathognomonic of Whipple's disease [18].

6.2.2 Ocular Manifestations

Ocular manifestations of this disease are rare and generally occur late in the disease. Almost 10% of patients with classic Whipple's disease have ocular involvement. In some cases, the patients may not have extraocular manifestations [20]. Ocular findings may be uni- or bilateral.

Symptoms include mild vision loss, floaters, blurred vision, or metamorphopsia.

On slit-lamp examination, keratitis may be present, and anterior chamber cells, keratic precipitates, and vitreous cells may also be found [20–24]. Anterior or posterior uveitis are the predominant features of Whipple's disease.

Fundus findings are consistent with chronic inflammation as: vitritis, vitreous strands, retinitis, retinal vasculitis, RPE changes, choroiditis characterized by multiple round white lesions, optic disk swelling, and macular edema. Retinal hemorrhages, cotton wool spots, and peripapillary exudates may be also present [20, 21, 25] (Figs. 6.3, 6.4 and 6.5).

6.2.3 Imaging

6.2.3.1 Fundus Fluorescein Angiography

On FFA disk hyperfluorescence is present, and in most cases it is found bilaterally; also cystoid macular edema and vasculitis are seen. Vasculitis is predominantly seen as periphlebitis [20, 21].

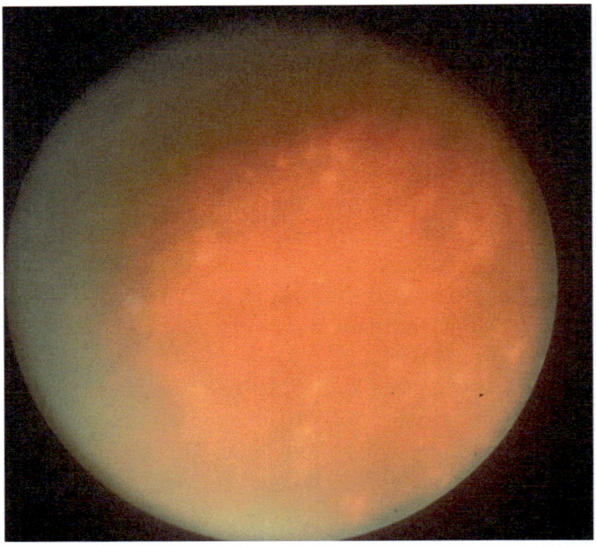

Fig. 6.3 Patient with Whipple's disease. Photograph shows multiple faint, white choroidal lesions (Courtesy of Lawrence A. Yanuzzi, MD)

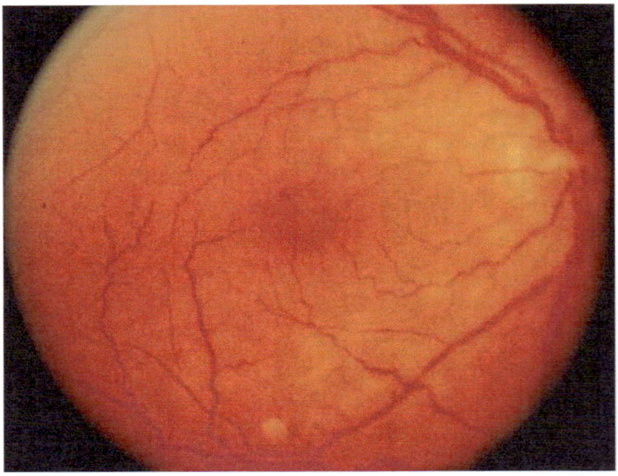

Fig. 6.4 Patient with Whipple's disease. Photograph shows multiple faint, white choroidal lesions (Reprinted with permission from Ref. [21])

Multiple hyperfluorescent spots in the venous phase may be seen, with discrete leakage located in the posterior pole [22].

Diagnosis is generally difficult; in ocular Whipple's disease, vitreous PCR is a helpful diagnostic tool, since it can confirm the presence of the organism in the vitreous. Treatment is based on long-term antibiotic therapy with TMP-SMX; other therapies include tetracycline or doxycycline, however.

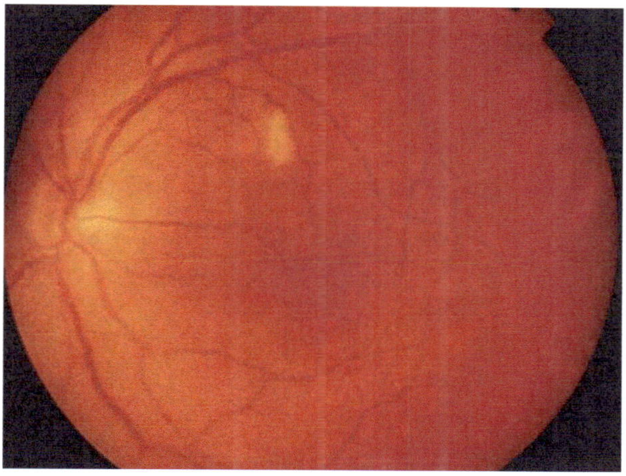

Fig. 6.5 Patient with Whipple's disease. Cotton-wool spot in superior macula (Reprinted with permission from Ref. [21])

6.3 Avitaminosis A

6.3.1 Introduction

Avitaminosis A is a rare disease, secondary to multiple etiologies, including malnourishment, malabsorption secondary to gastrointestinal surgery, or liver disease that leads to fat malabsorption [26]. Because of increasing gastrointestinal procedures, especially bariatric surgery, this deficiency is becoming more common. The prevalence varies from 52% at 1 year after the surgery to 69% after 4 years [27].

Vitamin A is a key factor in normal retinal metabolism. Vitamin A deficiency produces decreased levels of rhodopsin, rod sensitivity loss, and slowed dark adaptation that patients notice as night blindness [28, 29].

6.3.2 Ocular Manifestations

Xerophthalmia is a common manifestation of avitaminosis A, but it is not always present.

Night blindness or nyctalopia is one of the first clinical symptoms of this disease.

On slit-lamp examination, conjunctival and corneal xeroses may be present [26, 30]. On fundus examination, flecked retina is a common finding associated to multiple yellow-white retinal spots in the mid-periphery and posterior pole [31] (Figs. 6.6 and 6.7). Papilledema has also been described in association with vitamin A deficiency, but it is extremely rare [30].

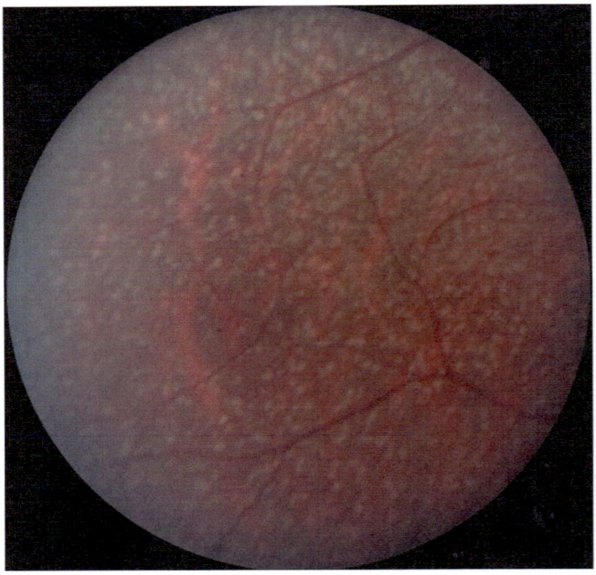

Fig. 6.6 Patient with A avitaminosis, note multiple white flecks in the mid periphery. (Courtesy of William F. Mieler, MD)

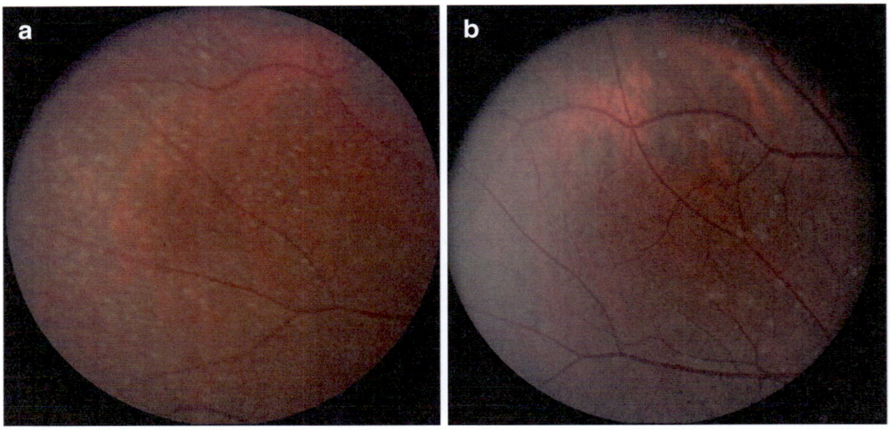

Fig. 6.7 Patient with A avitaminosis. A: multiple white flecks in the mid periphery. (Courtesy of William F. Mieler, MD). B: Same patient after treatment of vitamin A deficiency, note the white flecks disappeared and left hyperpigmented spots. (Courtesy of William F. Mieler, MD)

Diagnosis of vitamin A deficiency is confirmed by blood levels of vitamin A under 0.3 mg/dl (normal levels 0.3–1.2 mg/dl) [28]. Retinal disease is confirmed by electroretinogram (ERG) findings such as non-detectable rod function, borderline reduced cone function, and normal response on photopic single flash and flicker [28, 29, 32].

Visual field testing may show mild to moderate concentric restriction to II-2-e target, on Goldmann kinetic perimetry 940, or mild to moderate decreased sensibility on computerized Goldmann perimetry. Patients may not notice visual field changes.

6.3.3 Imaging

6.3.3.1 Fundus Fluorescein Angiography and Autofluorescence

On FFA, multiple hyperfluorescent spots are seen with no late leakage, mostly located in the mid-periphery [29].

Short-wave autofluorescence imaging (SW-AF) demonstrates the lesions as hypoautofluorescent [28].

6.3.3.2 Optical Coherence Tomography

SD-OCT shows hyperreflective material above the RPE bulging the ellipsoid zone, corresponding to the yellow fleck lesions in the fundus [26, 28]. Retina around these lesions may be normal. RPE under the hyperreflective zones may be intact, and EZ band over the hyperreflective lesions may be normal as well [28].

Ophthalmological findings are reversible, with adequate supplementation and when normal Vitamin A levels are reached. Also ERG abnormalities and fundus appearance are reversible.

6.4 Pancreatitis: Purtscher's-Like Retinopathy

6.4.1 Introduction

Purtscher's retinopathy was first described in 1910, by Othmar Purtscher, associated to closed thoracic trauma [33]. In 1975, Purtscher's-like retinopathy was first described in association with pancreatitis [34]. Besides pancreatitis other diseases can produce Purtscher-like retinopathy such as renal failure, autoimmune disease, amniotic fluid embolism, collagen-vascular disorders, and coagulation disorders [33, 35].

It is a rare condition, with an estimated incidence of 0.24 cases per year including Purtscher's and Purtscher-like retinopathies, but an underestimation is possible because many patients can be visually asymptomatic [35].

Purtscher-like retinopathy is a severe and self-limited complication of pancreatitis, with no established treatment. Associated visual loss can vary from mild to severe, but improvement can be spontaneous from partial to complete visual recovery. It is also considered as an indicator of multi-organ failure and has been associated with fatal outcome [36].

The pathophysiology is still to be elucidated, but it is believed that leukocytic embolus occludes retinal arterioles and choroidal vessels. This emboli result from pancreatic damage that releases proteolytic enzymes that activate the complement C5a-induced leukocyte, platelet, and fibrin aggregates [37].

6.4.2 Ocular Manifestations

It is characterized by sudden visual loss of variable severity, between hours and days from the onset of the pancreatic disease. Bilateral disease is expected in 60% of

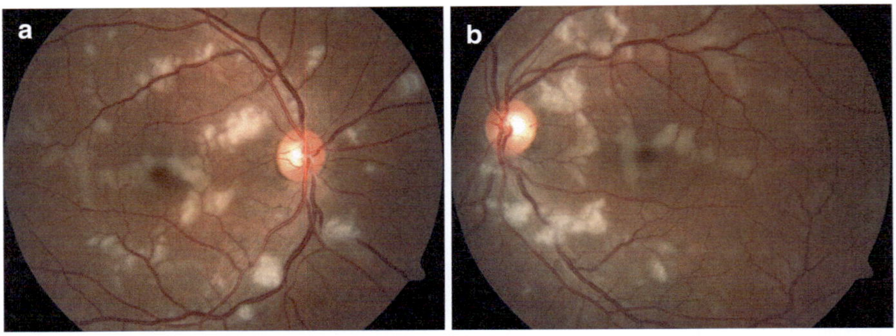

Fig. 6.8 Patient with purtscher like retinopathy. A right and B left eye. Images show cotton-wool spots, retinal flecken, macular whitening and a pseudo cherry red spot

patients. Fundus exam shows posterior pole lesions that appear in 83–92% of cases, and these include cotton wool spots and intraretinal hemorrhages [33]. Purtscher flecken occur in 50% of patients and are the result of precapillary artery occlusions; they are seen as macular retinal whitening that spare 50 μm of retinal arterioles, different from cotton wool spots that can be over retinal vessels [38, 39]. Disk swelling and pseudo-cherry red spot can also appear in Purtscher's and Purtscher-like retinopathies [35] (Fig. 6.8).

Follow-up findings in the chronic phase include normalization of retinal appearance in 40% of patients, optic atrophy in 64%, retinal thinning, and retinal mottling of the RPE [33].

6.4.3 Imaging

6.4.3.1 Fundus Fluorescein Angiography

Fundus fluorescein angiography (FFA) manifestations result from occlusive disease. Images show leakage of dye from retinal arterioles, venules, and capillaries; delayed arterial filling, multiple ischemic areas, and arteriolar obstruction occur in more severe cases. Choroidal hypoperfusion and disk staining have been described [33, 37, 40, 41].

In the late venous phase, hypofluorescence due to ischemia and macular edema can be seen as well as perivenous staining [33] (Fig. 6.9).

On indocyanine green angiography (ICG-A), areas of choroidal hypofluorescence have been described [41, 42].

6.4.3.2 Optical Coherence Tomography

In acute phase, severe edema and hyperreflectivity of the inner plexiform, inner nuclear, and outer plexiform layers have been reported [43].

In the follow-up, macular atrophy [43], reduction of retinal nerve fiber layer secondary to cotton wool spots, can be seen [35].

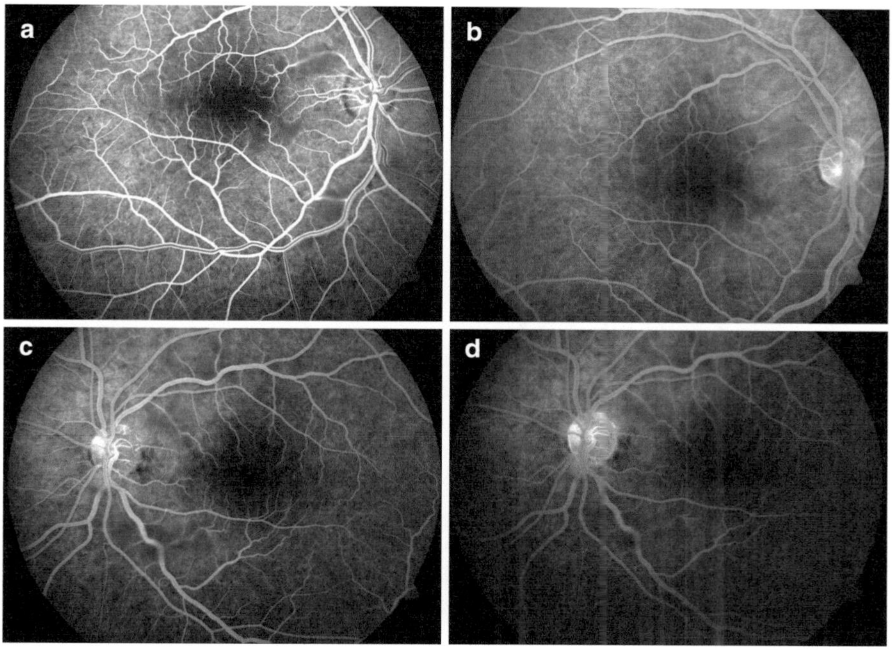

Fig. 6.9 Fundus Fluorescein angiography from the same patient in figure 8. A and B multiple hypofluorescent lesions in the macular and perivascular area, that do not progress during late phases (C and D)

6.5 Behçet's Disease

6.5.1 Introduction

Behçet's disease is a multisystemic chronic and recurrent vasculitis of unknown etiology, characterized by endothelial dysfunction. Clinical characteristics include a recurrent triple-symptom complex of oral aphthous ulcers, genital ulcers, and uveitis [44]. The disease shows a variable prevalence related to geographic factors, being higher between countries among the ancient Silk Route. The mean age of onset is between the third and fourth decade of life, and it is more common among men in endemic countries, while females are more frequently affected in North America and North European countries [45, 46].

Diagnosis is based on clinical criteria; there is no specific ancillary laboratory test to confirm the disease [45]. Clinical manifestations are defined as major and minor. Mucous membrane lesions (oral and genital ulcers), skin lesions (pseudofolliculitis, erythema nodosum), and ocular involvement are major manifestations [47]. Joint, neurological, pulmonary, cardiac, vascular, and gastrointestinal manifestations are minor lesions, although some of them can cause major morbidity and worse vital prognosis [46].

Behçet's disease is characterized histopathologically by necrotizing leukocytoclastic vasculitis that results in the obliteration of the endothelial lumen and intensive lymphocytic and monocytic cellular infiltration of retinal vessels with diffuse or focal infiltration of the choroid without vasculitis in acute phases [46, 48]. In chronic phases the choroid shows edema and fibrosis [49].

6.5.2 Ocular Manifestations

Ocular involvement occurs in approximately 70–90% of the patients, and it has been reported that 50 to 93% have posterior segment involvement [48, 50]. The most common form of ocular manifestation is a non-granulomatous anterior uveitis with hypopyon, present in 19–31% of the cases [51]. Male patients are more susceptible to ocular involvement and have worse visual prognosis [46, 52].

Posterior inflammation may affect the vitreous, retina, optic nerve, and choroid. The more frequent form is necrotizing occlusive vasculitis, which can result in vascular occlusion and subsequent ischemia and retinal atrophy in the areas of occluded vessels. Both, inflammation and decreased blood flow, lead to retinal nerve fiber loss and optic nerve damage, followed by retinal and optic disk atrophy or neovascularization [48].

Patients with inactive Behçet's disease show cataract, secondary glaucoma, cyclitic membranes, epiretinal membrane (ERM), narrowing of retinal vessels or ghost retinal vessels (that correlate with longer duration of the disease), macular hole, retinal detachment, retinal and optic nerve atrophy, and phthisis bulbi. Other fundus changes include vitreous hemorrhages, vascular sheathing, retinal vascular occlusions, retinal exudates, and hemorrhages [46, 48, 49, 51] (Figs. 6.10 and 6.11).

6.5.3 Imaging

6.5.3.1 Fundus Fluorescein Angiography and Indocyanine Green Angiography

Fundus fluorescein angiography typical finding is diffuse capillary leakage of the retinal vasculature, as a consequence of inflammation, obstructive retinal vasculitis, and ischemia [49]. Leakage may be present before obvious ophthalmoscopic signs of retinal vasculitis [53]. Because of chronic and permanent damage of blood vessels, mild and persistent leakage can be seen for a long time after the resolution of active inflammation [54].

Other FFA findings are staining and dye leakage of the optic disc, macular ischemia, macular edema, retinal and optic nerve neovascularization, and angiographic changes due to nonischemic central retinal or branch vein retinal occlusion [49, 54, 55]. On ultrawide-field imaging (UWFI) FFA, peripheral retinal non-perfusion, vessel leakage, and neovascularization are evident [56].

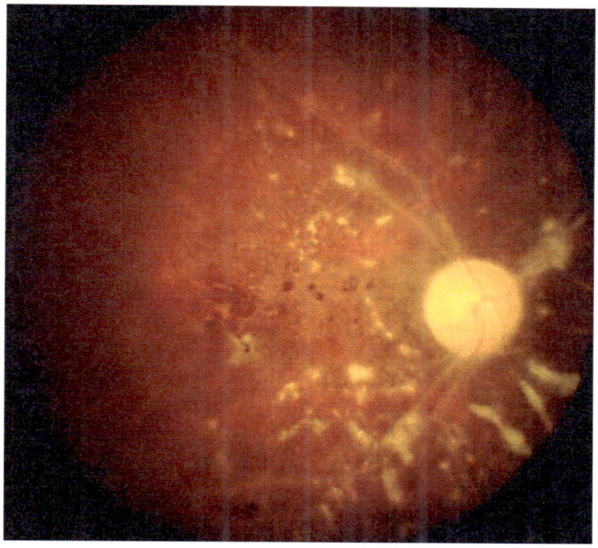

Fig. 6.10 Patient with Behçet disease, right eye color photograph showing severe occlusive disease, pale disc, vascular sheating, macular hemorrhages, and exudates

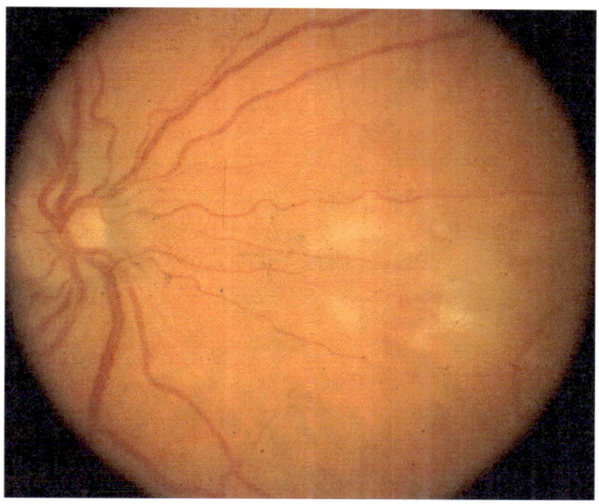

Fig. 6.11 Patient with Behçet disease, right eye color photograph, nasal area with multiple hemorrhages and vascular sheating.

ICG angiography findings suggest that choroidal inflammation is an etiologic factor related to the vasculitis episode [48]. These include hypofluorescent well-defined plaque lesions, hyperfluorescent spots, hyper- and/or hypofluorescent irregular filling of the choriocapillaris, choroidal filling defects, delayed choroidal filling, and diffuse leakage from choroidal vessels. In the late phases, this leakage is due to the damage of the wall of large vessels [50, 53, 55, 57]. Hypofluorescent plaques could be due to edema, fibrosis, or atrophy of the choroidal tissue [49].

6.5.3.2 Multimodal Imaging

Ultrawide-field fundus autofluorescence image findings suggest that active vasculitis also induces distinct patterns of retinal pigment epithelium alterations. FAF findings described in the literature are limited. A report found hyperautofluorescent spots and chorioretinal atrophic hypoautofluorescent lesions adjacent to retinal vessels and surrounding the optic disk [56].

6.5.3.3 Optical Coherence Tomography

SD-OCT

Macular thickness analysis is helpful in the diagnosis and follow-up of macular edema and macular atrophy [58]. Usually the macula is thinner in patients with chronic disease and recurrent posterior segment involvement [48]. Other OCT findings are epiretinal membranes, loss of external layers of the retina, loss of integrity of ellipsoid zone (ELZ) and external limiting membrane (ELM), and intraretinal fluid [49, 50]. Loss of integrity and definition of the ELZ and ELM lines appear to be associated with best-corrected visual acuity (BCVA) in patients with BD as in other diseases, although other irreversible changes of sensory retina may also affect visual prognosis [59, 60].

On EDI-OCT, the choroid shows a significant increase in thickness in active phases. During the active phase, dilation of choroidal vessels is observed, and the choroidal thickness is greater than that in remission phase. After systemic treatment for BD, choroidal thickness decreases and maintains thereafter [61]. In patients with active posterior uveitis, increase in choroidal thickness is related with retinal vascular leakage in fundus fluorescein angiography [62]. In longer disease duration, choroidal fibrosis can be seen with subsequent thickness decrease [49].

6.6 Familial Adenomatous Polyposis: Gardner's Syndrome

6.6.1 Introduction

Familial adenomatous polyposis (FAP), also known as familial polyposis coli (FPC), is a hereditary autosomal dominant condition that has a mutation of the APC gene in chromosome 5, and it is characterized by the presence of multiple adenomatous lesions in the large bowel and/or duodenal tract polyps, with high risk of malignant transformation into colon cancer [63, 64]. Frequency is 1 in 12,000. Eighty percent of the patients have a positive family history, and 20% arise from spontaneous mutations. Usually this syndrome manifests between 20 and 40 years [65].

Gardner's syndrome is a variant of familial adenomatous polyposis. Clinical findings include colorectal adenomatous polyps, with extracolonic manifestations such as dermoid cysts, teeth abnormalities, epidermoid cysts, thyroid masses, and also abnormalities in the retinal pigment epithelium (RPE) [63, 65, 66].

6.6.2 Ocular Manifestations

Ocular findings distinguish this syndrome from other forms of FAP. Congenital hypertrophy of the retinal pigment epithelium (CHRPE) is the typical manifestation and is present in over 85% of the patients. The presence of CHRPE has a sensitivity that ranges from 65% to 84% and specificity greater than 94% for FAP, when the patient has an affected relative [65, 67].

Gardner-related CHRPE are multiple, flat, pigmented, well-defined ovoid RPE lesions, located in the equator or mid-periphery of both eyes, and appear early after birth, being the first clinical sign of the syndrome [65, 68, 69]. These lesions may have a depigmented halo, a fishtail-shaped hypopigmented change at one or both ends, and/or depigmented lacunae [67, 70]. Choroidal vessels can be seen within the depigmented areas around the lesion [71] (Fig. 6.12).

Histological findings are hyperplastic RPE cells and densely pigmented cells between Bruch's membrane and the basement membrane with degenerated photoreceptors [72].

Other pigmented lesions not associated with extraocular abnormalities can be found in the fundus examination in 8–13% of patients with FAP, as solitary CHRPE, bear tracks, retinal pigment hyperplasia after trauma or inflammation, or choroidal nevi [73–75].

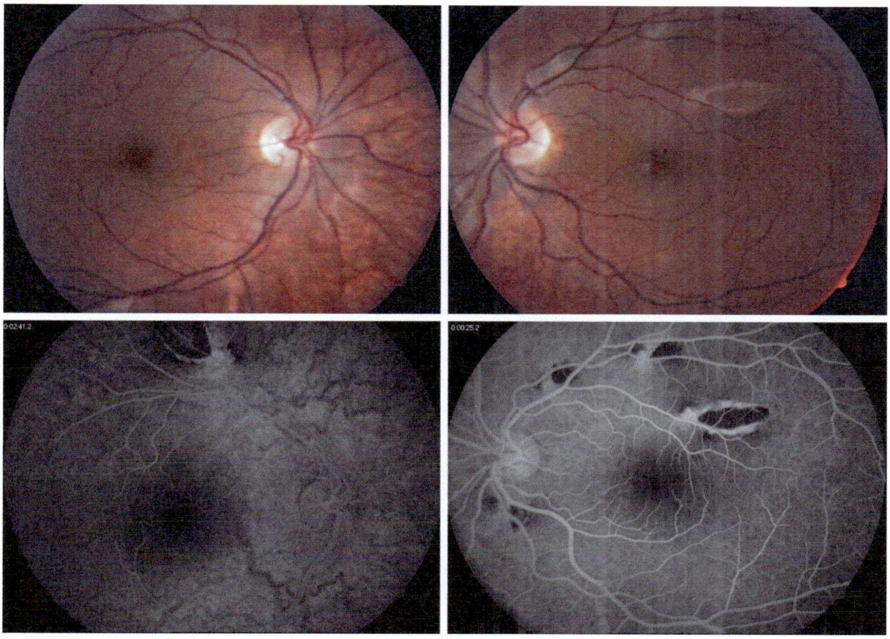

Fig. 6.12 Multiple lesions of congenital hypertrophy of the RPE, associated with familiar adenomatous polyposis and Gardner's Syndrome in a 19 years old male. (Courtesy of Ricardo Infante, MD)

6.6.3 Imaging

6.6.3.1 Fundus Fluorescein Angiography

Fundus fluorescein angiography (FFA) is useful to confirm the diagnosis and detect additional changes of Gardner-related CHRPE. These lesions present an angiographic pattern characterized by hypofluorescent block defect that corresponds to hyperpigmented areas, and hyperfluorescent window defects in the areas of atrophy and in the depigmented marginal streaks, that show no leakage during the study [70].

Capillary irregularities such as non-perfusion areas and reduction of the capillary network can be seen on FFA. Other vascular changes found are microaneurysms, chorioretinal anastomosis, partial block of retinal arteries crossing the lesion (vascular strangulation), visualization of the capillary vessels, and entwined choriocapillary vessel. Satellite small hypofluorescent lesions near bigger lesions can be found in FFA, not seen in ophthalmoscopy [70].

6.6.3.2 Multimodal Imaging

Fundus autofluorescence (FAF) features a hypoautofluorescent lesion due to the absence of lipofuscin between the pigmented RPE cells, with lacunae showing isoautofluorescence or hypoautofluorescence, corresponding to the segmental absence of RPE. On IR (infrared) reflectance imaging, CHRPE displays hyporeflectivity in the hyperpigmented areas of the lesion and hyperreflectivity within the lacunae [74, 76].

6.6.3.3 Optical Coherence Tomography

RPE Gardner lesions show a characteristic pattern on spectral domain-optical coherence tomography (SD-OCT), although the acquisition of the image is technically difficult because most of the lesions are localized in the equator and periphery. On OCT, CHRPE is seen as a flat lesion of the RPE with absent, thickened, or irregular RPE and an overlying retinal thinning with photoreceptor atrophy that begins at the margin of the lesion [77]. Subretinal cleft, intralesional lacunae (absent RPE with bright transmission of light through the defect), and other unusual findings such as hyperreflective spots and cystoid edema can also be seen. Choroidal thickness and vascular pattern are usually normal. Bruch's membrane can be normal or thickened [69, 76].

Future Remarks

- Although uncommon, a differential diagnosis of retinal vasculitis and vaso-occlusive disease may include gastrointestinal diseases.
- Gastrointestinal specialist should also be involved in the management.
- Underdiagnosis is due to low prevalence.
- Some of the retinal and choroidal findings may serve as markers of disease activity.
- New available technology, such as Angio-OCT, swept source, and microperimetry, may show new patterns associated with gastrointestinal diseases.

Conclusions

Gastrointestinal disease can manifest in various forms in the eye.

Inflammatory bowel disease, Behçet's disease, and Whipple's disease have common ocular features, such as uveitis, vasculitis, and vaso-occlusive disease. On imaging these diseases have similar behavior and cannot be differentiated from other causes of ocular disease but may indicate activity of the pathology.

Pancreatitis presents as Purtscher-like syndrome, and vaso-occlusive changes with retinal edema, retinal flecken, and hemorrhages characterize the disease.

Avitaminosis A is rare and may be underdiagnosed, but it is increasing in frequency due to surgical treatment for obesity, as bariatric surgery. Night blindness and retinal flecks are typical features of the disease, and the flecks have a characteristic hypoautoflurescent pattern on FAF and hyperreflective lesions between RPE and EZ on SD-OCT. Adaptive optics can be useful to study changes on photoreceptor layers.

Gardner-related RPE lesions have no functional visual impact but are important findings in the diagnosis of the disease. Multimodal imaging aids in the differentiation of Gardner-related lesions from other fundus-pigmented lesions.

Available and new emerging technology will show us with better details more information about these diseases, can help us explain better the pathophysiology and prognosis, and may be characterized as biomarkers of either disease activity or progression.

Key Learning Points

- FFA, ICG angiography, and SD-OCT complement each other as diagnostic tools. Findings are not specific or pathognomonic of these diseases but appear to be helpful in the evaluation of posterior segment compromise, ocular complications that can cause visual impairment, and treatment follow-up.
- FFA is useful to assess and monitor activity of ocular inflammation. In addition to OCT, they will allow the evaluation of morphological and functional changes inside the retina and choroid, even before fundus ophthalmoscopic signs develop.
- Ultrawide-field and multimodal imaging can be used for the diagnosis, extent treatment, and follow-up of patients with gastrointestinal disease and ocular involvement.
- Gastrointestinal diseases related with ocular inflammation, such as anterior uveitis, posterior uveitis, and retinal vasculitis, cannot be differentiated from other systemic causes, but rarely they are the first clinical manifestation.

References

1. Su CG, Judge TA, Lichtenstein GR. Extraintestinal manifestations of inflammatory bowel disease. Gastroenterol Clin N Am. 2002;31(1):307–27.
2. Ghanchi FD, Rembacken BJ. Inflammatory bowel disease and the eye. Surv Ophthalmol. 2003;48(6):663–76.

3. Vavricka SR, Brun L, Ballabeni P, Pittet V, Prinz Vavricka BM, Zeitz J, et al. Frequency and risk factors for extraintestinal manifestations in the Swiss inflammatory bowel disease cohort. Am J Gastroenterol. 2011;106(1):110–9.
4. Onal IK, Yuksel E, Bayrakceken K, Demir MM, Karaca EE, Ibis M, et al. Measurement and clinical implications of choroidal thickness in patients with inflammatory bowel disease. Arq Bras Oftalmol. 2015;78(5):278–82.
5. Figueiredo L, Rothwell R, Brandão A, Fonseca S. Central retinal vein occlusion in a patient with retinal vasculitis and Crohn's disease. Case Rep Ophthalmol Med. 2014;2014:967878.
6. Saatci OA, Koçak N, Durak I, Ergin MH. Unilateral retinal vasculitis, branch retinal artery occlusion and subsequent retinal neovascularization in Crohn's disease. Int Ophthalmol. 2001;24(2):89–92.
7. Yilmaz S, Aydemir E, Maden A, Unsal B. The prevalence of ocular involvement in patients with inflammatory bowel disease. Int J Color Dis. 2007;22(9):1027–30.
8. Felekis T, Katsanos K, Kitsanou M, Trakos N, Theopistos V, Christodoulou D, et al. Spectrum and frequency of ophthalmologic manifestations in patients with inflammatory bowel disease: a prospective single-center study. Inflamm Bowel Dis. 2009;15(1):29–34.
9. Loftus EV. Clinical epidemiology of inflammatory bowel disease: incidence, prevalence, and environmental influences. Gastroenterology. 2004;126(6):1504–17.
10. Ernst BB, Lowder CY, Meisler DM, Gutman FA. Posterior segment manifestations of inflammatory bowel disease. Ophthalmology. 1991;98(8):1272–80.
11. Larsson J, Hansson-Lundblad C. Central retinal vein occlusion in two patients with inflammatory bowel disease. Retina Phila Pa. 2000;20(6):681–2.
12. Ishihara K, Tsujikawa A, Yodoi Y, Kameda T, Yoshimura N. Choroidal neovascularization in a patient with ulcerative colitis. Jpn J Ophthalmol. 2008;52(6):515–8.
13. Unal A, Sipahioglu MH, Akgun H, Yurci A, Tokgoz B, Erkilic K, et al. Crohn's disease complicated by granulomatous interstitial nephritis, choroidal neovascularization, and central retinal vein occlusion. Intern Med Tokyo Jpn. 2008;47(2):103–7.
14. Whipple GH. A hitherto undescribed disease characterized anatomically by deposits of fat and fatty acids in the intestinal and mesenteric lymphatic tissues. Bull Johns Hopkins Hosp. 1907;18(198):382–91.
15. Schöniger-Hekele M, Petermann D, Weber B, Müller C. Tropheryma whipplei in the environment: survey of sewage plant influxes and sewage plant workers. Appl Environ Microbiol. 2007;73(6):2033–5.
16. Maiwald M, Schuhmacher F, Ditton HJ, von Herbay A. Environmental occurrence of the Whipple's disease bacterium (Tropheryma whippelii). Appl Environ Microbiol. 1998;64(2): 760–2.
17. Fenollar F, Lepidi H, Gérolami R, Drancourt M, Raoult D. Whipple disease associated with giardiasis. J Infect Dis. 2003;188(6):828–34.
18. Schneider T, Moos V, Loddenkemper C, Marth T, Fenollar F, Raoult D. Whipple's disease: new aspects of pathogenesis and treatment. Lancet Infect Dis. 2008;8(3):179–90.
19. Durand DV, Lecomte C, Cathébras P, Rousset H, Godeau P. Whipple disease. Clinical review of 52 cases. The SNFMI research group on Whipple disease. Medicine. 1997;76(3):170–84.
20. Touitou V, Fenollar F, Cassoux N, Merle-Beral H, LeHoang P, Amoura Z, et al. Ocular Whipple's disease: therapeutic strategy and long-term follow-up. Ophthalmology. 2012;119(7): 1465–9.
21. Chan RY, Yannuzzi LA, Foster CS. Ocular Whipple's disease: earlier definitive diagnosis. Ophthalmology. 2001;108(12):2225–31.
22. Razonable RR, Pulido JS, Deziel PJ, Dev S, Salomão DR, Walker RC. Chorioretinitis and vitreitis due to Tropheryma whipplei after transplantation: case report and review. Transpl Infect Dis Off J Transplant Soc. 2008;10(6):413–8.
23. Thaler S, Grisanti S, Klingel K, Raible A, Kempf VA, Schulte B. Intermediate uveitis and arthralgia as early symptoms in Whipple's disease. Int J Infect Dis. 2010;14(Suppl 3): e388–9.
24. Williams JG, Edward DP, Tessler HH, Persing DH, Mitchell PS, Goldstein DA. Ocular manifestations of Whipple disease: an atypical presentation. Arch Ophthalmol. 1998;116(9):1232–4.

25. Playford RJ, Schulenburg E, Herrington CS, Hodgson HJ. Whipple's disease complicated by a retinal Jarisch-Herxheimer reaction: a case report. Gut. 1992;33(1):132–4.
26. Chow CC, Mieler WF. Vitamin a deficiency and xerophthalmic fundus in autoimmune hepatitis and cirrhosis. Retin Cases Brief Rep. 2014;8(3):164–6.
27. Slater GH, Ren CJ, Siegel N, Williams T, Barr D, Wolfe B, et al. Serum fat-soluble vitamin deficiency and abnormal calcium metabolism after malabsorptive bariatric surgery. J Gastrointest Surg Off. 2004;8(1):48–55. discussion 54–5
28. Aleman TS, Garrity ST, Brucker AJ. Retinal structure in vitamin a deficiency as explored with multimodal imaging. Doc Ophthalmol. 2013;127(3):239–43.
29. Genead MA, Fishman GA, Lindeman M. Fundus white spots and acquired night blindness due to vitamin a deficiency. Doc Ophthalmol Adv Ophthalmol. 2009;119(3):229–33.
30. Panozzo G, Babighian S, Bonora A. Association of xerophthalmia, flecked retina, and pseudotumor cerebri caused by hypovitaminosis a. Am J Ophthalmol. 1998;125(5):708–10.
31. De Laey JJ. Flecked retina disorders. Bull Soc Belge Ophtalmol. 1993;249:11–22.
32. Elison JR, Friedman AH, Brodie SE. Acquired subretinal flecks secondary to hypovitaminosis a in a patient with hepatitis C. Doc Ophthalmol Adv Ophthalmol. 2004;109(3):279–81.
33. Miguel AIM, Henriques F, Azevedo LFR, Loureiro AJR, Maberley D. A. L. systematic review of Purtscher's and Purtscher-like retinopathies. Eye Lond Engl. 2013;27(1):1–13.
34. Inkeles DM, Walsh JB. Retinal fat emboli as sequela to acute pancreatitis. Am J Ophthalmol. 1975;80(5):935–8.
35. Massa R, Vale C, Macedo M, Furtado MJ, Gomes M, Lume M, et al. Purtscher-like retinopathy. Case Rep Ophthalmol Med. 2015;2015:421329.
36. Holló G. Frequency of Purtscher's retinopathy. Br J Ophthalmol. 2008;92(8):1159.
37. Carrera CRL, Pierre LM, Medina FMC, Pierre-Filho P d TP. Purtscher-like retinopathy associated with acute pancreatitis. São Paulo Med J. 2005;123(6):289–91.
38. Proença Pina J, Ssi-Yan-Kai K, de Monchy I, Charpentier B, Offret H, Labetoulle M. Purtscher-like retinopathy: case report and review of the literature. J Fr Ophtalmol. 2008;31(6 Pt 1): 609–13.
39. Kincaid MC, Green WR, Knox DL, Mohler C. A clinicopathological case report of retinopathy of pancreatitis. Br J Ophthalmol. 1982;66(4):219–26.
40. Campo SM, Gasparri V, Catarinelli G, Sepe M. Acute pancreatitis with Purtscher's retinopathy: case report and review of the literature. Dig Liver Dis Off. 2000;32(8):729–32.
41. Agrawal A, McKibbin MA. Purtscher's and Purtscher-like retinopathies: a review. Surv Ophthalmol. 2006;51(2):129–36.
42. Gomez-Ulla F, Fente B, Torreiro MG, Salorio MS, Gonzalez F. Choroidal vascular abnormality in Purtscher's retinopathy shown by indocyanine green angiography. Am J Ophthalmol. 1996;122(2):261–3.
43. Wright EM, Liang MM, Reichel EM. Man referred for sudden onset decline in vision in left eye. Ocular Surgery News [Internet]. 2015. Cited 01 Dec 2015. Available from: http://www.healio.com/ophthalmology/retina-vitreous/news/print/ocular-surgery-news/%7B06f12fe0-1b0a-4326-baf6-9f59b8ee8e71%7D/man-referred-for-sudden-onset-decline-in-vision-in-left-eye
44. Hatemi G, Seyahi E, Fresko I, Talarico R, Hamuryudan V. Behçet's syndrome: a critical digest of the 2013-2014 literature. Clin Exp Rheumatol. 2014;32(4 Suppl 84):S112–22.
45. Skef W, Hamilton MJ, Arayssi T. Gastrointestinal Behçet's disease: a review. World J Gastroenterol. 2015;21(13):3801–12.
46. Evereklioglu C. Current concepts in the etiology and treatment of Behçet disease. Surv Ophthalmol. 2005;50(4):297–350.
47. Davatchi F, Chams-Davatchi C, Shams H, Nadji A, Faezi T, Akhlaghi M, et al. Adult Behcet's disease in Iran: analysis of 6075 patients. Int J Rheum Dis. 2015;19(1):95–103.
48. Ataş M, Yuvacı I, Demircan S, Güler E, Altunel O, Pangal E, et al. Evaluation of the macular, peripapillary nerve fiber layer and choroid thickness changes in Behçet's disease with spectral-domain OCT. J Ophthalmol. 2014;2014:865394.
49. Coskun E, Gurler B, Pehlivan Y, Kisacik B, Okumus S, Yayuspayı R, et al. Enhanced depth imaging optical coherence tomography findings in Behçet disease. Ocul Immunol Inflamm. 2013;21(6):440–5.

50. Corrêa TP, Arantes TE, Lima VC, Muccioli C. Structural evaluation of posterior pole in patients with Behçet's disease. Arq Bras Oftalmol. 2011;74(6):395–9.
51. Tekeli O, Ozdemir O. Heidelberg retina tomograph in ocular Behçet's disease. Eye. 2004;18(2): 143–6.
52. Davatchi F, Shahram F, Shams H, Nadji A, Chams-Davatchi C, Akhlaghi M, et al. Gender influence on ocular manifestations and their outcome in Behcet's disease. A long-term follow-up of up to 20 years. Clin Rheumatol. 2011;30(4):541–7.
53. Atmaca LS, Sonmez PA. Fluorescein and indocyanine green angiography findings in Behçet's disease. Br J Ophthalmol. 2003;87(12):1466–8.
54. Kang HM, Lee SC. Long-term progression of retinal vasculitis in Behçet patients using a fluorescein angiography scoring system. Graefes Arch Clin Exp Ophthalmol. 2014;252(6):1001–8.
55. Gedik S, Akova Y, Yilmaz G, Bozbeyoğlu S. Indocyanine green and fundus fluorescein angiographic findings in patients with active ocular Behcet's disease. Ocul Immunol Inflamm. 2005;13(1):51–8.
56. Mesquida M, Llorenç V, Fontenla JR, Navarro MJ, Adán A. Use of ultra-wide-field retinal imaging in the management of active Behçet retinal vasculitis. Retina. 2014;34(10):2121–7.
57. Bozzoni-Pantaleoni F, Gharbiya M, Pirraglia MP, Accorinti M, Pivetti-Pezzi P. Indocyanine green angiographic findings in Behçet disease. Retina. 2001;21(3):230–6.
58. Iaccarino G, Cennamo G, Forte R, Cennamo G. Evaluation of posterior pole with echography and optical coherence tomography in patients with Behçet's disease. Ophthalmol J Int Ophtalmol. 2009;223(4):250–5.
59. Unoki N, Nishijima K, Kita M, Hayashi R, Yoshimura N. Structural changes of fovea during remission of Behçet's disease as imaged by spectral domain optical coherence tomography. Eye. 2010;24(6):969–75.
60. Yuksel K, Goker YS, Yazici AT, Ozkaya A, Cosar G. Can perifoveal pseudocyst area be a prognostic factor in macular hole surgery?: a prospective study with quantitative data. Medicine. 2014;93(28):e182.
61. Ishikawa S, Taguchi M, Muraoka T, Sakurai Y, Kanda T, Takeuchi M. Changes in subfoveal choroidal thickness associated with uveitis activity in patients with Behçet's disease. Br J Ophthalmol. 2014;98(11):1508–13.
62. Kim M, Kim H, Kwon HJ, Kim SS, Koh HJ, Lee SC. Choroidal thickness in Behcet's uveitis: an enhanced depth imaging-optical coherence tomography and its association with angiographic changes. Invest Ophthalmol Vis Sci. 2013;54(9):6033–9.
63. Juhn E, Khachemoune A. Gardner syndrome: skin manifestations, differential diagnosis and management. Am J Clin Dermatol. 2010;11(2):117–22.
64. Kennedy RD, Potter DD, Moir CR, El-Youssef M. The natural history of familial adenomatous polyposis syndrome: a 24 years review of a single center experience in screening, diagnosis, and outcomes. J Pediatr Surg. 2014;49(1):82–6.
65. Butler J, Healy C, Toner M, Flint S. Gardner syndrome—review and report of a case. Oral Oncol Extra. 2005;41(5):89–92.
66. Cristofaro MG, Giudice A, Amantea M, Riccelli U, Giudice M. Gardner's syndrome: a clinical and genetic study of a family. Oral Surg Oral Med Oral Pathol Oral Radiol. 2013;115(3):e1–6.
67. Nusliha A, Dalpatadu U, Amarasinghe B, Chandrasinghe PC, Deen KI. Congenital hypertrophy of retinal pigment epithelium (CHRPE) in patients with familial adenomatous polyposis (FAP); a polyposis registry experience. BMC Res Notes. 2014;7:734.
68. Gómez García EB, Knoers NVAM. Gardner's syndrome (familial adenomatous polyposis): a cilia-related disorder. Lancet Oncol. 2009;10(7):727–35.
69. Schwartz SG, Hickey M, Flynn HW. Congenital hypertrophy of the retinal pigment epithelium: choroidal cavitation demonstrated on spectral-domain OCT. Ophthalmic Surg Lasers Imaging Retina. 2013;44(3):301–2.
70. Touriño R, Rodríguez-Ares MT, López-Valladares MJ, Gómez-Ulla F, Gómez-Torreiro M, Capeans C. Fluorescein angiographic features of the congenital hypertrophy of the retinal pigment epithelium in the familial adenomatous polyposis. Int Ophthalmol. 2005;26(1-2):59–65.

71. Coleman P, Barnard NAS. Congenital hypertrophy of the retinal pigment epithelium: prevalence and ocular features in the optometric population. Ophthalmic Physiol Opt J Br Coll Ophthalmic Opt Optom. 2007;27(6):547–55.
72. Islam S, Islam E, Attaya H, Parupudi S, Shami M, Gonzalez MF, et al. Congenital hypertrophy retinal pigment epithelium as a manifestation of colon cancer. Am J Gastroenterol. 2010;105(11):2510–1.
73. Chen CS, Phillips KD, Grist S, Bennet G, Craig JE, Muecke JS, et al. Congenital hypertrophy of the retinal pigment epithelium (CHRPE) in familial colorectal cancer. Familial Cancer. 2006;5(4):397–404.
74. Touriño R, Conde-Freire R, Cabezas-Agrícola JM, Rodríguez-Aves T, López-Valladares MJ, Otero-Cepeda JL, et al. Value of the congenital hypertrophy of the retinal pigment epithelium in the diagnosis of familial adenomatous polyposis. Int Ophthalmol. 2004;25(2):101–12.
75. Villegas VM, Schwartz SG, Flynn HW, Capó H, Berrocal AM, Murray TG, et al. Distinguishing torpedo maculopathy from similar lesions of the posterior segment. Ophthalmic Surg Lasers Imaging Retina. 2014;45(3):222–6.
76. Fung AT, Pellegrini M, Shields CL. Congenital hypertrophy of the retinal pigment epithelium: enhanced-depth imaging optical coherence tomography in 18 cases. Ophthalmology. 2014;121(1):251–6.
77. Shields CL, Manalac J, Das C, Saktanasate J, Shields JA. Review of spectral domain-enhanced depth imaging optical coherence tomography of tumors of the retina and retinal pigment epithelium in children and adults. Indian J Ophthalmol. 2015;63(2):128–32.

Ocular Sarcoidosis

7

David Ehmann and Sunir Garg

Abstract

Sarcoidosis is a multisystem granulomatous disease that can involve any organ in the body, however it most commonly affects the lungs, lymphatic system, skin, and eye. The diagnostic histopathologic hallmark of sarcoidosis is the presence of non-caseating epithelioid granulomas. Although the etiology of sarcoidosis is unknown, potential infectious sources such as mycobacteria and propionibacteria have been proposed.

Ocular sarcoidosis occurs in up to 83% of patients with systemic sarcoidosis and uveitis is the most common ocular manifestation occurring in 50% of patients with ocular sarcoidosis. Both gender and ethnic variance is seen in ocular sarcoidosis with females affected more than males and African Americans more commonly affected than Caucasians. Although 70% of ocular sarcoid presents before age 40, a bimodal distribution in patients aged 20–40 years and 50–60 years occurs. In addition, African American patients generally have an earlier disease onset than Caucasian patients. Patients typically present with symptoms of pain, photophobia, blurred vision, and floaters. After excluding infectious etiologies, the diagnosis of ocular sarcoidosis can be made following the IWOS guidelines, which consist of a combination of ocular signs, blood tests, and imaging modalities. The most common presenting sign of anterior uveitis includes anterior chamber cell and flare with granulomatous ("mutton fat") keratic precipitates, however 15% present with non-granulomatous keratic precipitates. Early treatment with corticosteroids alone or in combination with immunomodulatory agents can restore vision and prevent blinding complications. As a significant proportion of patients develop chronic disease, regular follow-up with both ophthalmology and internal medicine is required.

D. Ehmann • S. Garg (✉)
Wills Eye Hospital, Philadelphia, PA, USA
e-mail: dehmann@midatlanticretina.com; sgarg@midatlanticretina.com; sunirgarg@yahoo.com

J. Chhablani et al. (eds.), *Retinal and Choroidal Imaging in Systemic Diseases*,
https://doi.org/10.1007/978-981-10-5461-7_7

7.1 Introduction

Sarcoidosis is a multisystem granulomatous disease of unknown origin. It can involve any organ in the body, however it most commonly affects the lungs, lymphatic system, skin, and eye [1–4]. The diagnostic histopathologic hallmark of sarcoidosis is the presence of non-caseating epithelioid granulomas, a key distinguishing factor from other granulomatous diseases such as tuberculosis (Fig. 7.1).

Ocular sarcoidosis has been recognized since the early 1900s [5] and its prevalence among patients with known systemic sarcoidosis has been reported to range from 13–83% [1–4]. Although sarcoidosis can involve any part of the eye and surrounding tissue, uveitis is the most common manifestation and occurs in up to 50% of patients [4]. Because 30% of patients with sarcoidosis initially present with uveitis [3] it is important both to be aware of the various ways in which ocular sarcoidosis can present and to maintain a high level of suspicion in patients with uveitis. This can help establish an early diagnosis which can lead to prompt therapy [2].

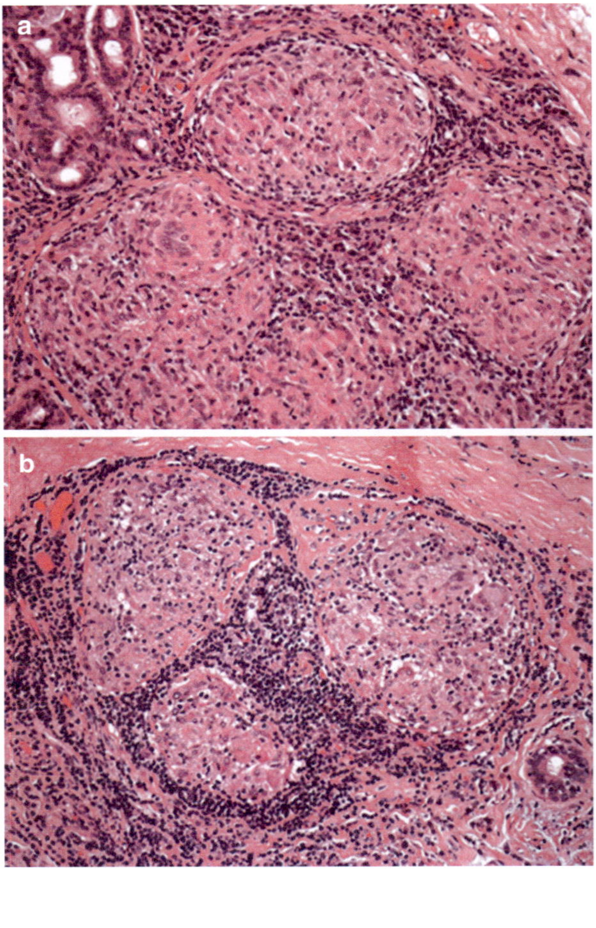

Fig. 7.1 This photomicrograph of a patient with sarcoid dacryoadenitis demonstrates a non-caseating granuloma (**a**, **b**). *(Image courtesy of Dr. Ralph Eagle, MD)*

7.2 Etiology

Although the etiology of sarcoidosis is unknown, potential infectious sources have been proposed [6–8]. Both mycobacteria and propionibacteria are known to induce granulomatous inflammation consistent with sarcoidosis. Propionibacteria acnes has been cultured from biopsy samples of patients with sarcoidosis [6]. Polymerase chain reaction (PCR) testing of tissue samples from patients with sarcoidosis has revealed mycobacterium tuberculosis DNA [7]. Non-infectious agents such as tattoo die have also been implicated as a causative trigger [9, 10]. Genetic factors are known to contribute to the development of sarcoidosis with familial cases reported [2]. Children of parents with sarcoidosis have been reported to have a four times higher risk of developing sarcoidosis than those without [11]. In addition, HLA-DRB1 alleles are strongly associated with ocular sarcoidosis [12, 13].

7.3 Clinical Manifestations of Ocular Sarcoid

Both gender and ethnic variance are seen in ocular sarcoidosis with females affected more than males and African Americans more commonly affected than Caucasians [1–4]. Although 70% of ocular sarcoid presents before age 40 [4], a bimodal distribution in patients aged 20–40 years and 50–60 years occurs [3]. African American patients generally have an earlier disease onset than Caucasian patients [3]. The majority (90%) of cases are bilateral with some experiencing spontaneous remission within 3–5 years, however, the majority develop chronic disease requiring long-term suppression [4].

Although ocular sarcoidosis can manifest in any ocular structure, uveitis is the most common manifestation and occurs in up to 50% of cases [4]. In one report of 112 eyes with sarcoid uveitis, 28% had anterior uveitis, 38% had intermediate uveitis, 12% had posterior uveitis, and 22% had panuveitis [14]. Patients often present with symptoms of pain, photophobia, blurred vision, and floaters. The most common presenting sign of anterior uveitis includes anterior chamber cell and flare with granulomatous ("mutton fat") keratic precipitates, however 15% present with non-granulomatous keratic precipitates [14] (Fig. 7.2). In severe cases, posterior segment spillover of anterior chamber cells can be seen. Other signs include ciliary flush, conjunctival nodules, tented peripheral anterior synechiae, posterior synechiae, and iris nodules (Koeppe nodules are at the iris border, and Busacca nodules are in the iris stroma, and Berlin's nodules are in the angle). In chronic cases, inflammatory sequelae include band keratopathy, glaucoma, and cataract formation.

The hallmark of intermediate uveitis is the presence of anterior vitreous cells, vitreous snowballs, and/or an inferior snowbank. Vitreous snowballs consist of aggregates of inflammatory cells whereas a snowbank represents pars plana exudation.

In posterior uveitis, perivascular sheathing and midperipheral periphlebitis can be seen. The phlebitis associated with sarcoidosis is classically termed "candle wax drippings" or "taches de bougies" and is seen in up to 70% of patients [4] (Fig. 7.3). Retinal and choroidal lesions can be seen together or in isolation (Fig. 7.4).

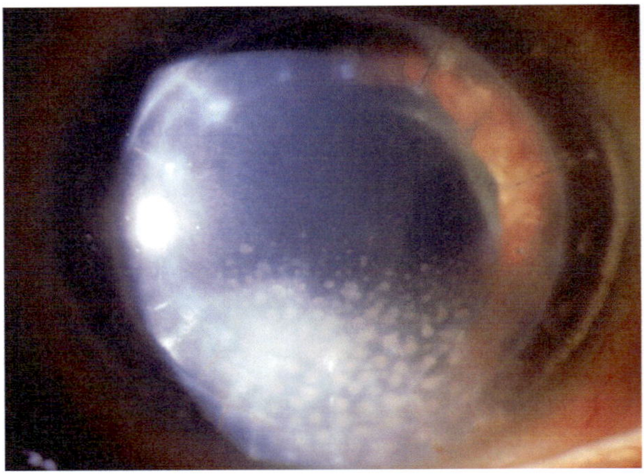

Fig. 7.2 Granulomatous "Mutton fat" keratic precipitates in a patient with sarcoid uveitis. *(Image courtesy of Dr. Christopher Rapuano)*

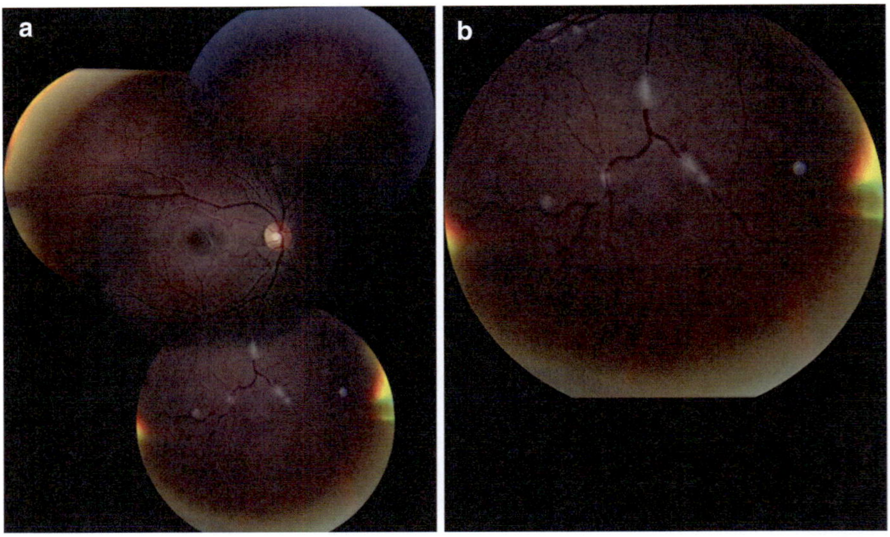

Fig. 7.3 Sarcoid vasculitis (**a**). Enlarged view demonstrating phlebitis with candle wax drippings (**b**). *(Image courtesy of Dr. Jayanth Sridhar, MD)*

Choroidal granulomas vary in size and can be unifocal or multifocal. In multifocal sarcoid choroiditis small creamy white lesions (Dalen-Fuchs-like nodules) can be seen in the mid to far periphery (most commonly inferiorly) and usually spare the macula. As they resolve, punched out chorioretinal scars develop. Disc edema and rarely vascular occlusions can be seen in cases of posterior uveitis (Fig. 7.5). In addition, capillary closure and ischemia can result in peripheral retinal neovascularization with vitreous hemorrhage.

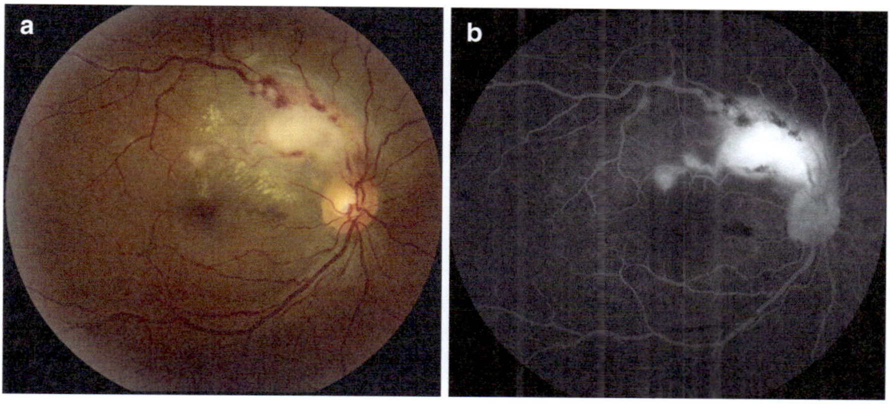

Fig. 7.4 Retinal sarcoid granuloma with macular edema (**a**) and corresponding fluorescein angiogram demonstrating hyperfluorescent staining (**b**). *(Image courtesy of Dr. Murtaza Adam, MD)*

Fig. 7.5 Ischemic superior hemiretinal vein occlusion in a patient with sarcoid vasculitis. *(Image courtesy of Dr. Sundeep Kasi, MD)*

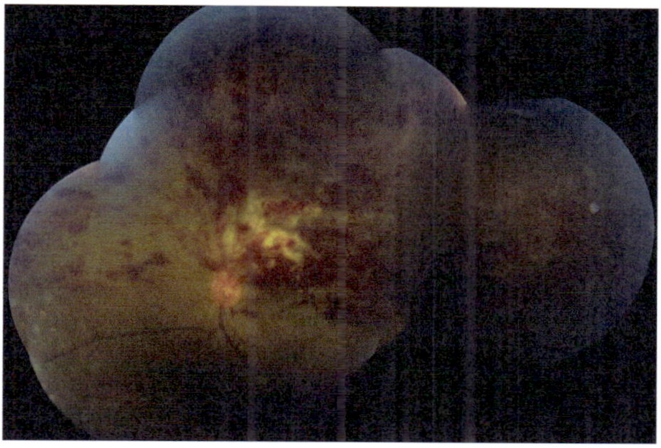

Although uveitis is the most common ocular manifestation in sarcoidosis, any ocular structure can be involved [3]. Other manifestations of ocular sarcoidosis include eyelid or orbital granulomas, cicatrizing conjunctivitis, conjunctival nodules, keratoconjunctivitis sicca secondary to dacryoadenitis, peripheral ulcerative keratitis, and interstitial keratitis [3]. Cranial neuropathy is the most frequent manifestation of neurosarcoidosis, and most commonly involves the optic and facial nerves. Optic nerve involvement reveals the presence of an infiltrative granuloma, disc edema, or disc atrophy. The symptoms associated with neurosarcoidosis depend on the location of an inflammatory granuloma along the visual pathway and include decreased vision and various patterns of visual field loss. Manifestations of neurological involvement include encephalopathy, meningitis, hydrocephalus, myopathy, seizures, and psychosis [3].

7.4 Diagnosis

The diagnostic gold standard for sarcoidosis is a tissue biopsy that demonstrates non-caseating granulomas. In ocular sarcoidosis, conjunctival nodules can be biopsied and have a positive diagnostic yield of 43–75% [15, 16]. In the absence of diagnostic tissue, the diagnosis is made using a combination of clinical signs, laboratory tests, and imaging. Angiotensin converting enzyme (ACE) and lysozyme are serological tests that reflect active granulomatous disease. Although both ACE and lysozyme levels are commonly ordered, they are poor screening tests due to their low sensitivity and specificity [17]. Pulmonary involvement is seen in 90% of patients with sarcoidosis. A chest radiograph (CXR) demonstrating bilateral hilar lymphadenopathy can be a useful screening test for sarcoidosis with a reported sensitivity of up to 79%, however many specialists report rates lower than this [18]. In cases where a CXR is negative yet the clinical suspicion remains high, a spiral computed tomogram (CT) and/or Gallium scan should be ordered [18, 19]. CT allows for better evaluation of the lung parenchyma and is more sensitive and specific than a CXR [19]. 18-flurodeoxyglucose PET (18-FDG PET) scan is used to detect occult sites of disease and has become the preferred nuclear imaging technique for sarcoidosis [20]. Compared to Gallium scans, 18-FDG PET is more sensitive, faster, safer, and demonstrates lower interobserver variability [20]. Diagnostic vitrectomy can also be used to assess the CD4 to CD8 ratio, with higher ratios demonstrating a sensitivity of 100% and specificity of 96.3%, however this is generally used as a test of last resort and only when the results would alter management [21, 22].

In 2009, the results from the first International Workshop on Ocular Sarcoidosis (IWOS) which identified seven clinical signs, five laboratory investigations, and four diagnostic terms for ocular sarcoidosis were published [23]. These guidelines have since been validated for use in clinical practice [24, 25], with a reported sensitivity of 100%, specificity of 95.6%, a positive predictive value of 79.1%, and a negative predictive value of 100% [25]. The ocular signs suggestive of ocular sarcoidosis include mutton fat keratic precipitates and/or iris nodules, trabecular meshwork nodules and/or tented peripheral anterior synechiae, vitreous snowballs, active or inactive multifocal chorioretinal lesions, periphlebitis, granulomas of the optic disk and/or choroid, and bilateral involvement. The laboratory investigations include a negative tuberculin skin test, elevated serum angiotensin converting enzyme (ACE) levels, elevated lysozyme levels, elevated liver enzymes, a chest radiograph demonstrating bilateral symmetric hilar adenopathy, or a positive chest CT in patients with a negative chest radiograph.

A definite diagnosis of ocular sarcoidosis is confirmed with a positive tissue biopsy with a compatible uveitis. A presumed diagnosis of ocular sarcoidosis is confirmed with a chest radiograph demonstrating bilateral hilar adenopathy with a compatible uveitis if a biopsy is not done. A probable diagnosis of ocular sarcoidosis is made with the presence of three ocular signs and two positive laboratory tests if a biopsy was not done and a CXR does not show bilateral hilar adenopathy. A possible diagnosis is made with the presence of at least four ocular signs and two positive laboratory tests if a lung biopsy was done and was negative [23].

7.5 Treatment

The ultimate goal of treating ocular sarcoidosis is to restore vision and prevent inflammation-related complications. For most forms of ocular sarcoidosis, corticosteroids are first line therapy and can be administered either topically, locally, or systemically depending on the degree and location of inflammation. For anterior uveitis, topical agents such as prednisolone acetate 1% or difluprednate are effective and should be titrated to the amount of anterior chamber inflammation. A cycloplegic agent such as cyclopentolate or atropine is also typically used to reduce ciliary spasm and prevent posterior synechiae formation. For intermediate uveitis, local or systemic therapy is often required. Sub-Tenon triamcinolone injection is an effective option and can provide therapy for 3–4 months in many eyes. Oral prednisone (0.5–1 mg/kg daily) is also effective, however, carries a risk of systemic side effects, particularly at more than 7.5 mg daily. Posterior uveitis and panuveitis often require both local and systemic therapy. For severe cases, initial pulse therapy with intravenous methylprednisolone can be considered. Longer acting steroid implants such as dexamethasone (Ozurdex, Allergan) and fluocinolone acetonide (Retisert, Bausch & Lomb) have both demonstrated efficacy in randomized control trials for the treatment of non-infectious posterior uveitis [26, 27]. Although less common in eyes that received the dexamethasone implant, cataract surgery and ocular hypertension >10 mmHg was reported in 95% and 70% of patients, respectively, who were treated with fluocinolone acetonide [26, 28].

In patients who do not tolerate corticosteroids, immunomodulatory agents such as methotrexate [29], azathioprine [29], leflunomide [30], and mycophenolate mofetil [31] have demonstrated both safety and efficacy. Biologic agents, specifically anti-TNF-α agents such as infliximab and adalimumab [32], have demonstrated efficacy in treating chronic refractory uveitis, however they are limited by high cost and adverse drug events [29, 32]. Etanercept has not shown benefit for the treatment of refractory ocular sarcoidosis [33]. In addition, iatrogenic sarcoidosis has been reported to occur in rheumatoid arthritis patients treated with etanercept [34]. Full resolution was seen upon discontinuation of etanercept, suggesting a possible triggering effect for this agent [34].

7.6 Prognosis

In ocular sarcoid, visual outcomes vary depending on disease severity, chronicity, time to presentation, and the development of ocular complications such as glaucoma, cataracts, and cystoid macular edema [3, 14]. In one study of 75 patients with sarcoid uveitis, 54% maintained visual acuity better than 20/40 at 10 years [35].

In the same study, 17% of patients developed extraocular sarcoidosis after 10 years and the visual prognosis was not found to be related to the presence of extraocular disease [35].

Conclusion

Sarcoidosis is a systemic granulomatous disease with many ocular manifestations of which uveitis is the most common. After excluding infectious etiologies, the diagnosis of ocular sarcoidosis can be made following the IWOS guidelines, which consist of a combination of ocular signs, blood tests, and imaging modalities [23]. Early treatment with corticosteroids alone or in combination with immunomodulatory agents can restore vision and prevent blinding complications. As a significant proportion of patients develop chronic disease, regular follow-up with both ophthalmology and internal medicine is required.

Key Learning Points

- Ocular sarcoidosis is seen in up to 83% of patients with systemic sarcoidosis.
- Thirty percent of patients with sarcoidosis initially present with ocular disease.
- Uveitis is the most common ocular manifestation of sarcoidosis.
- The diagnosis of ocular sarcoidosis can be made following the IWOS guidelines, which consist of a combination of ocular signs, blood tests, and imaging modalities.
- Treatment with corticosteroids or immunomodulatory agents is effective at controlling inflammation and preventing long-term complications.

References

1. Patel S. Ocular sarcoidosis. Int Ophthalmol Clin. 2015;55:15–24. DOI: 10.1097/IIO.0000000000000069.
2. Liu D, Birnbaum AD. Update on sarcoidosis. Curr Opin Ophthalmol. 2015;26:512–6. DOI: 10.1097/ICU.0000000000000207.
3. Pasadhika S, Rosenbaum JT. Ocular sarcoidosis. Clin Chest Med. 2015;36:669–83. DOI: 10.1016/j.ccm.2015.08.009.
4. Jamilloux Y, Kodjikian L, Broussolle C, Sève P. Sarcoidosis and uveitis. Autoimmun Rev. 2014;13:840–9. DOI: 10.1016/j.autrev.2014.04.001.
5. Crick RP, Hoyle C, Smellie H. The eyes in SARCOIDOSIS. Br J Ophthalmol. 1961;45:461–81.
6. Abe C, Iwai K, Mikami R, Hosoda Y. Frequent isolation of Propionibacterium acnes from sarcoidosis lymph nodes. Zentralbl Bakteriol Mikrobiol Hyg A. 1984;256:541–7.
7. Mohapatra PR, Garg K, Singhal N, et al. Tuberculosis lymphadenitis in a well managed case of sarcoidosis. Indian J Chest Dis Allied Sci. 2013;55:217–20.
8. Surat G, Wallace WA, Laurenson IF, Seagar A-L. Rapid real-time PCR for detection of mycobacterium tuberculosis complex DNA in formalin-fixed paraffin embedded tissues: 16% of histological "sarcoid" may contain such DNA. J Clin Pathol. 2014;67:1084–7. DOI: 10.1136/jclinpath-2014-202307.
9. Antonovich DD, Callen JP. Development of sarcoidosis in cosmetic tattoos. Arch Dermatol. 2005;141:869–72. DOI: 10.1001/archderm.141.7.869.

10. Psaltis NM, Gardner RG, Denton WJ. Systemic sarcoidosis and red dye granulomatous tattoo inflammation after influenza vaccination: a case report and review of literature. Ocul Immunol Inflamm. 2014;22:314–21. DOI: 10.3109/09273948.2014.891041.
11. Rybicki BA, Major M, Popovich J, et al. Racial differences in sarcoidosis incidence: a 5-year study in a health maintenance organization. Am J Epidemiol. 1997;145:234–41.
12. Darlington P, Tallstedt L, Padyukov L, et al. HLA-DRB1* alleles and symptoms associated with Heerfordt's syndrome in sarcoidosis. Eur Respir J. 2011;38:1151–7. DOI: 10.1183/09031936.00025011.
13. Rossman MD, Thompson B, Frederick M, et al. HLA-DRB1*1101: a significant risk factor for sarcoidosis in blacks and whites. Am J Hum Genet. 2003;73:720–35. DOI: 10.1086/378097.
14. Dana MR, Merayo-Lloves J, Schaumberg DA, Foster CS. Prognosticators for visual outcome in sarcoid uveitis. Ophthalmology. 1996;103:1846–53.
15. Bui KM, Garcia-Gonzalez JM, Patel SS, et al. Directed conjunctival biopsy and impact of histologic sectioning methodology on the diagnosis of ocular sarcoidosis. J Ophthalmic Inflamm Infect. 2014;4:8. DOI: 10.1186/1869-5760-4-8.
16. Merritt JC, Ross G, Avery A. Conjunctival biopsy in sarcoidosis: 4 year NCMH experience. N C Med J. 1983;44:636–7.
17. Govender P, Berman JS. The diagnosis of sarcoidosis. Clin Chest Med. 2015;36:585–602. DOI: 10.1016/j.ccm.2015.08.003.
18. Klech H, Köhn H, Pohl W, et al. Diagnosis in sarcoidosis. Sensitivity and specificity of 67-gallium scintigraphy, serum angiotensin converting enzyme levels, thoracic radiography and blood lymphocyte subpopulations. Wien Med Wochenschr. 1983;133:425–32.
19. Kaiser PK, Lowder CY, Sullivan P, et al. Chest computerized tomography in the evaluation of uveitis in elderly women. Am J Ophthalmol. 2002;133:499–505.
20. Keijsers RGM, van den Heuvel DAF, Grutters JC. Imaging the inflammatory activity of sarcoidosis. Eur Respir J. 2013;41:743–51. DOI: 10.1183/09031936.00088612.
21. Kojima K, Maruyama K, Inaba T, et al. The CD4/CD8 ratio in vitreous fluid is of high diagnostic value in sarcoidosis. Ophthalmology. 2012;119:2386–92. DOI: 10.1016/j.ophtha.2012.05.033.
22. Scott AW, Mruthyunjaya P, McCallum RM, Jaffe GJ. Diagnostic yield of vitreous biopsy in presumed sarcoidosis-related posterior segment inflammation. Graefes Arch Clin Exp Ophthalmol. 2012;250:1379–85. DOI: 10.1007/s00417-012-1993-9.
23. Herbort CP, Rao NA, Mochizuki M, Members of Scientific Committee of First International Workshop on Ocular Sarcoidosis. International criteria for the diagnosis of ocular sarcoidosis: results of the first international workshop on ocular Sarcoidosis (IWOS). Ocul Immunol Inflamm. 2009;17:160–9. DOI: 10.1080/09273940902818861
24. Agrawal R, Gonzalez-Lopez JJ, Meier F, et al. Ocular and systemic features of sarcoidosis and correlation with the international workshop for ocular Sarcoidosis diagnostic criteria. Sarcoidosis Vasc Diffuse Lung Dis. 2015;32:237–45.
25. Takase H, Shimizu K, Yamada Y, et al. Validation of international criteria for the diagnosis of ocular sarcoidosis proposed by the first international workshop on ocular sarcoidosis. Jpn J Ophthalmol. 2010;54:529–36. DOI: 10.1007/s10384-010-0873-2.
26. Sangwan VS, Pearson PA, Paul H, Comstock TL. Use of the fluocinolone acetonide intravitreal implant for the treatment of noninfectious posterior uveitis: 3-year results of a randomized clinical trial in a predominantly asian population. Ophthalmol Therapy. 2015;4:1–19. DOI: 10.1007/s40123-014-0027-6.
27. Lowder C, Belfort R, Lightman S, et al. Dexamethasone intravitreal implant for noninfectious intermediate or posterior uveitis. Arch Ophthalmol. 2011;129:545–53. DOI: 10.1001/archophthalmol.2010.339.
28. Multicenter Uveitis Steroid Treatment (MUST) Trial Research Group, Kempen JH, Altaweel MM, et al. Benefits of systemic anti-inflammatory therapy versus fluocinolone acetonide intraocular implant for intermediate uveitis, posterior uveitis, and panuveitis: fifty-four-month results of the multicenter uveitis steroid treatment (MUST) trial and follow-up study. Ophthalmology. 2015;122:1967–75. DOI: 10.1016/j.ophtha.2015.06.042.

29. Baughman RP, Lower EE, Ingledue R, Kaufman AH. Management of ocular sarcoidosis. Sarcoidosis Vasc Diffuse Lung Dis. 2012;29:26–33.
30. Baughman RP, Lower EE. Leflunomide for chronic sarcoidosis. Sarcoidosis Vasc Diffuse Lung Dis. 2004;21:43–8.
31. Bhat P, Cervantes-Castañeda RA, Doctor PP, et al. Mycophenolate mofetil therapy for sarcoidosis-associated uveitis. Ocul Immunol Inflamm. 2009;17:185–90. DOI: 10.1080/09273940902862992.
32. Erckens RJ, Mostard RLM, Wijnen PA, et al. Adalimumab successful in sarcoidosis patients with refractory chronic non-infectious uveitis. Graefes Arch Clin Exp Ophthalmol. 2012;250:713–20. DOI: 10.1007/s00417-011-1844-0.
33. Baughman RP, Lower EE, Bradley DA, et al. Etanercept for refractory ocular sarcoidosis: results of a double-blind randomized trial. Chest. 2005;128:1062–47. DOI: 10.1378/chest.128.2.1062.
34. Verschueren K, Van Essche E, Verschueren P, et al. Development of sarcoidosis in etanercept-treated rheumatoid arthritis patients. Clin Rheumatol. 2007;26:1969–71. DOI: 10.1007/s10067-007-0594-1.
35. Edelsten C, Pearson A, Joynes E, et al. The ocular and systemic prognosis of patients presenting with sarcoid uveitis. Eye. 1999;13(Pt 6):748–53. DOI: 10.1038/eye.1999.221.

Autoimmune Retinopathy

8

David Ehmann and Sunir Garg

Abstract

Autoimmune retinopathy (AIR) is a general term for rare disease entities that include cancer associated retinopathy (CAR), melanoma-associated retinopathy (MAR), bilateral diffuse uveal melanocytic proliferation (BDUMP), and non-paraneoplastic autoimmune retinopathies (npAIR). Although the exact pathophysiology is unknown, autoimmune retinopathy occurs when a tumor expresses protein antigens that are normally present in the retina. This results in molecular mimicry and immunologic cross reactivity leading to retinal degeneration. AIR typically presents with progressive bilateral or asymmetric, painless, vision loss occurring over days to years. Visual symptoms are usually worse than the clinical findings and include photo aversion, prolonged glare after light exposure, decreased visual acuity, dyschromatopsia, central scotomas, nyctalopia, shimmering lights, photopsias, prolonged dark adaptation, midperipheral (ring) scotomas, and more extensive peripheral visual field defects. Although the initial retinal examination is often unremarkable, clinical findings may include subtle retinal pigment epithelial (RPE) changes to marked RPE bone spicules, arterial sheathing or attenuation, periphlebitis, disc pallor, and rarely low-grade inflammation in the vitreous and/or anterior chamber.

The diagnosis can be made using a combination of the patient's history, clinical exam, and a multitude of diagnostic tests including spectral domain optical coherence tomography (SD-OCT), electrophysiology, fundus autofluorescence, visual field testing, and serology for antiretinal antibodies. All patients suspected of having AIR require a thorough work-up for malignancy. Early diagnosis and treatment can prolong life and prevent or reverse visual acuity loss in some patients.

D. Ehmann • S. Garg (✉)
Wills Eye Hospital, Philadelphia, PA 19107, USA
e-mail: dehmann@midatlanticretina.com; sgarg@midatlanticretina.com; sunirgarg@yahoo.com

J. Chhablani et al. (eds.), *Retinal and Choroidal Imaging in Systemic Diseases*,
https://doi.org/10.1007/978-981-10-5461-7_8

8.1 Introduction

Autoimmune retinopathy (AIR) is a general term for rare disease entities that include cancer associated retinopathy (CAR), melanoma-associated retinopathy (MAR), bilateral diffuse uveal melanocytic proliferation (BDUMP), and non-paraneoplastic autoimmune retinopathies (npAIR).

Although the exact pathophysiology is unknown, AIR occurs when a tumor expresses protein antigens that are normally present in the retina [1–4]. This results in molecular mimicry and immunologic cross reactivity leading to retinal degeneration [1–4].

In 1976 Sawyer first reported CAR in three patients with an anaplastic tumor [5]. All three patients presented with rapid painless visual loss, positive visual phenomenon, and visual field defects secondary to a degenerative retinopathy [5]. The serum from CAR patients was later found to react with recoverin, a 23 kDa calcium binding protein found in photoreceptors [6]. CAR is most often associated with tumors of the lung, gynecological system (uterus, ovaries, cervix), and breast [4], however, it has also been reported in cancers involving the blood, prostate, colon, and thymus [1–4, 7]. MAR was first described in 1988 in a patient with cutaneous malignant melanoma who developed night blindness and shimmering photopsias [8]. MAR has also been reported in cases of choroidal and ciliary body melanoma [9]. BDUMP, a condition in which the primary tumor stimulates proliferation of uveal melanocytes [4], was first described by Bahar [10] and is associated with tumors of the reproductive tract, lung, colon, and pancreas [4].

Non-paraneoplastic autoimmune retinopathies (npAIR) have been reported in patients without a known history of malignancy who display similar phenotypes and electrophysiological findings to patients with CAR.

Although paraneoplastic syndromes have been reported to occur in 10–15% of all malignancies [11], the prevalence of retinal involvement remains unknown. The overlap of clinical features with other degenerative retinal disorders such as retinitis pigmentosa and acute zonal occult outer retinopathy (AZOOR) combined with the lack of standardized clinical and laboratory diagnostic criteria makes AIR prevalence estimations difficult [2].

8.2 Presentation and Clinical Findings

AIR typically presents with progressive bilateral or asymmetric, painless, vision loss occurring over days to years. Visual symptoms are usually worse than the clinical findings, however symptoms can help elucidate which visual system (cone, rod, or both) is most severely affected. Presenting symptoms of cone dysfunction include photo aversion, prolonged glare after light exposure, decreased visual acuity, dyschromatopsia, and central scotomas. Rod dysfunction often presents as nyctalopia, shimmering lights, photopsias, prolonged dark adaptation, midperipheral (ring) scotomas, and more extensive peripheral visual field defects.

Although the initial retinal examination is often unremarkable, clinical findings may include subtle retinal pigment epithelial (RPE) changes to marked RPE bone spicules, arterial sheathing or attenuation, periphlebitis, disc pallor, and rarely low-grade inflammation in the vitreous and/or anterior chamber [3, 4] (Fig. 8.1).

CAR typically affects women twice as frequently as men and has been reported to develop at an average age of 65 years (range 24–85 years) [12]. In approximately half of affected individuals, the visual symptoms and signs of CAR precede the diagnosis of malignancy by weeks to years in approximately ½ of all cases [12].

In contrast to CAR, MAR typically affects men more than women and has been reported to develop at an average age of 58 years (range 30–78 years) [13]. The average time from melanoma diagnosis to onset of MAR has been reported to be 3.6 years (range 2 months to 19 years) [7]. Unlike CAR, MAR usually presents after a diagnosis of melanoma has been established and typically indicates metastatic

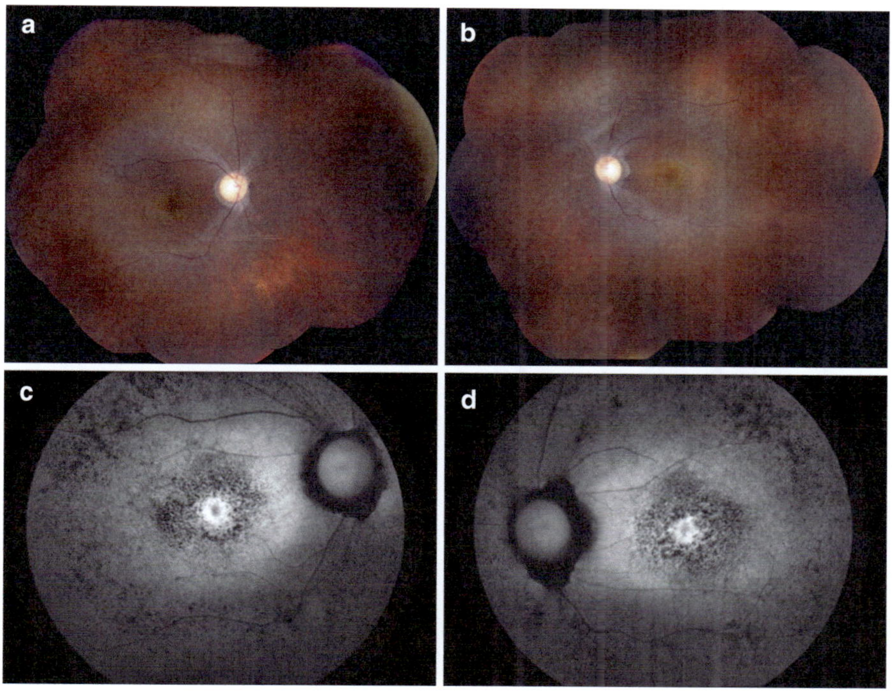

Fig. 8.1 Color fundus photos (**a**, **b**) with corresponding fundus autofluorescence (FAF) (**c**, **d**) from a 63-year-old female with non-metastatic breast cancer and a 2-year history of progressive bilateral visual loss. The fundus images show symmetric findings consistent with end-stage retinal disease with waxy pallor of the optic nerves, and retinal vascular attenuation with sclerotic vessels (**a**, **b**). Diffuse retinal atrophy was supported by the prominent visualization of the choroidal capillary bed and a bull's eye maculopathy with a "beaten-metal" appearance (**a**, **b**). FAF shows a corresponding perifoveal hyperautofluorescent ring and granular/speckled hypoautofluorescence along the arcades (**c**, **d**). (Images courtesy of Maggie M. Wei and H. Nida Sen, MD, NEI, NIH)

disease [7]. Recently, the presence of serum transient receptor potential melastatin 1 (TRPM1) autoantibodies was used to diagnose an occult melanoma in a patient with MAR [14]. Paraneoplastic vitelliform maculopathy (PVM), a possible variant of MAR has been associated with both choroidal and cutaneous melanoma. In PVM, a serous or vitelliform detachment of the neurosensory retina occurs in the posterior pole [4, 15].

Non-paraneoplastic autoimmune retinopathies (npAIR), the most common type of AIR, generally affects women twice as frequently as men and has been reported to develop at an average age of 55 years [16]. In addition, npAIR is associated with a history of autoimmune disorders in as many as 70% of cases [17]. All cases of suspected npAIR should have a thorough work-up to rule out malignancy (Figs. 8.2 and 8.3).

BDUMP affects women and men equally and typically precedes the diagnosis of cancer by months to years. Five characteristic signs have been described: bilateral multiple subtle round or oval subretinal round red patches in the RPE, early

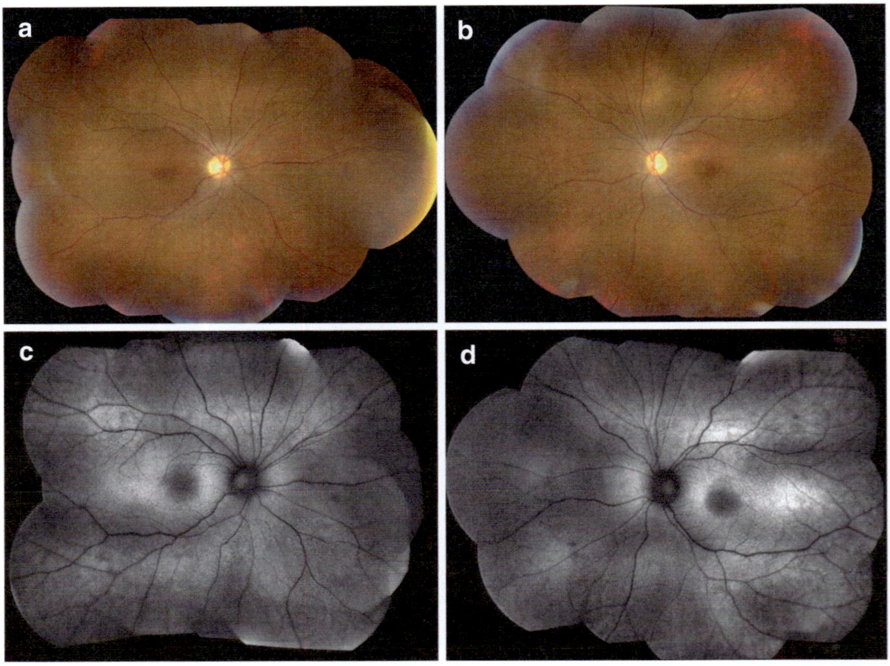

Fig. 8.2 Color fundus photos (**a**, **b**) and fundus autofluorescence (FAF) (**c**, **d**) of a 35-year-old male with a history of progressive vision loss over several years and positive anti-retinal and anti-optic nerve antibodies. Fundus images show mild to moderate pallor of the optic nerves with otherwise unremarkable retinas (**a**, **b**). FAF shows no specific pattern or abnormality (**c**, **d**). (Image courtesy of Maggie M. Wei and H. Nida Sen, MD, NEI, NIH)

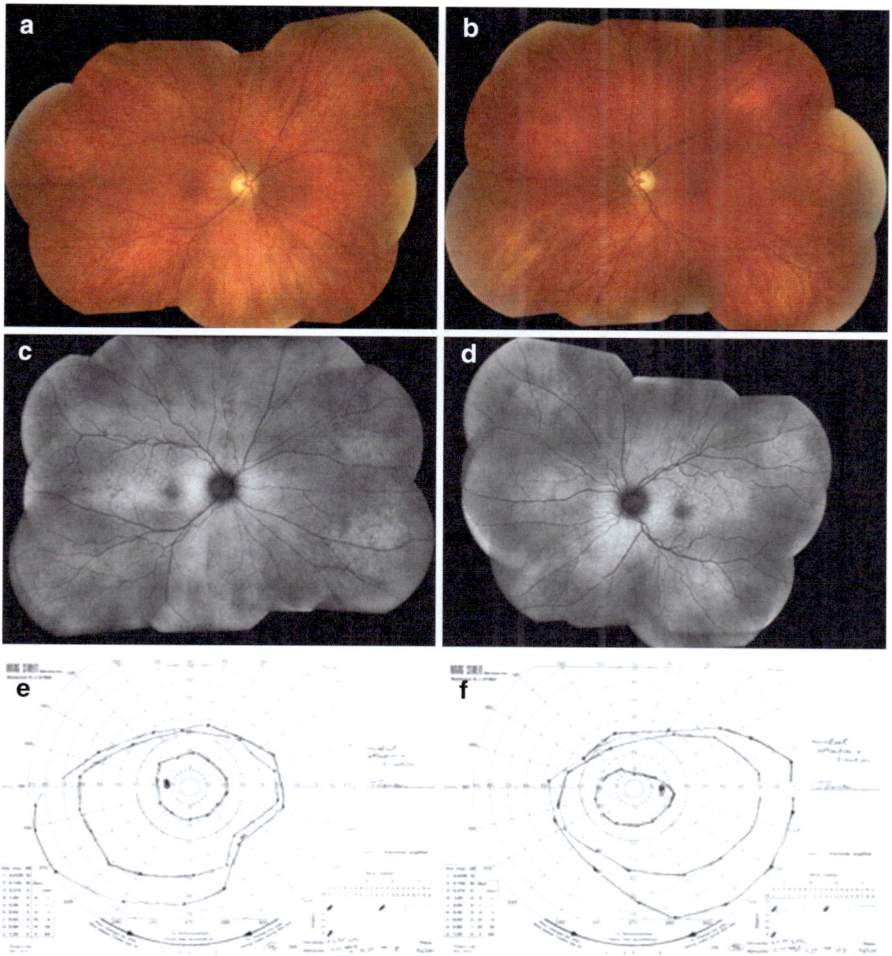

Fig. 8.3 Color fundus photos (**a**, **b**), fundus autofluorescence (FAF) (**c**, **d**) and Goldmann visual fields (GVF) (**e**, **f**) of a 56-year-old male with progressive vision loss over 18 months and positive antiretinal antibodies. Fundus images show a mildly increased cup-to-disc ratio with otherwise unremarkable retinas OU (**a**, **b**). FAF shows nonspecific changes including hypoautofluorescent patches OU, a speckled hypoautofluorescent patch temporal to macula OD, and foveal mottling OS (**c**, **d**). GVF showed superior central constriction OD and nasal peripheral constriction OS (**e**, **f**). (Images courtesy of Maggie M. Wei and H. Nida Sen, MD, NEI, NIH)

hyperfluorescence of these lesions on fluorescein angiography (FA), multiple elevated pigmented and non-pigmented uveal melanocytic tumors with diffuse uveal tract thickening, exudative retinal detachment, and rapid cataract development [18] (Fig.8.4). Furthermore, periocular pigmentation and palmar fasciitis can be seen [19, 20].

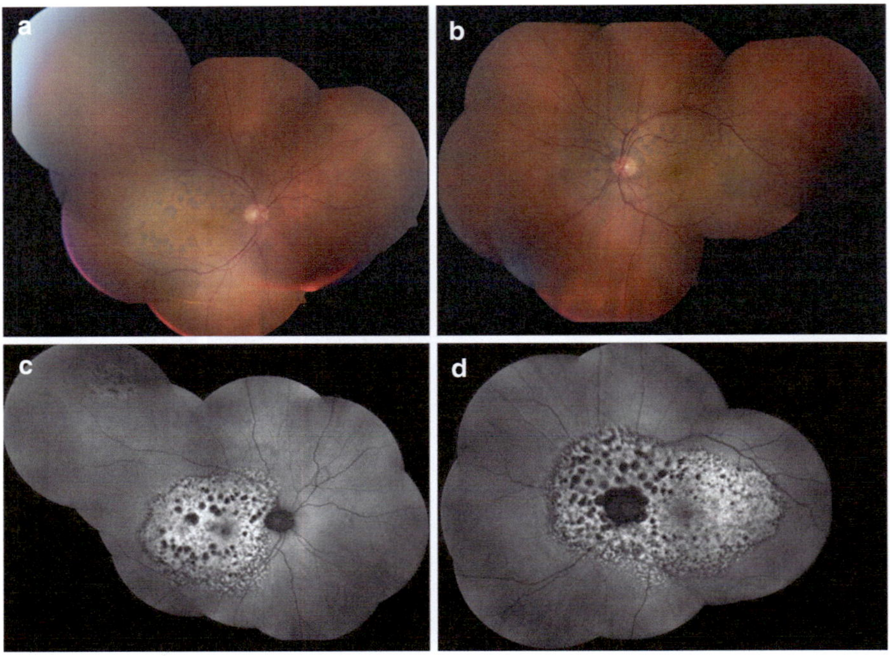

Fig. 8.4 Color fundus photos (**a**, **b**) with corresponding fundus autofluorescence (FAF) (**c**, **d**) in a patient with bilateral diffuse uveal melanocytic proliferation. Note the bilateral, round or ovoid, subretinal, elevated pigmented uveal melanocytic tumors (**a**, **b**) with corresponding hypoautofluorescence on FAF (**c**, **d**). (Images courtesy of Dr. Carol Shields, MD)

8.3 Diagnostic Tests

Several diagnostic tests are essential to establish the diagnosis of AIR. These include serology for antiretinal antibodies (ARA), fundus autofluorescence (FAF), spectral domain optical coherence tomography (SD-OCT), electrophysiological tests including full field electroretinogram (ffERG) and multifocal electroretinogram (mfERG), visual fields (VF), and fluorescein angiography (FA).

8.3.1 Antiretinal Antibodies (ARA)

To date, at least 18 different anti-retinal antibodies have been reported with antibodies to recoverin the most specific [1, 3, 4, 12, 16]. Other antibodies include alpha enolase, transferrin, interphotoreceptor retinoid binding protein, neurofilament proteins, tubby-like protein 1, heat shock cognate protein 70, glyceraldyhyde-3-phosphate-dehydrogenase, carbonic anhydrase II, arrestin, bestrophin, and myelin basic protein [3]. In CAR, variations in disease phenotype have been linked to specific ARAs [21]. CAR associated with anti-recoverin antibodies demonstrates a very rapid disease onset and visual decline, whereas cases associated with anti-enolase antibodies demonstrate a more subacute presentation with less severe visual loss [21].

ARA can be detected using laboratory techniques such as immunohistochemistry, western blot, as well as enzyme linked immunosorbent assay, however, all these techniques lack standardization and therefore their diagnostic yield can vary significantly. The detection of ARA is not sufficient alone for a diagnosis of AIR nor can detection confirm an antibody to be pathogenic. Seropositivity ranges from 65% in CAR and MAR [12] to 41% in npAIR [16]. When detected, most patients with AIR are found to have three or more autoantibodies [3]. ARAs have been found in up to 62% of normal human serum used in commercial diagnostic labs [22]. Furthermore, ARAs have been found in several retinal diseases including retinitis pigmentosa, Vogt-Koyanagi-Harada disease, Behcet's, sympathetic ophthalmia, toxoplasmosis, onchocerciasis, age-related macular degeneration, diabetic retinopathy, idiopathic vasculitis, and uveitis [2, 4, 7]. As a result it is important to correlate ARA testing within the clinical context. Validation studies are required before the true sensitivity and specificity of ARAs can be determined and contribute to reliable diagnostic criteria [2, 3].

8.4 Fundus Autofluorescence (FAF)

On FAF, AIR occasionally demonstrates a characteristic parafoveal ring of hyperautofluorescence with normal autofluorescence inside the ring and progressive hypoautofluorescence outside the ring [23] (Fig. 8.1c, d). SD-OCT confirms loss of the ellipsoid layer and thinning of the outer nuclear layer (ONL) over the hyperautofluorescent transition zone. This correlates with an extensive scotoma on visual field testing. Within the ring, thinning of the ONL is seen [23].

8.4.1 Spectral Domain Optical Coherence Tomography (SD-OCT)

Outer retinal abnormalities on SD-OCT have been reported in the majority of patients with CAR and npAIR. These include loss of the outer nuclear layer, external limiting membrane, ellipsoid layer, and a general reduction in central macular thickness [3, 7, 23]. Although less common, cystoid macular edema (CME) and mild schisis-like changes can also be seen [3]. All findings are more evident in the later stages of disease (Fig. 8.5).

8.4.2 Full Field and Multifocal Electroretinogram (ffERG, mfERG)

Electrophysiological tests such as full field ERG (ffERG) and multifocal ERG (mfERG) are important to diagnose AIR. Early in the disease, abnormalities in rod, cone, or bipolar cell responses can be seen resulting in severely diminished or extinguished a and b waves (Fig. 8.6). CAR predominantly affects the photoreceptors

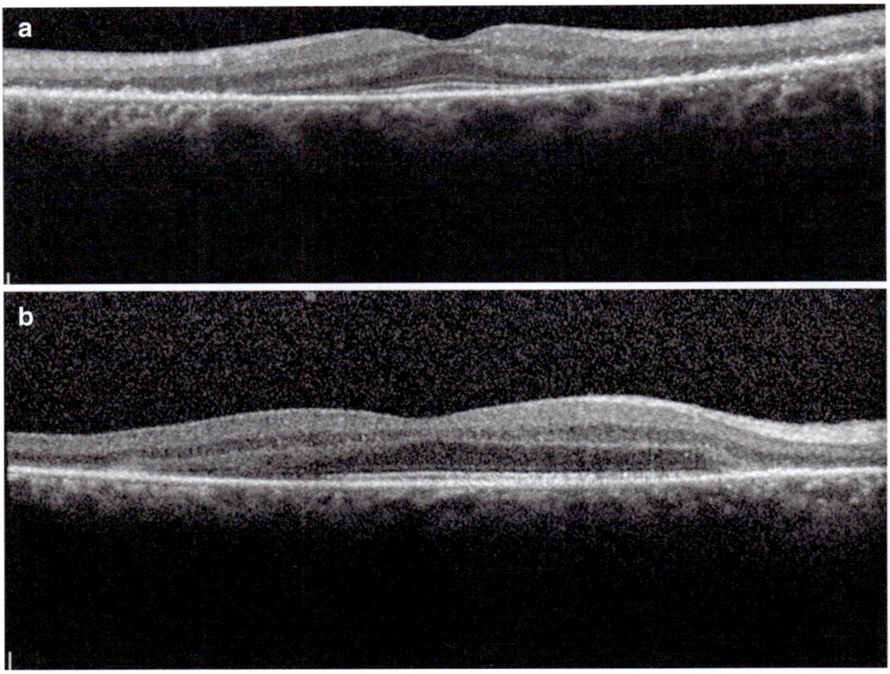

Fig. 8.5 Spectral domain optical coherence tomography (SD-OCT) images for the right (**a**) and left (**b**) eyes of a patient with CAR. Note the diffuse atrophy with loss of the outer retinal bands. (Images courtesy of Dr. Murtaza Adam, MD)

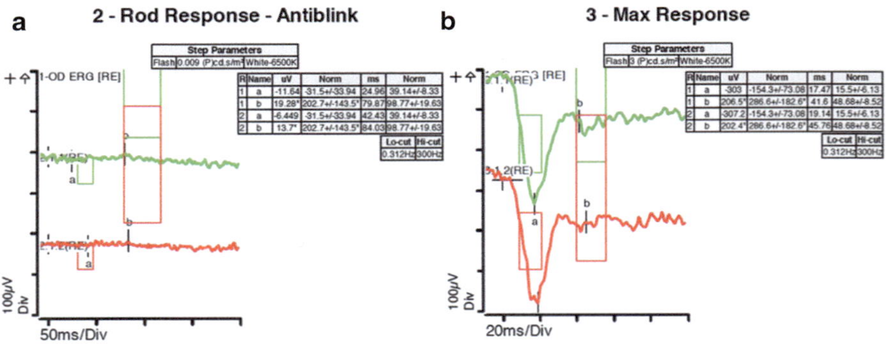

Fig. 8.6 Scotopic full field electroretinogram (ffERG) rod response (**a**) and combined maximal response (**b**) for the right eye of a patient with CAR. Note the flat ERG (**a**) and negative B wave (**b**). (Images courtesy of Elizabeth Affel)

and thus the a-wave is severely reduced particularly in the macula; this can be confirmed with mfERG [1, 3, 7]. MAR typically affects ON-bipolar cell function and therefore results in an electronegative ERG characterized by a markedly reduced dark-adapted b-wave (Fig. 8.6b) [1, 3, 7]. ERG findings in npAIR are similar to CAR but can be highly variable [3, 7].

8.5 Visual Fields

AIR is associated with variable patterns of visual field loss. CAR is most commonly associated with a central scotoma while MAR is more commonly associated with a peripheral ring scotoma [3, 4, 7] (Fig. 8.3e, f). NpAIR is associated with generalized sensitivity loss and peripheral constriction [7].

8.6 Fluorescein Angiography

Fluorescein angiography is typically unremarkable in AIR, however, it is helpful in order to rule out other retinal diseases. Perivascular leakage, optic nerve staining, and CME have been reported [2, 7].

8.7 Treatment

As a rare disease, there is no established treatment protocol for AIR. Currently the evidence for therapeutic intervention stems from case reports and small case series [17]. Despite this, early, long-term systemic immunosuppression is recommended as treatment is likely to have little effect once photoreceptor degeneration has occurred [17].

Several different treatments for AIR have been reported each with varying success. These include cytoreductive procedures (such as radiation or surgery), corticosteroids, immunomodulatory agents, IVIG, and plasmapheresis [1–4, 7]. Cytoreductive procedures are thought to work by decreasing ARA production through a decrease in tumor burden. Corticosteroids have been administered periocularly, orally, intraocularly, and intravenously. Immunomodulatory agents used include cyclosporine, azathioprine, mycophenolate mofetil, rituximab, and alemtuzumab [1–4]. A recent retrospective review of long-term immunosuppression for AIR in 30 patients found that immunosuppression resulted in clinical improvement in all subgroups of AIR, however, patients with CAR were the most responsive and those with npAIR the least responsive. Furthermore, patients with a family history of autoimmune disease were less responsive to immunosuppression therapy [17]. Treatment outcomes for MAR overall have been disappointing, but plasmapheresis has demonstrated some promise [4, 13]. Treatment response is best followed by serial visual field testing and ERG. ARA levels have also been proposed as a useful marker for monitoring treatment response [1, 4].

Conclusion

AIR is a rare yet potentially blinding condition that encompasses CAR, MAR, BDUMP, and npAIR. All patients suspected of having AIR require a thorough work-up for malignancy. The diagnosis can be made using a combination of the patient's history, clinical exam, and a multitude of diagnostic tests including SD-OCT, ERG, fundus autofluorescence, visual field testing, and serology for ARA. Early diagnosis and treatment can prolong life and prevent or reverse visual acuity loss in some patients.

Key Learning Points

- Autoimmune retinopathy (AIR) is a general term for rare disease entities that include cancer associated retinopathy (CAR), melanoma-associated retinopathy (MAR), bilateral diffuse uveal melanocytic proliferation (BDUMP), and non-paraneoplastic autoimmune retinopathies (npAIR).
- In AIR, visual symptoms are typical worse than the clinical findings.
- A diagnosis can be made using a combination of tests including spectral-domain optical coherence tomography (SD-OCT), visual field testing, electrophysiology (ERG), and anti-retinal antibody (ARA) testing.
- All patients suspected of having non-paraneoplastic autoimmune retinopathy (npAIR) require a thorough work-up to rule out malignancy.
- Treatment with corticosteroids or immunomodulatory agents has demonstrated efficacy, however visual prognosis is typically poor.

References

1. Shildkrot Y, Sobrin L, Gragoudas ES. Cancer-associated retinopathy: update on pathogenesis and therapy. Semin Ophthalmol. 2011;26:321–8. DOI: 10.3109/08820538.2011.588657.
2. Grange L, Dalal M, Nussenblatt RB, Sen HN. Autoimmune retinopathy. Am J Ophthalmol. 2014;157:266–272.e1. DOI: 10.1016/j.ajo.2013.09.019.
3. Grewal DS, Fishman GA, Jampol LM. Autoimmune retinopathy and antiretinal antibodies: a review. Retina. 2014;34:827–45. DOI: 10.1097/IAE.0000000000000119.
4. Rahimy E, Sarraf D. Paraneoplastic and non-paraneoplastic retinopathy and optic neuropathy: evaluation and management. Surv Ophthalmol. 2013;58:430–58. DOI: 10.1016/j.survophthal.2012.09.001.
5. Sawyer RA, Selhorst JB, Zimmerman LE, Hoyt WF. Blindness caused by photoreceptor degeneration as a remote effect of cancer. Am J Ophthalmol. 1976;81:606–13.
6. Polans AS, Burton MD, Haley TL, et al. Recoverin, but not visinin, is an autoantigen in the human retina identified with a cancer-associated retinopathy. Invest Ophthalmol Vis Sci. 1993;34:81–90.
7. Braithwaite T, Vugler A, Tufail A. Autoimmune retinopathy. Ophthalmologica. 2012;228:131–42. DOI: 10.1159/000338240.
8. Berson EL, Lessell S. Paraneoplastic night blindness with malignant melanoma. Am J Ophthalmol. 1988;106:307–11.
9. Lu Y, Jia L, He S, et al. Melanoma-associated retinopathy: a paraneoplastic autoimmune complication. Arch Ophthalmol. 2009;127:1572–80. DOI: 10.1001/archophthalmol.2009.311.
10. Bahar I, Weinherger D, Kremer MR, et al. Ocular manifestation of bronchogenic carcinoma: simultaneous occurrence of diffuse uveal melanocytic proliferation and uveal metastases. Harefuah. 2007;146(2–3):80.
11. Pelosof LC, Gerber DE. Paraneoplastic syndromes: an approach to diagnosis and treatment. Mayo Clin Proc. 2010;85:838–54. DOI: 10.4065/mcp.2010.0099.
12. Adamus G. Autoantibody targets and their cancer relationship in the pathogenicity of paraneoplastic retinopathy. Autoimmun Rev. 2009;8:410–4. DOI: 10.1016/j.autrev.2009.01.002.
13. Keltner JL, Thirkill CE, Yip PT. Clinical and immunologic characteristics of melanoma-associated retinopathy syndrome: eleven new cases and a review of 51 previously published cases. J Neuroophthalmol. 2001;21:173–87.
14. Dalal MD, Morgans CW, Duvoisin RM, et al. Diagnosis of occult melanoma using transient receptor potential melastatin 1 (TRPM1) autoantibody testing: a novel approach. Ophthalmology. 2013;120:2560–4. DOI: 10.1016/j.ophtha.2013.07.037.

15. Jampol LM, Kim HH, Bryar PJ, et al. Multiple serous retinal detachments and subretinal deposits as the presenting signs of metastatic melanoma. Retina. 2004;24:320–2.
16. Adamus G, Ren G, Weleber RG. Autoantibodies against retinal proteins in paraneoplastic and autoimmune retinopathy. BMC Ophthalmol. 2004;4:5. DOI: 10.1186/1471-2415-4-5.
17. Ferreyra HA, Jayasundera T, Khan NW, et al. Management of autoimmune retinopathies with immunosuppression. Arch Ophthalmol. 2009;127:390–7. DOI: 10.1001/archophthalmol.2009.24.
18. Gass JD, Gieser RG, Wilkinson CP, et al. Bilateral diffuse uveal melanocytic proliferation in patients with occult carcinoma. Arch Ophthalmol. 1990;108:527–33.
19. Rohrbach JM, Roggendorf W, Thanos S, et al. Simultaneous bilateral diffuse melanocytic uveal hyperplasia. Am J Ophthalmol. 1990;110:49–56.
20. Sen J, Clewes AR, Quah S-A, et al. Presymptomatic diagnosis of bronchogenic carcinoma associated with bilateral diffuse uveal melanocytic proliferation. Clin Experiment Ophthalmol. 2006;34:156–8. DOI: 10.1111/j.1442-9071.2006.01145.x.
21. Weleber RG, Watzke RC, Shults WT, et al. Clinical and electrophysiologic characterization of paraneoplastic and autoimmune retinopathies associated with antienolase antibodies. Am J Ophthalmol. 2005;139:780–94. DOI: 10.1016/j.ajo.2004.12.104.
22. Shimazaki K, Jirawuthiworavong GV, Heckenlively JR, Gordon LK. Frequency of anti-retinal antibodies in normal human serum. J Neuroophthalmol. 2008;28:5–11. DOI: 10.1097/WNO.0b013e318167549f.
23. Lima LH, Greenberg JP, Greenstein VC, et al. Hyperautofluorescent ring in autoimmune retinopathy. Retina. 2012;32:1385–94. DOI: 10.1097/IAE.0b013e3182398107.

Systemic Infectious Diseases

9

Aniruddha Agarwal and Vishali Gupta

Abstract

Systemic infectious diseases can affect various organ systems including the ocular tissue. Organisms such as bacteria, viruses, fungi, and parasites can disseminate from their systemic foci of infection and involve the retinal and the choroid. Retinochoroidal involvement due to systemic infectious conditions can present with protean clinical manifestations and can often result in a diagnostic challenge. Often, these entities can present with unusual ocular findings. Thus, the clinician may need advanced laboratory support including analysis of ocular fluids and/or tissues to establish accurate diagnosis. In the past few decades, there have been numerous advances in the field of ocular imaging. With the introduction of newer imaging modalities such as enhanced-depth imaging optical coherence tomography and ultrawide-field fundus photography, it is possible to obtain high-quality near-histological images of the retina and choroid. Such observations can greatly aid the clinician in establishing the diagnosis early. In the index chapter, infectious chorioretinal diseases such as tuberculosis, toxoplasmosis, Lyme disease, and syphilis have been described with an emphasis on their clinical and imaging features.

A. Agarwal
Department of Ophthalmology, Advanced Eye Center, Post Graduate Institute of Medical Education and Research (PGIMER), Sector 12, Chandigarh 160012, India

V. Gupta (✉)
Department of Ophthalmology, Advanced Eye Center, Post Graduate Institute of Medical Education and Research (PGIMER), Sector 12, Chandigarh 160012, India
e-mail: vishalisara@yahoo.co.in

J. Chhablani et al. (eds.), *Retinal and Choroidal Imaging in Systemic Diseases*,
https://doi.org/10.1007/978-981-10-5461-7_9

9.1 Introduction

A number of systemic infections can result in ocular disease that may be associated with severe visual morbidity. Often, ocular findings may be the presenting feature of these conditions. On the other hand, delay in the diagnosis of infectious posterior uveitis and chorioretinitis may be associated with permanent visual impairment [1]. While systemic infections caused by bacteria, viruses, fungi, and parasites are more common in developing countries, many pathogens are endemic throughout the world, and thus, conditions such as tuberculosis can present in developed countries as well [2]. Therefore, a clinician must rule out infectious etiologies when evaluating every case of chorioretinitis because immunosuppressive therapy in the absence of appropriate antibiotic cover can lead to life-threatening fulminant disease. In addition, ocular infection can rapidly spread resulting in sight-threatening sequelae.

Apart from direct invasion of the ocular tissues, systemic infectious agents can result in retinochoroidal inflammation due to altered immunological response of the host due to various mechanisms such as molecular mimicry [3]. Hypersensitivity reaction to the proteins of such infectious microorganisms can also result in tissue damage and inflammation. Thus, immunological response of the host plays an important role in pathogenesis of the disease.

With advancing biomedical engineering techniques, a number of state-of-the-art imaging devices have been introduced in the field of ophthalmology in the past few decades. It is now possible to image various ocular tissues noninvasively.

With the help of multimodal imaging techniques, staging, treatment response, and prognosis of various entities such as tubercular serpiginous-like choroiditis (SLC) and toxoplasmosis can be accurately assessed. In the following sections, a comprehensive overview of imaging features for each of these conditions is presented.

9.2 Tuberculosis

Tuberculosis (TB) is a leading infectious cause of morbidity and mortality. Worldwide, one-third of the population is estimated to be infected with *Mycobacterium tuberculosis* (*latent TB*). Nearly 10% of individuals with latent TB are likely to develop the disease at some time in their lives [4]. In 2014, 9.6 million individuals the world over suffered from TB-related disease with over 1.5 million TB-related deaths [5]. During the same year, the rate of decline of TB cases decreased in the USA, suggesting that the disease may potentially reemerge even in non-endemic areas.

9.2.1 Systemic Features of Tuberculosis

The spread of TB occurs through the aerial route. When infectious mycobacteria are inhaled, primary infection may occur in the lung. Involvement of lung parenchyma, regional lymph nodes, and pleural tissue may result in the formation of *Ghon focus*. If the host's immune system is capable of destroying the multiplying mycobacteria, the patient may not manifest the disease. However, reactivation of the disease is possible in the future during states of immunosuppression. Pulmonary TB may present with cavitatory lesions and destruction of lung parenchymal tissue. Pleural effusion may accompany lesions in the lung [6].

Dissemination of the organism may occur and extrapulmonary sites may be affected due to TB. Commonly affected organs include the central nervous system (*tubercular meningitis*), cardiovascular system, liver, gastrointestinal system, vertebrae (*Pott's spine*), joints (*tubercular arthritis*), and lymph nodes, among others. Extrapulmonary involvement with TB may be very severe, especially in the presence of HIV coinfection [7]. Highly virulent form of the disease may ensue, leading to rapid weight loss, wasting, and death of the patient [8].

9.2.2 Intraocular Tuberculosis

Intraocular TB represents an extrapulmonary form of the disease, which may occur in 1.4–6.8% of patients with pulmonary TB [9, 10]. However, often intraocular TB may not be accompanied by pulmonary disease making the diagnosis challenging. Moreover, the paucibacillary nature of ocular infection makes the microbiological diagnosis challenging [11]. Therefore, diagnosis of intraocular TB is based on a multitude of clinical findings, systemic TB, chorioretinal imaging, and supportive laboratory tests evaluating tubercular hypersensitivity (such as tuberculin skin test and interferon gamma release assay).

Although posterior segment uveitis is the most common form of intraocular TB, patients may present with chronic, recurrent anterior uveitis. Anterior uveitis is usually granulomatous inflammation with cells, flare, rarely hypopyon, mutton-fat keratic precipitates, iris nodules (Koeppe's or Busacca's), and broad-based posterior synechiae. TB-related granulomas may be found in the angle of the anterior chamber. Chronic anterior uveitis may be associated with development of posterior subcapsular cataract, pupillary block, and secondary glaucoma. Other features include iris neovascularization and band-shaped keratopathy. Intermediate uveitis may be seen due to spillover of the inflammation into the vitreous cavity. There may be severe vitritis, snow balls, snow banking, peripheral vascular sheathing, and cystoid macular edema. There may be presence of tuberculomas of the ciliary body detectable on ultrasound biomicroscopy [11].

Posterior segment manifestations of ocular TB include *serpiginous-like choroiditis* (or *multifocal serpiginous choroiditis*), tubercular granulomas or tubercles, subretinal abscesses, neuroretinitis, retinal vasculitis, and rarely endophthalmitis or panophthalmitis [2, 11, 12]. The following sections describe clinical and imaging characteristics of tubercular lesions that primarily involve the retinochoroid.

9.2.2.1 Serpiginous-Like Choroiditis

Serpiginous-like choroiditis (SLC) typically affects young to middle-aged adults from TB-endemic areas (Fig. 9.1) [13, 14]. Unlike autoimmune serpiginous choroiditis, tubercular serpiginous-like choroiditis occurs at a younger age, associated

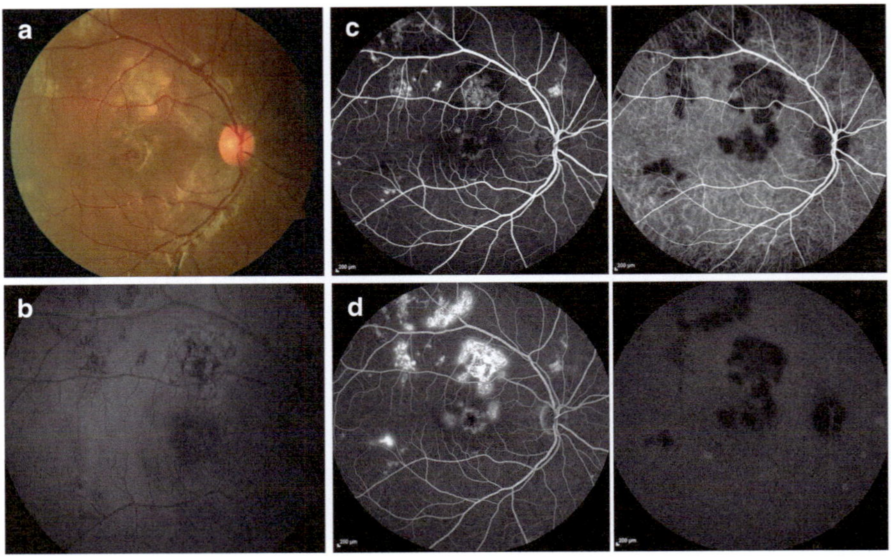

Fig. 9.1 Multimodal imaging of a 24-year-old male diagnosed with tubercular serpiginous-like choroiditis (SLC). (**a**) Color fundus photography shows presence of multifocal yellowish-white perivascular choroiditis lesions involving the posterior pole and mid-periphery. On fundus autofluorescence, the lesions show central areas of hypo-autofluorescence. Active edges appear hyperautofluorescent (**b**). Simultaneous fluorescein angiography (FA) and indocyanine green angiography (ICGA) in the early phase (**c**) show RPE window defects in the healed areas. Active lesions appear hypofluorescent on FA. ICGA shows diffuse hypofluorescence. In the late phase (**d**), the active lesions show intense hyperfluorescence on FA and hypofluorescence on ICGA

with mild vitritis, and is bilateral in majority of the cases [15]. TB SLC may have different morphological patterns [13]:

1. Multifocal choroiditis: This phenotype presents with discreet lesions, is yellowish white in color, measures about ¼–1 disk diameter in size with well-defined margins and slightly raised edges which are noncontiguous to begin with, and shows a wavelike progression over a period of 1–4 weeks and gradually becomes confluent (Fig. 9.1).
2. Placoid chorioretinitis: This phenotype presents with a diffuse plaque-like lesion with an amoeboid pattern and active serpiginous-like edge at the initial presentation. The edges are yellowish white and elevated, whereas the center of the lesion is less elevated with pigmentary changes suggestive of a healing process in the center of the lesion.
3. Mixed pattern: These lesions present with overlapping features of both multifocal and placoid chorioretinitis.

9.2.2.2 Choroidal Granulomas, Tubercles, and Subretinal Abscesses

Choroidal granulomas and tubercles occur as a result of hematogenous dissemination of TB bacilli from pulmonary and extrapulmonary sites [2, 16]. The tubercles may be unilateral or bilateral, usually multiple, discreet grayish-white to yellowish subretinal lesions with indistinct borders. The lesions are usually seen in the posterior pole but may be present in the mid-periphery [10]. A choroidal granuloma may clinically resemble non-inflammatory condition such as central serous chorioretinopathy, choroidal metastases, melanoma of the choroid, and age-related macular degeneration (Fig. 9.2).

On the other hand, solitary choroidal granuloma may present as a large, elevated yellowish *subretinal mass* often associated with exudative retinal detachment. The lesion is associated with rapid necrosis and tissue destruction [17]. These patients often have disseminated systemic TB [18]. TB-related subretinal abscess appears distinct and more yellowish in color compared to a small choroidal granuloma. They usually have overlying retinal hemorrhages and have a tendency to develop retinal angiomatous proliferation over a period of time.

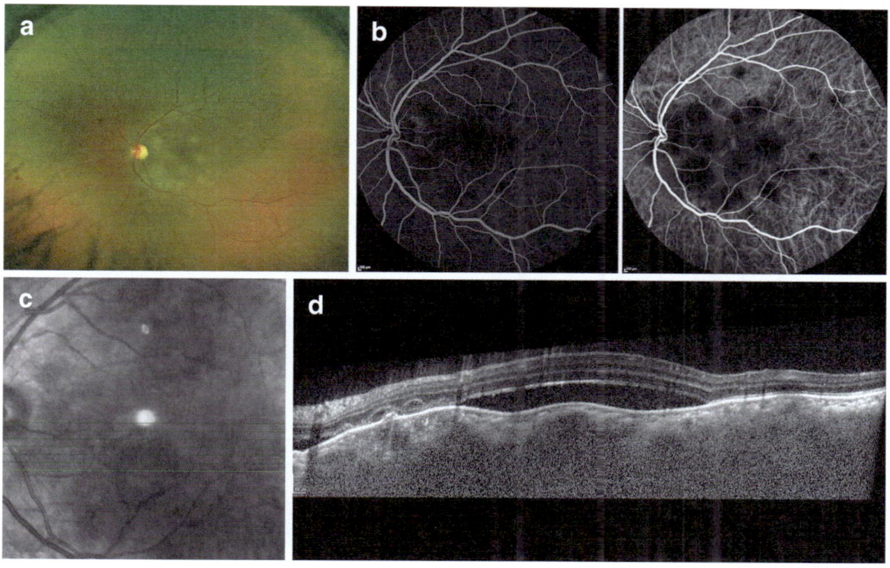

Fig. 9.2 Imaging features of a 40-year-old male with tubercular granulomas in the *left* eye. On ultrawide-field fundus photography (**a**), the lesions appear yellow-white, subretinal, and multiple, involving the posterior pole. Simultaneous fluorescein angiography (FA) and indocyanine green angiography (ICGA) in the early phase (**b**) show hypofluorescence of the lesions. On infrared imaging (**c**), the granulomas are clearly demarcated. Enhanced-depth imaging optical coherence tomography through the subretinal granuloma shows elevation of RPE due to the granulomas, subretinal fluid, and atrophy of the inner choroidal vasculature (**d**)

9.2.2.3 Tubercular Retinitis

Rarely, intraocular TB may present with atypical features mimicking other etiologies of infectious necrotizing retinitis such as viral (herpetic) retinitis or atypical toxoplasma retinochoroiditis. Often, these patients may be immunocompromised due to HIV coinfection. Such cases may be accompanied by retinal periphlebitis [19].

9.2.3 Imaging Features

9.2.3.1 Fundus Photography, Autofluorescence, and Ultra-wide field Fundus Imaging

Since the diagnosis of TB SLC depends upon the clinical appearance and morphology of the choroiditis lesions, adequate assessment of the disease phenotype using high-quality color fundus photography is essential. Serial fundus photography (from acute stage to the stage of healing) is very useful in the assessment of morphological evolution of the lesions [13]. In addition, color fundus photography can enable detection of vitreous haze among patients with intraocular TB.

FAF is a very useful noninvasive imaging modality in the management of TB SLC. Characteristic changes are observed on FAF as the lesions evolve from active to healed stage. Lesions of TB SLC can be staged using FAF to determine the response of therapy (Fig. 9.3) [20]. Active lesions demonstrate ill-defined hyper-autofluorescence throughout the lesions giving them a diffuse, amorphous appearance (stage 1). In the stage of early healing, a thin rim of hypo-autofluorescence is seen surrounding the lesion which remains predominantly hyper-autofluorescent with a stippled pattern (stage 2). With further healing, the lesion becomes predominantly hypo-autofluorescent (stage 3). On complete healing, the lesions become uniformly hypo-autofluorescent (stage 4) (Fig. 9.3; Table 9.1) [20].

Ultrawide-field fundus imaging can provide new insights into the disease pathophysiology. In a recent study, using ultrawide-field imaging, additional features such as peripheral choroiditis, active retinal vasculitis, and neovascularization were observed among patients with TB SLC compared to conventional imaging [21]. Using this technology, it is possible to simultaneously document posterior and peripheral TB SLC lesions in one image and monitor the overall response to treatment on successive visits. Therefore, ultrawide-field imaging may be superior to conventional imaging in identifying changes such as *peripheral paradoxical worsening* which may be otherwise missed (Fig. 9.4) [21].

9.2.3.2 Fluorescein Angiography

On FA, active lesions of TB SLC are hypofluorescent in the early phase. Active lesions show late hyperfluorescence. As the lesions progress and become confluent, the advancing edge shows early hypofluorescence with late hyperfluorescence. Areas of resolution show retinal pigment epithelial transmission defects. Choroidal tubercles and granulomas are hypofluorescent in the phase of early dye transit and become hyperfluorescent in the late frames (Fig. 9.1) [13].

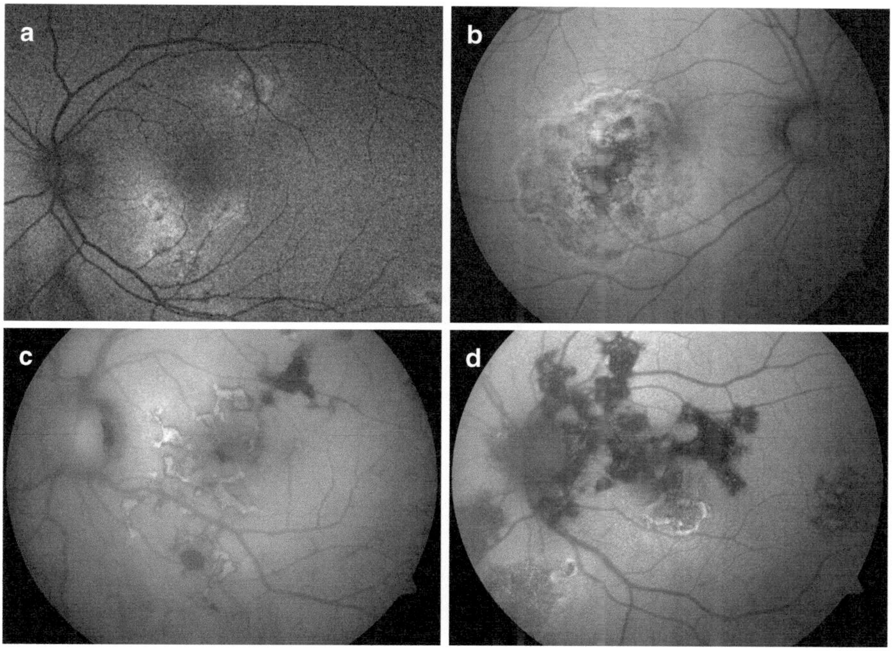

Fig. 9.3 Fundus autofluorescence of tubercular serpiginous-like choroiditis (SLC) lesions in various stages of the disease. In the early active stage (**a**), there is diffuse hyper-autofluorescence of the lesions (stage 1). Stage 2 is characterized by a thin rim of hypo-autofluorescence surrounding the hyper-autofluorescent lesions (**b**). Stage 3 is characterized by stippled appearance with mixed hyper- and hypo-autofluorescence, but predominant hypo-autofluorescence (**c**). In the stage 4, the lesions appear uniformly hypo-autofluorescent (**d**)

Ultrawide-field FA is very useful in the management of intraocular TB. In comparison with conventional FA, ultrawide-field imaging can reveal additional information such as peripheral capillary non-perfusion areas, retinal neovascularization, and retinal vascular leakage. Such findings may alter treatment decisions such as the need for scatter laser photocoagulation [21].

9.2.3.3 Indocyanine Green Angiography

Active lesions of TB SLC remain hypofluorescent from early to late phase on ICGA. ICGA is very useful in detecting choriocapillaritis among patients with tubercular choroiditis. On the other hand, choroidal tubercles show early and intermediate hypofluorescence on ICGA. In the late phase, the lesions may become hyperfluorescent (type 1) indicating active choroidal lesions or remain hypofluorescent (type 2) indicating areas of atrophy. There may be presence of numerous hyperfluorescent spots, fuzzy appearance of choroidal vessels in the intermediate phase, and late choroidal hyperfluorescence due to dye leakage which tends to regress after completion of treatment with antitubercular therapy and corticosteroids. The ICGA

Table 9.1 Imaging features of lesions of tubercular serpiginous-like choroiditis

Stage of lesions	FAF features	Features on EDI-OCT	Appearance on ICGA	Features on FA
1	Ill-defined hyper-autofluorescence throughout the lesions	Outer retinal hyper-reflectivity, sub-RPE hyper-reflective deposits, IS-OS disruption, decreased choroidal reflectance	Early and late hypofluorescence; fuzzy margins	Early hypofluorescence with late hyperfluorescence
2	Thin rim of hypo-autofluorescence surrounding the lesion which remains predominantly hyper-autofluorescent	Irregular hyper-reflective elevations in the RPE, IS-OS and ELM disruption, mildly decreased choroidal reflectance	Early hypofluorescence with discrete margins	Early hypofluorescence with late hyperfluorescence
3	Predominantly hypo-autofluorescence of the lesions	Outer retinal hyper-reflective deposits with knob-like elevations of RPE, IS-OS and ELM disruption, atrophy of RPE-Bruch's complex, increased choroidal reflectance	Early hypofluorescence with discrete margins	Early and late hyperfluorescence due to RPE window defects
4	Uniform hypo-autofluorescence of the lesions	Atrophy of outer retinal layers and RPE, IS-OS, and ELM disruption, increased choroidal reflectance, choroidal thinning, loss of choriocapillaris layer	Early and late hypofluorescence	Early and late hyperfluorescence due to RPE window defects

EDI-OCT enhanced-depth imaging optical coherence tomography, *ELM* external limiting membrane, *FA* fluorescein angiography, *ICGA* indocyanine green angiography, *IS-OS* photoreceptor inner segment-outer segment, *OCTA* optical coherence tomography angiography, *RPE* retinal pigment epithelium

changes are usually reversible and may be used to monitor the response to therapy (Figs. 9.1 and 9.2) [22–24].

9.2.3.4 Optical Coherence Tomography

Optical Coherence Tomography Features of Tubercular Serpiginous-Like Choroiditis

OCT features of TB SLC include peripapillary retinal atrophy, disruption of the photoreceptor layer, thinning of retinal pigment epithelium (RPE), mild cystic changes, as well as subretinal fibrosis in the area of old choroidal neovascularization and marked attenuation of the interdigitation zone in the outer retina [25, 26]. In the

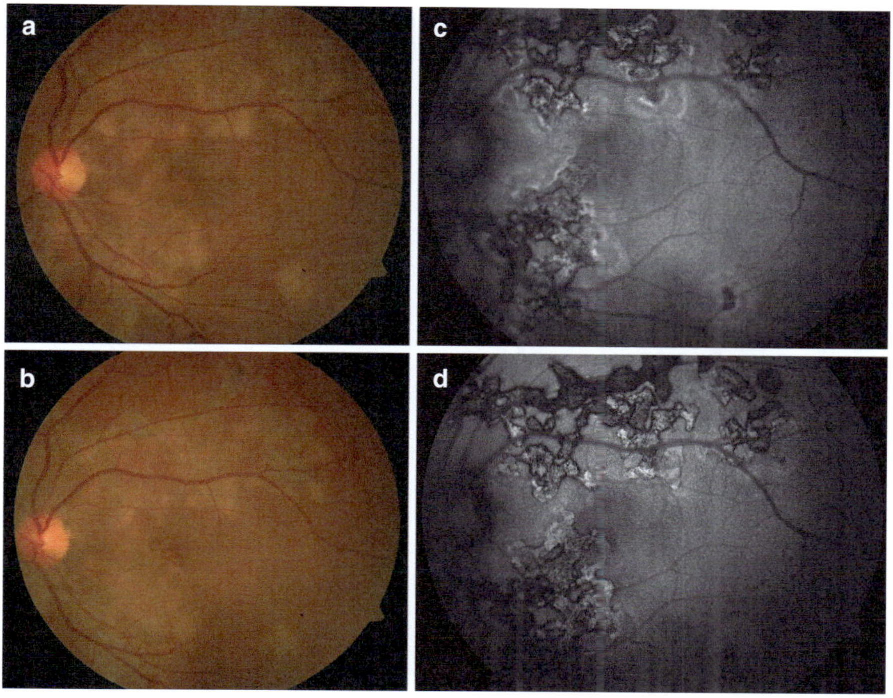

Fig. 9.4 Paradoxical worsening of tubercular serpiginous-like choroiditis (SLC) lesions after initiation of antitubercular therapy (ATT). At presentation, color fundus photography (**a**) shows presence of multifocal choroiditis lesions along the superior vascular arcade and in the inferior macula. Three weeks after initiation of ATT, there is continuous progression of SLC lesions and coalescence in the macula, threatening central vision (**b**). At presentation fundus autofluorescence (FAF) shows presence of hyper-autofluorescence within the lesion indicating active disease (**c**). Repeat FAF imaging shows increase in the size of the lesions and persistent hyper-autofluorescence (**d**)

acute stage of TB SLC, active edge of the lesions shows a localized, fuzzy area of hyper-reflectivity in the outer retinal layers involving the RPE, photoreceptor outer segment tips, ellipsoid and myoid zones, external limiting membrane, and the outer nuclear layer with no increased backscattering from the inner choroid. As the lesions begin to heal from the center, the hyper-reflective fuzzy areas begin to disappear from OCT scans and are replaced by irregular, hyper-reflective knobbly elevations of the outer retinal layers. The RPE, ellipsoid and myoid zones, and the external limiting membrane cannot be distinguished at this stage. There is an increased reflectance from the choroidal layers due to attenuation of the RPE-photoreceptor complex. As the lesions continue to heal further, there is loss of RPE and outer retinal layers and persistent increased reflectance from the choroid on OCT [27].

The technology of enhanced-depth imaging (EDI)-OCT has provided new insights into the choroidal involvement in TB SLC. Using EDI-OCT, choroidal infiltration, elevation of the RPE-Bruch's membrane complex, and focal increase in choroidal thickness have been observed in patients with active TB SLC [27].

Optical Coherence Tomography Features of Tubercular Granulomas
OCT is very useful in the diagnosis and management of tubercular granulomas. Findings on OCT among patients with subretinal granulomas correlate well with ICGA, obviating the need for an invasive procedure. On OCT, an area of localized adhesion between the choriocapillaris-RPE and the overlying neurosensory retina may be observed (*contact sign*) due to inflammatory adhesions overlying the granuloma [28]. Thus, OCT can help to differentiate tubercular choroidal granulomas from other non-inflammatory lesions. In addition, OCT is useful in confirming the presence of exudative retinal detachment associated with choroidal granulomas. On EDI-OCT, active choroidal granulomas generate an increased transmission of the OCT signal toward the sclera. Granulomas in patients affected by TB-related uveitis were more likely to have a lobulated shape and nonhomogeneous internal pattern compared to granulomas related to other entities such as sarcoidosis (Fig. 9.2) [29].

9.2.3.5 Optical Coherence Tomography Angiography

Newer imaging modalities such as optical coherence tomography angiography (OCTA) are being increasingly used in the evaluation of posterior uveitides such as TB-related choroiditis. Using OCTA, choriocapillaris hypoperfusion in association with TB SLC is seen as flow void areas on en face OCTA. These correlate well with findings on ICGA. Thus, noninvasive tools such as OCTA may enable detailed evaluation of the retinochoroidal vasculature among patients with intraocular TB [30]. In a recent report, choroidal neovascularization was detected using OCTA in a patient with tubercular choroiditis [31]. Thus, further advances in imaging may enhance our knowledge of pathogenesis of intraocular TB.

9.2.4 Treatment of Tuberculosis

Treatment of systemic tuberculosis consists of multidrug therapy consisting of first-line antimycobacterial agents such as isoniazid, rifampin, ethambutol, and pyrazinamide, as well as second-line agents such as levofloxacin, streptomycin, and amikacin/kanamycin, among others. The duration and dosing regimen depend on the organ system involved, severity of disease, history of prior anti-TB therapy, and sensitivity of the mycobacteria. In the past decade, there have been increasing cases of multidrug-resistant TB (MDR TB) as well as extensively drug-resistant TB (XDR TB) reported in literature [32–34]. Rifampin resistance has also been recently demonstrated in ocular TB [35].

The treatment of ocular TB consists of four-drug regimen of isoniazid (5 mg/kg/day), rifampicin (10 mg/kg/day), ethambutol (15 mg/kg/day), and pyrazinamide (20–25 mg/kg/day) along with pyridoxine. The clinical features of ocular TB are assessed using retinal and choroidal imaging to assess the activity of the lesions. Ethambutol and pyrazinamide are stopped after a period of 2 months, while isoniazid and rifampin are usually continued for 1 year. Anti-TB therapy is usually given in combination with systemic steroids (oral prednisolone 1 mg/kg/day) which is tapered over the next 6–12 weeks depending upon the level of inflammation. Topical steroids may be employed in cases with anterior segment inflammation. Systemic immunosuppressants and steroid-sparing agents such as azathioprine may be added as and when required [11]. About 14% patients treated with anti-TB therapy may develop paradoxical worsening of ocular disease (*ocular Jarisch-Herxheimer reaction*) [36]. However, such cases are managed by increasing systemic immunosuppression and not by withholding anti-TB therapy. The role of anti-TB therapy in intraocular TB is to reduce the antigen load by eliminating the bacilli, which may prevent recurrence of the disease.

9.3 Syphilis

Syphilis is a sexually transmitted multisystem disease that is caused by a gram-negative spirochete, *Treponema pallidum*. Syphilis is highly contagious, and the infection can spread through small abrasions on the skin and mucous membranes. In addition, the disease spreads through sexual contact as well as through vertical transmission (transplacental route). The natural history of the acquired disease consists of four stages, namely, primary, secondary, latent, and tertiary syphilis.

9.3.1 Systemic Features of Syphilis

Primary syphilis manifests with a characteristic syphilitic *chancre* that appears as a painless, small ulcer with a hard base in the genital area. Syphilitic chancres are highly contagious and most commonly occur 2–6 weeks after infectious exposure. Although painless, the infective organisms spread from the lesion to involve regional lymph nodes resulting in painless nonsuppurative lymphadenopathy. The chancres usually heal without treatment. However, if left untreated, the organisms spread through the hematogenous route, and the disease often manifests with *secondary syphilis*. During this stage of the disease, the patient may develop fever and maculopapular rash involving the palms and soles. Other common features during this stage include headache, myalgia, and sore throat. Clinical features of secondary syphilis may spontaneously resolve, and the patient may develop *latent syphilis*. Latent syphilis is characterized by disappearance of primary and secondary symptoms though the patient continues to have systemic infection with treponema organisms. Latent syphilis can last for years before the patient develops tertiary disease [37, 38].

Approximately 30–40% patients develop involvement of other organ systems such as the central nervous system and cardiovascular system (*tertiary syphilis*) if left untreated. Tertiary syphilis is characterized by formation of *gumma*. These represent inflammatory infiltrates in the form of a granuloma and appear soft, swollen, rubbery lesions in the skin and other tissues. Tertiary syphilis manifests with *neurosyphilis* [39] that includes cranial nerve palsies, vascular occlusions presenting as strokes or focal neurological deficits, *tabes dorsalis* (syphilitic myelopathy resulting in loss of coordination), and generalized paresis. Patients may also develop severe dementia and neurological impairment. Cardiovascular involvement presents with aortitis, aortic aneurysms, and valvular insufficiencies. Other organ systems commonly affected include musculoskeletal system, liver, and joints. However, these manifestations have become increasingly rare with antibiotic therapy [38, 40].

With the availability of antibiotics such as penicillin and cephalosporins, the incidence of syphilis dramatically decreased. However, there have been higher numbers of cases reported recently from developed countries like the USA. This may be related to the increasing prevalence of HIV infection [41]. Syphilis coinfection among patients with HIV may result in a highly virulent form of the disease that may rapidly lead to death of the patient.

9.3.2 Ocular Features of Syphilis

Ocular syphilis is most commonly associated with secondary and tertiary syphilis. Ocular involvement occurs in approximately 4–5% of patients with secondary syphilis. The prevalence of syphilis among patients presenting to uveitis referral centers has been estimated to be between 1% and 8% [42].

Pathological manifestations of syphilis can affect any ocular tissue, and the disease can have protean manifestations (Table 9.2). Inflammation can involve the anterior segment, posterior segment, retinal vasculature, optic nerve, and orbit. Therefore, syphilis is referred to as the *great masquerader*. Syphilitic anterior uveitis is typically granulomatous and associated with anterior chamber cells, flare, keratic precipitates, and large iris nodules (Koeppe's or Busacca's nodules). Mild involvement can present with non-granulomatous anterior uveitis. Anterior segment inflammation may be associated with corneal involvement that manifests with interstitial keratitis. Interstitial keratitis is a non-ulcerative corneal stromal condition with sparing of the endothelium and epithelium. This condition presents with inflammation and vascularization with minimal loss of corneal tissue [42–44].

Posterior segment disease most commonly presents with focal or multifocal lesions of chorioretinitis. Lesions of chorioretinitis appear deep yellow-gray with a

Table 9.2 Ocular manifestations of syphilis

Cornea, conjunctiva	Interstitial keratitis, conjunctivitis
Episclera and sclera	Episcleritis, scleritis
Anterior chamber and iris	Anterior uveitis, iritis, iridocyclitis, iris nodules, hypopyon uveitis, iris roseola, gummas of the iris
Posterior segment	Panuveitis, intermediate uveitis, endophthalmitis/panophthalmitis, chorioretinitis, retinal vasculitis, acute syphilitic posterior placoid chorioretinitis, necrotizing retinitis, choroidal detachment, serous retinal detachment, macular edema
Optic nerve and neuro-ophthalmological structures	Optic neuritis, papilledema, neuroretinitis, optic perineuritis, optic atrophy, cranial nerve palsies, visual field defects, Argyll-Robertson pupil, cortical blindness

shallow serous retinal detachment and overlying vitreous inflammation. Severe infection may present with necrotizing retinitis that may mimic acute retinal necrosis [45]. Patients with *necrotizing retinitis* may present with single or multiple yellowish white patches of necrosis often associated with vasculitis, vitreous inflammation, and some anterior segment inflammation [42]. Other manifestations include retinal vasculitis with retinal ischemia. Both retinal veins and arteries may be involved in a focal or diffuse manner. Syphilitic retinal vasculitis may present as *frosted branch angiitis*. *Acute syphilitic posterior placoid chorioretinitis* (ASPPC) is a distinct entity originally described by Gass. Subsequently, a number of cases of ASPPC have been described in literature. The hallmark of ASPPC is presence of a large, placoid lesion in the posterior pole extending beyond the major arcades involving the outer retina and inner choroid (Fig. 9.5). In a series of 16 patients, Eandi et al. [46] have described ASPPC as pale yellowish, ill-defined lesions with a faded center and stippled hyperpigmentation of the RPE that coalesce to become large confluent lesions. These lesions may be associated with vitritis, superficial retinal hemorrhages, retinal vasculitis, disk edema, and serous detachment of the RPE. ASPPC is typically observed among the immunocompromised patients [46].

Syphilitic uveitis can also present with intermediate uveitis and panuveitis. Other ocular features include optic nerve inflammation (*syphilitic optic neuritis*) that may progress to optic atrophy and severe visual field defects. Patients with neurosyphilis may develop pupillary abnormalities (*Argyll-Robertson pupil*) (Table 9.2).

9.3.3 Imaging Features

9.3.3.1 Fundus Photography and Autofluorescence

Chorioretinal lesions of syphilis can be documented using color retinal photography. Color fundus photographs may be used in the follow-up of patients with vitritis, choroiditis, and other posterior segment diseases to document resolution with therapy. FAF imaging is very useful in the diagnosis of ASPPC. Matsumoto and Spaide have described FAF changes in two patients with FAF. In the area of the placoid lesion, there is usually a slightly increased autofluorescence in a geographic pattern. In addition, focal intensely hyper-autofluorescent spots may also be found [47]. Other features on FAF include punctate hypo-autofluorescent spots (Fig. 9.5) [46].

9.3.3.2 Fluorescein Angiography

FA provides useful information regarding the pathology of syphilitic posterior uveitis. On FA, lesions of chorioretinitis show early hypofluorescence followed by late staining. Lesions of ASPPC show early central hypofluorescence or faint hyperfluorescence followed by progressive hyperfluorescence in the area of the lesion. Variable or punctate hypofluorescence producing a classic *leopard spot* pattern may be seen in later stages of the disease. FA may also be useful in the detection of macular edema and optic nerve head inflammation among patients with syphilitic uveitis [46].

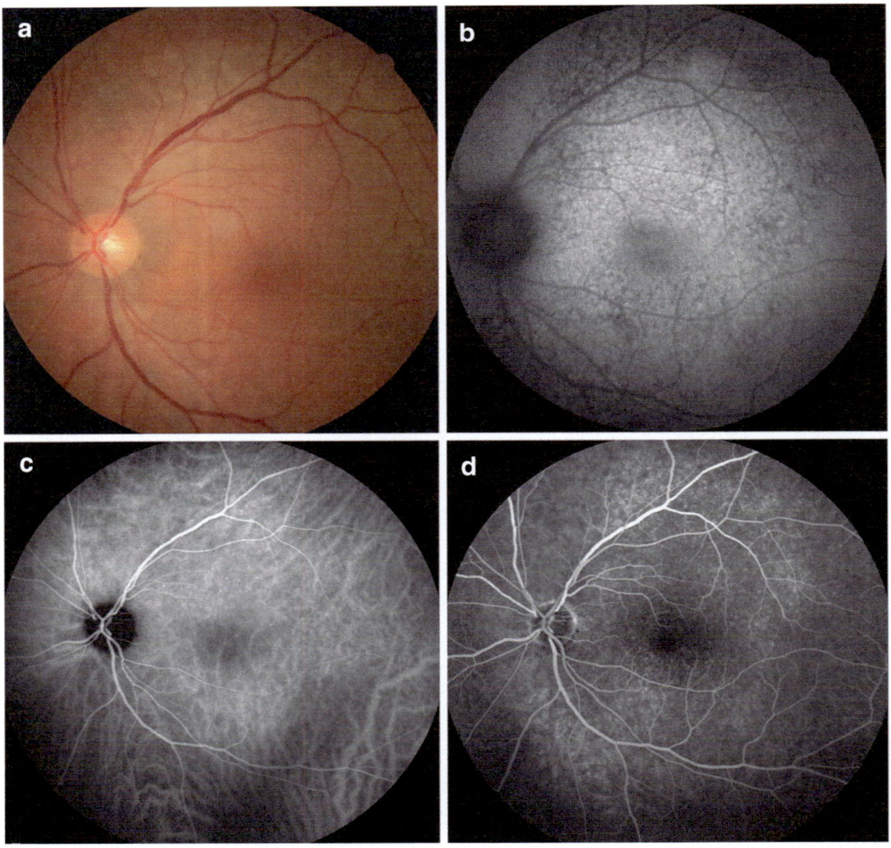

Fig. 9.5 Multimodal imaging of a patient with acute syphilitic posterior placoid chorioretinitis (ASPPC). Color fundus photography shows presence of a large, diffuse, placoid lesion involving the posterior pole and extending to the mid-periphery (**a**). Fundus autofluorescence shows presence of diffuse hyper-autofluorescence of the lesion with scattered focal areas of hypo-autofluorescence (**b**). Indocyanine green angiography (**c**) shows subtle hypofluorescence along the lesion. Fluorescein angiography (**d**) in the late phase shows punctate hyperfluorescence without any leakage. *(Image courtesy: Dr. Alessandro Invernizzi, MD, University of Milan, Italy)*

9.3.3.3 Indocyanine Green Angiography

Characteristic features of ICGA among patients with ASPPC have been described in various reports. Lesions of ASPPC show variable hypofluorescence in both early and late stages on ICGA. In some patients, there may be late hyperfluorescence on ICGA [42, 46]. ICGA is a useful tool to demonstrate choroidal vascular involvement among patients with syphilitic posterior uveitis (Fig. 9.5).

9.3.3.4 Optical Coherence Tomography

Serial imaging using OCT is very useful in the diagnosis and follow-up of patients with posterior segment manifestations associated with syphilis. Recent studies by Brito et al. and Pichi et al. have described the OCT features of ASPPC [48, 49]. During the early stage of the disease (within 1–2 days of presentation), OCT may show presence of a small amount of subretinal fluid, an intact external limiting membrane, disruption of the ellipsoid and myoid zone, and thickening and *granular hyper-reflectivity of the RPE* (without nodular elevations) (Fig. 9.6). Subsequently (7–10 days after presentation), subretinal fluid may resolve on OCT, but the scans may show an irregular thickening and hyper-reflectivity of the RPE with *prominent nodular elevations*, along with a loss of ellipsoid and myoid zones, and RPE bands. In addition, there may be areas of punctate hyper-reflectivity in the choroid.

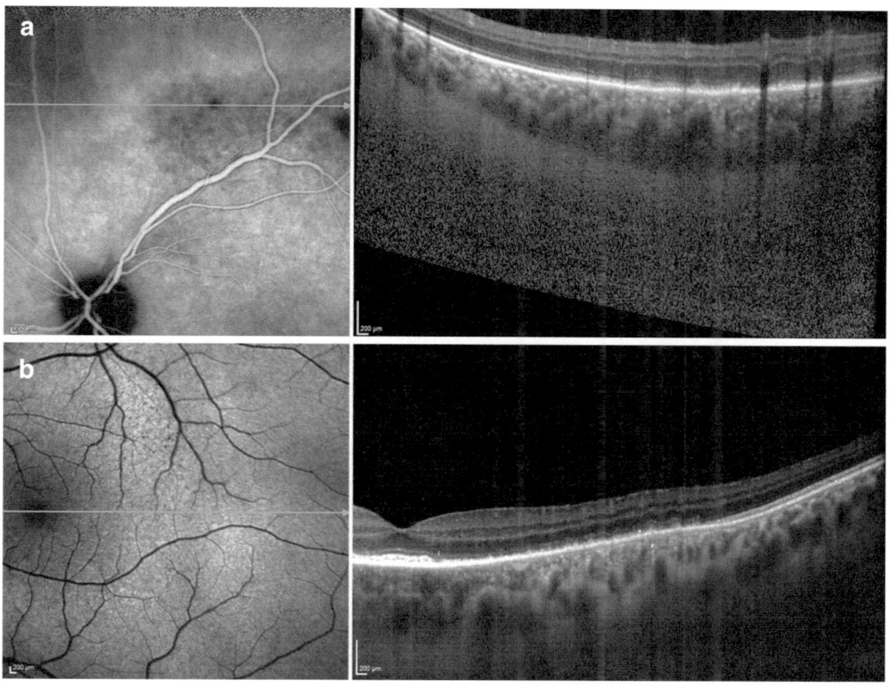

Fig. 9.6 Enhanced-depth imaging (EDI) optical coherence tomography (OCT) of a patient with acute syphilitic posterior placoid chorioretinitis (ASPPC). Combined indocyanine *green* angiography (ICGA) and EDI-OCT (**a**) show hypofluorescence on ICGA, and corresponding OCT B-scan shows granular hyper-reflectivity of the retinal pigment epithelium (RPE). There is mild choroidal thickening. Combined fundus autofluorescence and EDI-OCT B-scan passing through the macula in the same patient show macular RPE thickening and focal hyper-reflectivity in the region temporal to the fovea (**b**). *(Image courtesy: Dr. Alessandro Invernizzi, MD, University of Milan, Italy)*

Macular OCT may be useful in the detection of macular edema associated with syphilitic uveitis. OCT may also demonstrate presence of subretinal fluid along with outer retinal disruption. Retinal nerve fiber layer edema can be detected among patients with optic nerve head swelling using OCT.

9.3.3.5 Advanced Imaging Modalities

Newer imaging modalities such as the swept-source OCT may provide significant insights into the disease pathophysiology especially among cases presenting with ASPPC. Using swept-source OCT, superior imaging of the outer retina and inner choroid may be possible, leading to improved understanding of the nodular elevations and other changes observed on spectral-domain OCT. EDI-OCT imaging along with tools such as OCTA may provide information on inner choroidal changes among patients with syphilis.

9.3.4 Treatment of Ocular and Systemic Syphilis

Penicillin G is considered to be the preferred drug for the treatment of all stages of syphilis. Based on the stage of syphilis, preparation, dosage, and length of treatment may vary. Penicillin G is available in benzathine, aqueous, procaine, and crystalline preparations. Treatment of secondary and tertiary syphilis is typically longer compared to primary syphilis. Ocular syphilis is treated similar to neurosyphilis since these sites have relatively impermeable blood barriers. Aqueous penicillin G (18–24 million units/day intravenous for 10–14 days) or procaine penicillin G (2.4 million units intramuscular once a day for 10–14 days) in combination with probenecid (500 mg four times a day orally) is preferred for ocular syphilis. Alternatively, ceftriaxone (2 g/day intravenous for 10–14 days) can be employed for patients with penicillin allergy [50]. Topical steroids can be used for anterior segment inflammation and keratitis. Systemic steroids may be used adjunctively for posterior uveitis with significant intraocular inflammation and vitritis [45].

9.4 Lyme Disease

Lyme disease is a multisystem infectious disease caused by a spirochete, *Borrelia burgdorferi*, and transmitted by the ticks of *Ixodes ricinus* complex [51]. This condition is endemic in more than 20 states in the USA as well as in Europe and parts of Asia [52]. In the USA, more than 93% cases have been reported from *Northeastern states* such as Connecticut, Delaware, and Massachusetts [53]. The incidence of Lyme disease is highest among boys in the age range of 5–9 years and persons of both sexes in the age range of 60–64 years with an overall annual incidence of 106.6/100,000 persons in the USA [54]. A number of studies from European countries such as Italy, Bulgaria, and Belgium have also shown a variable incidence rate based on the local vector population [55–57]. A number of cases have been reported from India and China highlighting the need for continuous surveillance in non-endemic areas as well [58, 59].

9.4.1 Systemic Features of Lyme Disease

Lyme disease consists of three clinical stages: early infection with localized erythema migrans (stage 1); systemic dissemination that presents with cardiac, neurological, and articular involvement (stage 2); and late or persistent infection (stage 3) [60–62]. Early signs and symptoms may develop within 3–30 days after a tick bite. Common features include fever, chills, headache, and fatigue. *Erythema migrans* (EM) is a typical rash that occurs at the site of the tick bite. EM occurs in 70–80% individuals and can reach a size of 12 inches or more. EM has a bull's eye appearance with partial central clearing and a bright red border. Systemic dissemination may present months after a tick bite. Common clinical features include neurological involvement which presents with headache and neck stiffness. Patients may present with *bilateral facial palsy*, ataxia, and myelitis. *Lyme carditis* may present with myocarditis or atrioventricular block. There may be severe, disabling arthritis or persistent chronic articular inflammation [52]. Patients with Lyme disease may also develop posttreatment Lyme disease syndrome (*chronic Lyme disease*), an obscure entity that presents with fatigue, pain, and joint or muscle ache [63].

9.4.2 Ocular Features of Lyme Disease

Ocular features of Lyme disease can occur during the early stage or in the late stage, several months to years after primary infection [64]. Conjunctivitis is the most common manifestation of Lyme disease and presents during the early stage of the disease. It may be associated with periorbital edema. Neuro-ophthalmic manifestations also occur early during the course of the infection [65]. Other ocular features during stage 2 (stage of systemic dissemination) include blepharospasm, endophthalmitis/panophthalmitis, cystoid macular edema, optic neuritis (Fig. 9.7), retinal vasculitis, Horner's syndrome, and Argyll-Robertson pupil. Conditions such as stromal/nummular keratitis, episcleritis, and orbital myositis occur during stage 3 of the disease (Table 9.3) [65–68].

Intermediate uveitis or posterior uveitis in Lyme disease may be accompanied by retinal vasculitis. Patients with Lyme disease may also present with lesions of multifocal choroiditis that appear as small, round, and punched-out along with variable vitreous inflammation [69]. Other posterior segment findings in Lyme disease include acute exudative polymorphous vitelliform maculopathy (AEPVM) [70], neuroretinitis, and inflammatory choroidal neovascularization. Orbital myositis may present with thickening of extraocular muscles, lid edema, proptosis, ptosis, or dacryoadenitis.

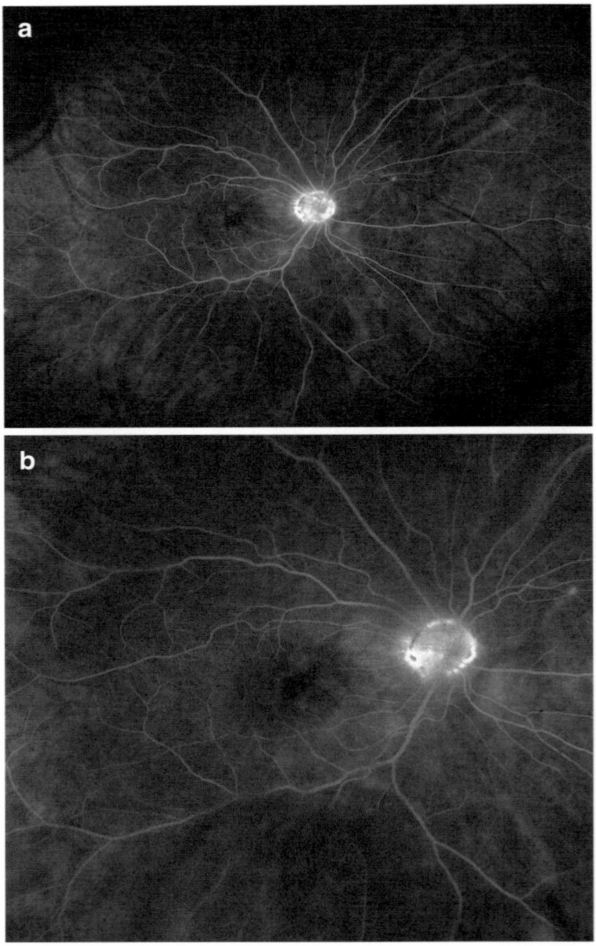

Fig. 9.7 Fluorescein angiography (FA) of a patient with Lyme disease-related optic neuritis, retinal vasculitis, and macular edema. Ultrawide-field FA (**a**) shows disk hyperfluorescence in the late phase, cystoid macular edema, and peripheral focal vascular leakage (predominantly venular). Magnified view (**b**) shows presence of optic neuritis and macular edema

Table 9.3 Ocular features of Lyme disease

Stage of the disease	Ocular features
1	Conjunctivitis, periorbital edema
2	Blepharospasm, uveitis (iridocyclitis/iritis), panophthalmitis, choroiditis, optic disk edema, macular edema, optic neuritis, pseudotumor cerebri, ischemic optic neuropathy, optic atrophy, Horner's syndrome, Argyll-Robertson pupil
3	Corneal involvement (stromal/nummular keratitis), episcleritis, orbital myositis, cortical blindness

9.4.3 Imaging Features

9.4.3.1 Fundus Photography

Among patients with Lyme disease, clinical fundus photography may be useful to document presence of vitreous haze. Choroidal lesions of Lyme disease appear as focal, punched-out lesions mostly involving the posterior pole and mid-periphery. There may be associated inflammatory choroidal neovascularization. Lesions of AEPVM present with multifocal serous retinal detachment and accumulation of deposits in the outer retinal layer [70].

9.4.3.2 Fluorescein Angiography

The appearance of chorioretinal lesions in Lyme disease on FA is similar to lesions of syphilis. Chorioretinal lesions demonstrate early hypofluorescence followed by late staining. Among patients with Lyme disease, FA may be useful to detect the presence of retinal vascular leakage due to vasculitis. Retinal vasculitis may be rarely associated with occlusion and ischemia. Optic nerve head hyperfluorescence suggests presence of optic neuritis (Fig. 9.7) [71, 72].

9.4.3.3 Optical Coherence Tomography

OCT imaging may help in characterizing the chorioretinal involvement in Lyme disease. OCT is useful in demonstrating swelling of the optic nerve head among patients with optic neuritis. Significant number of patients with Lyme disease may have cystoid macular edema that can be diagnosed and followed using OCT [67, 68].

9.4.4 Treatment of Lyme Disease

The treatment of Lyme disease consists of systemically administered antibiotics such as beta-lactams and tetracyclines along with corticosteroids [73]. Early Lyme disease that manifests with erythema migrans can be treated with oral doxycycline (100 mg twice a day), amoxicillin (500 mg three times a day), or cefuroxime axetil (500 mg twice a day) for 2 weeks. Macrolide antibiotics and first-generation cephalosporins such as cephalexin are not recommended for early Lyme disease. Drugs used in children include doxycycline (4–8 mg/kg/day) or amoxicillin (50 mg/kg/day) [73].

Intravenous route of administration may be employed for patients with neurological manifestations and advanced disease affecting the cardiovascular system. The treatment regimen consists of ceftriaxone or cefotaxime 2 g/day for 2–4 weeks [73–75]. There are no guidelines available in literature that guide therapy for ocular Lyme disease. Treatment of ocular disease depends on disappearance of serum antibody titers. Concomitant systemic or topical corticosteroids can be used to treat associated inflammation.

9.5 Cat Scratch Disease

Cat scratch disease (CSD) is also known as bartonellosis. CSD is a zoonotic infection caused by a gram-negative bacillus, *Bartonella henselae*. Domestic cats serve as the primary mammalian reservoir of this organism. *Ctenocephalides felis* (cat flea) is the arthropod vector that spreads the disease. Human infection is usually caused by scratch from an infected cat or contamination of surface wounds [76, 77]. The worldwide seroprevalence of this condition is estimated to be approximately 20%. Annual incidence of CSD based on national outpatient database in the USA is estimated to be 9.3/100,000 [78]. A pooled analysis of a large number of CSD cases was performed in Turkey [79]. In a small study conducted in Italy, 21% patients awaiting heart transplant were diagnosed to be seropositive for *B. henselae* [80].

9.5.1 Systemic Features of Cat Scratch Disease

CSD is commonly seen in children and young adults. The condition starts with a vesicular eruption at the site of inoculation. Following dissemination of the organism, tender regional lymphadenopathy develops within 1–2 weeks. Other systemic features include malaise, fever, anorexia, and arthralgia. Visceral involvement may present with hepatosplenomegaly. Rarely, CSD may present with meningoencephalitis, seizures, headache, and other neurological complaints. Cardiac involvement may present with endocarditis. Among immunocompromised subjects, CSD may present with a characteristic systemic features such as *bacillary angiomatosis* and peliosis. Bacillary angiomatoses are vascular proliferative lesions that appear red/purple papules on the skin and mucous membranes. These resemble vascular lesions of Kaposi's sarcoma [81, 82]. *Peliosis hepatitis* is an uncommon presentation with abdominal pain, nausea, and vomiting due to vascular lesions in the liver [83, 84].

9.5.2 Ocular Features of Cat Scratch Disease

Ocular manifestations of CSD can be divided into two categories: primary involvement (*Parinaud oculoglandular syndrome*) or secondary involvement due to systemic dissemination of the disease. Parinaud oculoglandular syndrome manifests with conjunctivitis, conjunctival granulomas, stromal keratitis, and orbital inflammation. Neuro-ophthalmic manifestations include optic nerve head edema, *neuroretinitis* [85], and inflammatory mass lesions involving the optic nerve. Retinochoroidal inflammation may manifest as juxtapapillary chorioretinitis that appear as cotton-wool spots. There may be accompanying satellite lesions in the retina. Vascular abnormalities such as angiomatous-like proliferation (similar to bacillary angiomatosis) (Fig. 9.8), branch retinal arteriole occlusion, or retinal vasculitis may be seen on careful examination. Other ocular features of CSD include serous retinal detachment, panuveitis, and intermediate uveitis [86, 87].

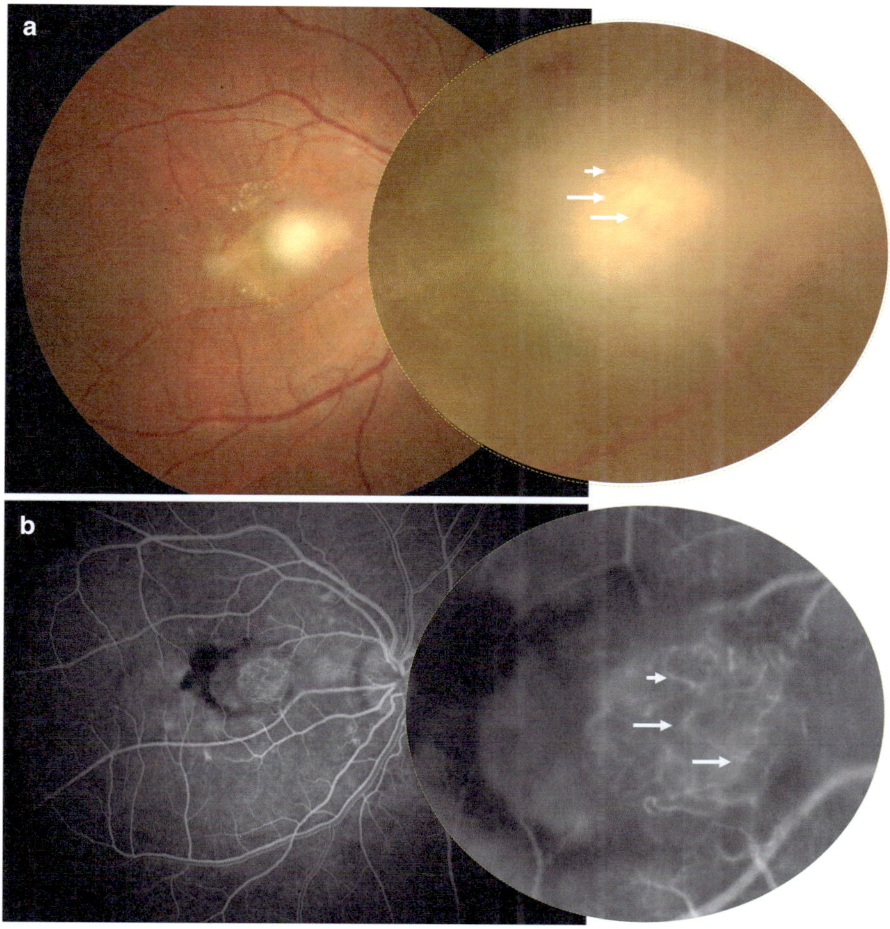

Fig. 9.8 Fundus photography and fluorescein angiography (FA) of a patient with cat scratch disease. A *yellowish-white* lesion with fuzzy edges, surrounding exudation, subretinal fluid, and internal limiting membrane wrinkling is seen on color fundus photography (**a**). Magnified view shows characteristic vascular pattern within the lesion. FA (early transit phase) (**b**) shows hyperfluorescence of the lesion with surrounding focal areas of hyperfluorescence (satellite lesions). Magnified view shows characteristic pattern of vascular proliferation reminiscent of bacillary angiomatosis

9.5.3 Imaging Features

9.5.3.1 Fundus Photography and Autofluorescence

Chorioretinal lesions of CSD can be documented using color fundus photography. Neuroretinitis presents with optic nerve head edema with a macular star formation due to exudation. In addition, internal limiting membrane wrinkling may be observed. Lesions of retinitis may appear dark on FAF because of blockade of the normal RPE autofluorescence due to the overlying retinitis lesion.

9.5.3.2 Fluorescein and Indocyanine Green Angiography

Lesions of CSD present with abnormal dye leakage on FA. In the early phase, juxtapapillary granulomas of CSD may present with dye leakage on FA. Abnormal retinal vascular patterns reminiscent of bacillary angiomatosis may be observed on FA [88]. Occasionally, chorioretinal lesions may present with only late leakage [89]. Other features seen on FA include cystoid macular edema, retinal vasculitis, and satellite lesions (Figs. 9.8 and 9.9). Atypical presentations of CSD on FA include retinal non-perfusion due to occlusive vasculitis [90]. Optic neuritis manifests as optic disk hyperfluorescence, which may be rarely associated with optic nerve neovascularization [91]. Serous retinal detachment may result in extensive pooling of the dye in the posterior pole or in the peripapillary region.

ICGA features of CSD include diffuse choroidal leakage and hypofluorescence in the region corresponding to the subretinal granulomas. However, the leakage observed on ICGA is typically lesser in amount compared to FA [88]. In addition, patients with optic neuritis may show hyperfluorescence of the optic nerve head on ICGA.

9.5.3.3 Optical Coherence Tomography

OCT is a useful imaging modality in the management of patients with CSD that helps in the characterization of retinitis lesions and detection of subretinal/choroidal neovascularization [92]. Serous retinal detachment or intraretinal fluid accumulation leading to macular edema can be seen on macular OCT. [93] Chorioretinal lesions of CSD appear as hyper-reflective deposits in the inner retinal layers with shadowing on the posterior retinal layers and the choroid (Fig. 9.10). Such changes are known to progressively diminish with antibiotic therapy [94].

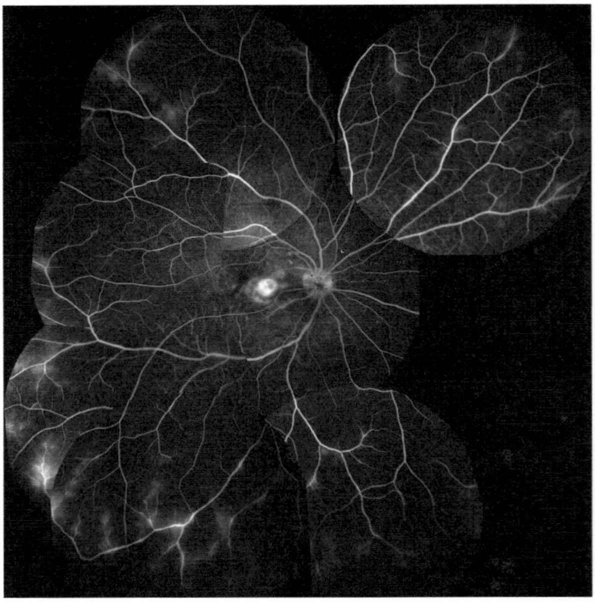

Fig. 9.9 Montage view of fluorescein angiography of a patient with cat scratch disease shows presence of significant peripheral vascular leakage suggestive of active vasculitis

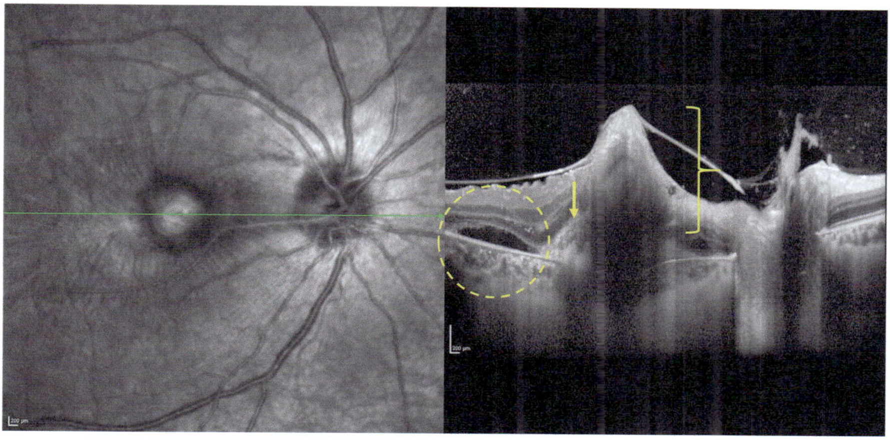

Fig. 9.10 Enhanced-depth imaging optical coherence tomography (EDI-OCT) of a patient with cat scratch disease shows presence of vitreous inflammation, full-thickness retinal involvement (*square bracket*), subretinal hyper-reflective material suggestive of choroidal neovascularization (*yellow arrow*), and subretinal fluid (*dashed circle*)

9.5.4 Treatment of Cat Scratch Disease

Treatment of CSD consists of systemic antibiotics. Concomitant corticosteroids (topical or oral prednisone) may be used for ocular CSD in the presence of severe inflammatory reaction. Antibiotics commonly employed in CSD include azithromycin, trimethoprim-sulfamethoxazole, ciprofloxacin, gentamicin, and rifampin [95]. Recommended therapy consists of azithromycin for patients with moderate to severe disease. For immunocompetent patients with mild to moderate disease, no antibiotic treatment may have a higher benefit-to-risk ratio. Among patients with severe disease, or immunocompromised status, combination of intravenous or oral doxycycline (100 mg twice daily) and rifampin (300 mg twice daily) may be used [96]. However, a recent report suggests that antibiotic therapy may not significantly affect the cure rate or the time to achieve cure among patients with CSD [95].

9.6 Future Directions

In the past decade, a number of advances have been made in the field of retinal and choroidal imaging. There has been an increasing trend toward the development of noninvasive and ultrahigh-speed imaging tools that can provide novel information about various uveitic entities. Systemic infections such as tuberculosis and syphilis commonly involve the choroid, which is often difficult to image using conventional modalities. Thus far, ICGA was the only tool to assess involvement of choroid and deeper structures. However, introduction of EDI-OCT, and more recently the swept-source OCT, is likely to greatly supplement conventional dye-based techniques such as ICGA in the evaluation of such clinical entities. The novel technology of OCTA also appears to be very useful in the management of intraocular tuberculosis. With the help of next-generation imaging technologies and availability of advanced image analysis software in the future, it is hoped that fast, noninvasive office procedures would provide detailed information regarding the pathology of ocular involvement in systemic infections.

Key Learning Points

- Systemic infectious diseases such as tuberculosis, syphilis, and cat scratch disease can have protean ophthalmic features that may lead to diagnostic challenges.
- Ancillary imaging tools such as fluorescein angiography, indocyanine green angiography, and optical coherence tomography, among others, are indispensable tools in the complete evaluation of patients with uveitis in order to establish accurate diagnosis and assess severity of the disease.
- Serial imaging using these techniques may enable precise assessment of response to therapy. This can be achieved noninvasively using modern techniques such as optical coherence tomography.
- With the development of advanced imaging technology such as swept-source optical coherence tomography and optical coherence tomography angiography, newer insights into the pathophysiology of diseases such as tuberculosis have been highlighted in literature.
- Further research in the field of retinal and choroidal imaging is likely to improve our understanding of the natural history of systemic infectious diseases that affect various ocular structures.

Financial Support The authors have no financial disclosure/proprietary interest. No conflicting relationship exists for any author.

This work was partly supported by a grant from the Department of Science and Technology, India, for the development of Centre of Excellence at the Advanced Eye Centre, PGIMER, Chandigarh.

References

1. Singh R, Gupta V, Gupta A. Pattern of uveitis in a referral eye clinic in north India. Indian J Ophthalmol. 2004;52(2):121–5.
2. Gupta A, Gupta V. Tubercular posterior uveitis. Int Ophthalmol Clin. 2005;45(2):71–88.
3. Hooper C, McCluskey P. Intraocular inflammation: its causes and investigations. Curr Allergy Asthma Rep. 2008;8(4):331–8.
4. WHO. Guidelines on the management of latent tuberculosis infection. Geneva: World Health Organization; 2015.
5. Global Health Observatory (GHO) data. 2014. http://www.who.int/gho/tb/en/. Accessed 27 Apr 2016.
6. Behr MA, Waters WR. Is tuberculosis a lymphatic disease with a pulmonary portal? Lancet. 2014;14(3):250–5.

7. Narendran G, Swaminathan S. TB-HIV co-infection: a catastrophic comradeship. Oral Dis. 2016;22(Suppl 1):46–52.
8. Balasubramanian V, Wiegeshaus EH, Taylor BT, Smith DW. Pathogenesis of tuberculosis: pathway to apical localization. Tuber Lung Dis. Jun 1994;75(3):168–78.
9. Lara LP, Ocampo V Jr. Prevalence of presumed ocular tuberculosis among pulmonary tuberculosis patients in a tertiary hospital in the Philippines. J Ophthal Inflamm Infect. 2013; 3(1):1.
10. Gupta V, Shoughy SS, Mahajan S, et al. Clinics of ocular tuberculosis. Ocul Immunol Inflamm. 2015;23(1):14–24.
11. Gupta V, Gupta A, Rao NA. Intraocular tuberculosis--an update. Surv Ophthalmol. 2007;52(6):561–87.
12. Gupta A, Bansal R, Gupta V, Sharma A, Bambery P. Ocular signs predictive of tubercular uveitis. Am J Ophthalmol. 2010;149(4):562–70.
13. Bansal R, Gupta A, Gupta V, Dogra MR, Sharma A, Bambery P. Tubercular serpiginous-like choroiditis presenting as multifocal serpiginoid choroiditis. Ophthalmology. 2012;119(11):2334–42.
14. Gupta V, Gupta A, Arora S, Bambery P, Dogra MR, Agarwal A. Presumed tubercular serpiginouslike choroiditis: clinical presentations and management. Ophthalmology. 2003;110(9):1744–9.
15. Nazari Khanamiri H, Rao NA. Serpiginous choroiditis and infectious multifocal serpiginoid choroiditis. Surv Ophthalmol. 2013;58(3):203–32.
16. Zhang M, Zhang J, Liu Y. Clinical presentations and therapeutic effect of presumed choroidal tuberculosis. Retina. 2012;32(4):805–13.
17. Biswas J, Madhavan HN, Gopal L, Badrinath SS. Intraocular tuberculosis. Clinicopathologic study of five cases. Retina. 1995;15(6):461–8.
18. Babu RB, Sudharshan S, Kumarasamy N, Therese L, Biswas J. Ocular tuberculosis in acquired immunodeficiency syndrome. Am J Ophthalmol. 2006;142(3):413–8.
19. Sudharshan S, Kaleemunnisha S, Banu AA, et al. Ocular lesions in 1,000 consecutive HIV-positive patients in India: a long-term study. J Ophthalm Inflamm Infect. 2013;3(1):2.
20. Gupta A, Bansal R, Gupta V, Sharma A. Fundus autofluorescence in serpiginouslike choroiditis. Retina. 2012;32(4):814–25.
21. Aggarwal K, Mulkutkar S, Mahajan S, et al. Role of ultra-wide field imaging in the management of tubercular posterior uveitis. Ocul Immunol Inflamm. 2016;6:1–6.
22. Wolfensberger TJ, Piguet B, Herbort CP. Indocyanine green angiographic features in tuberculous chorioretinitis. Am J Ophthalmol. 1999;127(3):350–3.
23. De Luigi G, Mantovani A, Papadia M, Herbort CP. Tuberculosis-related choriocapillaritis (multifocal-serpiginous choroiditis): follow-up and precise monitoring of therapy by indocyanine green angiography. Int Ophthalmol. 2012;32(1):55–60.
24. Invernizzi A, Agarwal A, Cozzi M, Viola F, Nguyen QD, Staurenghi G. Enhanced depth imaging optical coherence tomography features in areas of choriocapillaris hypoperfusion. Retina. 2016;36(10):2013–21.
25. Punjabi OS, Rich R, Davis JL, et al. Imaging serpiginous choroidopathy with spectral domain optical coherence tomography. Ophthalmic Surg Lasers Imaging. 2008;39(4 Suppl):S95–8.
26. Rifkin LM, Munk MR, Baddar D, Goldstein DA. A new OCT finding in tuberculous serpiginous-like choroidopathy. Ocul Immunol Inflamm. 2015;23(1):53–8.
27. Bansal R, Kulkarni P, Gupta A, Gupta V, Dogra MR. High-resolution spectral domain optical coherence tomography and fundus autofluorescence correlation in tubercular serpiginouslike choroiditis. J Ophthalm Inflamm Infect. 2011;1(4):157–63.
28. Salman A, Parmar P, Rajamohan M, Vanila CG, Thomas PA, Jesudasan CA. Optical coherence tomography in choroidal tuberculosis. Am J Ophthalmol. 2006;142(1):170–2.
29. Invernizzi A, Mapelli C, Viola F, et al. Choroidal granulomas visualized by enhanced depth imaging optical coherence tomography. Retina. 2015;35(3):525–31.
30. Mandadi SK, Agarwal A, Aggarwal K, Moharana B, Singh R, Sharma A, Bansal R, Dogra MR, Gupta V. For OCTA Study Group. Novel findings on optical coherence tomography

angiography in patients with tubercular serpiginous-like choroiditis. Retina. 2016 Dec 7. [Epub ahead of print].
31. Yee HYM, Keane PAF, Ho SLF, Agrawal RF. Optical coherence tomography angiography of choroidal neovascularization associated with tuberculous serpiginous-like choroiditis. Ocular Immunol Inflamm. 2016;30:1–3.
32. Marks SM, Hirsch-Moverman Y, Salcedo K, et al. Characteristics and costs of multidrug-resistant tuberculosis in-patient care in the United States, 2005–2007. IntJ Tuber Lung Dis. 2016;20(4):435–41.
33. Tiberi S, Sotgiu G, D'Ambrosio L, et al. Comparison of effectiveness and safety of imipenem/clavulanate- versus meropenem/clavulanate-containing regimens in the treatment of MDR- and XDR-TB. Eur Respir J. 2016;47(6):1758–66.
34. Sotgiu G, D'Ambrosio L, Centis R, et al. Carbapenems to treat multidrug and extensively drug-resistant tuberculosis: a systematic review. Int J Mol Sci. 2016;17(3):373.
35. Sharma K, Sharma A, Bansal R, Fiorella PD, Gupta A. Drug-Resistant Tubercular Uveitis. J Clin Microbiol. Nov 2014;52(11):4113–4.
36. Gupta V, Bansal R, Gupta A. Continuous progression of tubercular serpiginous-like choroiditis after initiating antituberculosis treatment. Am J Ophthalmol. 2011;152(5):857–863.e852.
37. Eickhoff CA, Decker CF. Syphilis. Dis Mon. 2016;62:280–6.
38. Mitja O, Asiedu K, Mabey D. Yaws. Lancet. 2013;381(9868):763–73.
39. Berger JR, Dean D. Neurosyphilis. Handb Clin Neurol. 2014;121:1461–72.
40. Lynn WA, Lightman S. Syphilis and HIV: a dangerous combination. Lancet. 2004;4(7):456–66.
41. Centers for Disease Control and Prevention (CDC). Outbreak of syphilis among men who have sex with men--Southern California, 2000. MMWR Morb Mortal Wkly Rep. 2001;50(7):117–20.
42. Davis JL. Ocular syphilis. Curr Opin Ophthalmol. 2014;25(6):513–8.
43. Yang P, Zhang N, Li F, Chen Y, Kijlstra A. Ocular manifestations of syphilitic uveitis in Chinese patients. Retina. 2012;32(9):1906–14.
44. Doris JP, Saha K, Jones NP, Sukthankar A. Ocular syphilis: the new epidemic. Eye. 2006;20(6):703–5.
45. Chao JR, Khurana RN, Fawzi AA, Reddy HS, Rao NA. Syphilis: reemergence of an old adversary. Ophthalmology. 2006;113(11):2074–9.
46. Eandi CM, Neri P, Adelman RA, Yannuzzi LA, Cunningham ET Jr. Acute syphilitic posterior placoid chorioretinitis: report of a case series and comprehensive review of the literature. Retina. 2012;32(9):1915–41.
47. Matsumoto Y, Spaide RF. Autofluorescence imaging of acute syphilitic posterior placoid chorioretinitis. Retinal Cases Brief Rep. 2007;1(3):123–7.
48. Brito P, Penas S, Carneiro A, Palmares J, Reis FF. Spectral-domain optical coherence tomography features of acute syphilitic posterior placoid chorioretinitis: the role of autoimmune response in pathogenesis. Case Rep Ophthalmol. 2011;2(1):39–44.
49. Pichi F, Ciardella AP, Cunningham ET Jr, et al. Spectral domain optical coherence tomography findings in patients with acute syphilitic posterior placoid chorioretinopathy. Retina. 2014;34(2):373–84.
50. Clement ME, Okeke NL, Hicks CB. Treatment of syphilis: a systematic review. JAMA. 2014;312(18):1905–17.
51. Lane RS, Piesman J, Burgdorfer W. Lyme borreliosis: relation of its causative agent to its vectors and hosts in North America and Europe. Annu Rev. Entomol. 1991;36:587–609.
52. Steere AC. Lyme disease. N Engl J Med. 2001;345(2):115–25.
53. Bacon RM, Kugeler KJ, Mead PS. Surveillance for Lyme disease--United States, 1992–2006. Morb Mortal Wkly Rep. 2008;57(10):1–9.
54. Nelson CA, Saha S, Kugeler KJ, et al. Incidence of clinician-diagnosed lyme disease, United States, 2005–2010. Emerg Infect Dis. 2015;21(9):1625–31.
55. Cimmino MA, Fumarola D, Sambri V, Accardo S. The epidemiology of Lyme borreliosis in Italy. Microbiologica. 1992;15(4):419–24.

56. Christova I, Komitova R. Clinical and epidemiological features of Lyme borreliosis in Bulgaria. Wien Klin Wochenschr. 2004;116(1–2):42–6.
57. Bleyenheuft C, Lernout T, Berger N, et al. Epidemiological situation of Lyme borreliosis in Belgium, 2003 to 2012. Arch Public Health. 2015;73(1):33.
58. Dou XF, Lyu YN, Jiang Y, et al. Lyme borreliosis-associated risk factors in residents of Beijing suburbs: a preliminary case-control study. Biomed Environ Sci. 2014;27(10):807–10.
59. Jairath V, Sehrawat M, Jindal N, Jain VK, Aggarwal P. Lyme disease in Haryana, India. Ind J Dermatol Venereol Leprol. 2014;80(4):320–3.
60. Sanchez JL. Clinical manifestations and treatment of lyme disease. Clin Lab Med. 2015;35(4):765–78.
61. Hoppa E, Bachur R. Lyme disease update. Curr Opin Pediatr. 2007;19(3):275–80.
62. Chomel B. Lyme disease. Rev Sci Tech. 2015;34(2):569–76.
63. Halperin JJ. Chronic Lyme disease: misconceptions and challenges for patient management. Infect Drug Resist. 2015;8:119–28.
64. Raja H, Starr MR, Bakri SJ. Ocular manifestations of tick-borne diseases. Surv Ophthalmol. 2016;61(6):726–44.
65. Winterkorn JM. Lyme disease: neurologic and ophthalmic manifestations. Surv Ophthalmol. 1990;35(3):191–204.
66. Balcer LJ, Winterkorn JM, Galetta SL. Neuro-ophthalmic manifestations of Lyme disease. J Neuroophthalmol. 1997;17(2):108–21.
67. Bergloff J, Gasser R, Feigl B. Ophthalmic manifestations in Lyme borreliosis. A review. J Neuroophthalmol. 1994;14(1):15–20.
68. Park M. Ocular manifestations of Lyme disease. J Am Optom Assoc. 1989;60(4):284–9.
69. Lardenoye CW, Van der Lelij A, de Loos WS, Treffers WF, Rothova A. Peripheral multifocal chorioretinitis: a distinct clinical entity? Ophthalmology. 1997;104(11):1820–6.
70. Singh RS, Tran LH, Kim JE. Acute exudative polymorphous vitelliform maculopathy in a patient with Lyme disease. Ophthal Surg Lasers Imag Retina. 2013;44(5):493–6.
71. Karma A, Mikkila H. Ocular manifestations and treatment of Lyme disease. Curr Opin Ophthalmol. 1996;7(3):7–12.
72. Karma A, Seppala I, Mikkila H, Kaakkola S, Viljanen M, Tarkkanen A. Diagnosis and clinical characteristics of ocular Lyme borreliosis. Am J Ophthalmol. 1995;119(2):127–35.
73. Wormser GP, Dattwyler RJ, Shapiro ED, et al. The clinical assessment, treatment, and prevention of lyme disease, human granulocytic anaplasmosis, and babesiosis: clinical practice guidelines by the Infectious Diseases Society of America. Clin Infect Dis. 2006;43(9):1089–134.
74. Wright WF, Riedel DJ, Talwani R, Gilliam BL. Diagnosis and management of Lyme disease. Am Fam Physician. 2012;85(11):1086–93.
75. Bratton RL, Whiteside JW, Hovan MJ, Engle RL, Edwards FD. Diagnosis and treatment of Lyme disease. Mayo Clin Proc. 2008;83(5):566–71.
76. Mogollon-Pasapera E, Otvos L Jr, Giordano A, Cassone M. Bartonella: emerging pathogen or emerging awareness? Int J Infect Dis. 2009;13(1):3–8.
77. Pretorius AM, Kelly PJ. An update on human bartonelloses. Central African J Med. 2000;46(7):194–200.
78. McElroy KM, Blagburn BL, Breitschwerdt EB, Mead PS, McQuiston JH. Flea-associated zoonotic diseases of cats in the USA: bartonellosis, flea-borne rickettsioses, and plague. Trends Parasitol. 2010;26(4):197–204.
79. Ulug M. Evaluation of cat scratch disease cases reported from Turkey between 1996 and 2013 and review of the literature. Cent Eur J Public Health. 2015;23(2):170–5.
80. Picascia A, Pagliuca C, Sommese L, et al. Seroprevalence of Bartonella henselae in patients awaiting heart transplant in southern Italy. J Microbiol Immunol Infect. 2017;50(2):239–44.
81. Maguina C, Guerra H, Ventosilla P. Bartonellosis. Clin Dermatol. 2009;27(3):271–80.
82. Batsakis JG, Ro JY, Frauenhoffer EE. Bacillary angiomatosis. Ann Otol Rhinol Laryngol. 1995;104(8):668–72.
83. Crocetti D, Palmieri A, Pedulla G, Pasta V, D'Orazi V, Grazi GL. Peliosis hepatis: personal experience and literature review. World J Gastroenterol. 2015;21(46):13188–94.

84. DeLeve LD. Vascular liver diseases. Curr Gastroenterol Rep. 2003;5(1):63–70.
85. Lezrek O, Laghmari M, Jait A, El Atiqi A, Lezrek M, Daoudi R. Neuroretinitis in ocular bartonellosis. J Pediatr. 2015;166(2):496–496.e491.
86. Ormerod LD, Skolnick KA, Menosky MM, Pavan PR, Pon DM. Retinal and choroidal manifestations of cat-scratch disease. Ophthalmology. 1998;105(6):1024–31.
87. Biancardi AL, Curi AL. Cat-scratch disease. Ocul Immunol Inflamm. 2014;22(2):148–54.
88. Matsuo T, Yamaoka A, Shiraga F, et al. Clinical and angiographic characteristics of retinal manifestations in cat scratch disease. Jpn J Ophthalmol. 2000;44(2):182–6.
89. Curi AL, Machado DO, Heringer G, Campos WR, Orefice F. Ocular manifestation of cat-scratch disease in HIV-positive patients. Am J Ophthalmol. 2006;141(2):400–1.
90. Gray AV, Reed JB, Wendel RT, Morse LS. Bartonella henselae infection associated with peripapillary angioma, branch retinal artery occlusion, and severe vision loss. Am J Ophthalmol. 1999;127(2):223–4.
91. Mason JO III. Retinal and optic nerve neovascularization associated with cat scratch neuroretinitis. Retina. 2004;24(1):176–8.
92. Latanza L, Viscogliosi F, Solimeo A, Calabro F, De Angelis V, De Rosa PS. Choroidal neovascularisation as an unusual ophthalmic manifestation of cat-scratch disease in an 8-year-old girl. Int Ophthalmol. 2015;35(5):709–16.
93. Manousaridis K, Peter S, Mennel S. Cat-scratch-disease-associated macular oedema treated with intravitreal ranibizumab. Acta Ophthalmol. 2015;93(2):e168–70.
94. Empeslidis T, Tsaousis KT, Konidaris V, Pradeep A, Deane J. Multifocal chorioretinitis caused by Bartonella henselae: imaging findings of spectral domain optical coherence tomography during treatment with trimethoprim-sulfamethoxazole. Eye. 2014;28(7):907–9.
95. Prutsky G, Domecq JP, Mori L, et al. Treatment outcomes of human bartonellosis: a systematic review and meta-analysis. Int J Infect Dis. 2013;17(10):e811–9.
96. Rolain JM, Brouqui P, Koehler JE, Maguina C, Dolan MJ, Raoult D. Recommendations for treatment of human infections caused by Bartonella species. Antimicrob Agents Chemother. 2004;48(6):1921–33.

Imaging of Retinal and Choroidal Metastases

10

Akshay Gopinathan Nair, David Fell, Sherief Raouf, and Swathi Kaliki

Abstract

The eye like any other organ in the body can harbor tumors of different types. Given the diverse anatomy of the eye, each distinct structure within the eye can be the site for primary tumors; that is, those tumors arising from the native tissue or metastatic tumors: those that arise from a distant site in the body. With reference to the eye and adnexa, metastatic tumors have been documented in the orbit, the extraocular muscles, conjunctiva, subconjunctival tissue, iris, and the retina with the most common site being the choroid [1]. This chapter presents in detail the clinical presentation, diagnosis, imaging findings, and treatment of retinal and choroidal metastases.

The eye like any other organ in the body can harbor tumors of different types. Given the diverse anatomy of the eye, each distinct structure within the eye can be the site for primary tumors; that is, those tumors arising from the native tissue or metastatic tumors: those that arise from a distant site in the body. With reference to the eye and adnexa, metastatic tumors have been documented in the orbit, the extraocular muscles, conjunctiva, subconjunctival tissue, iris, and the retina with the most common site being the choroid [1]. This chapter presents in detail the clinical presentation, diagnosis, imaging findings, and treatment of retinal and choroidal metastases.

A.G. Nair
Ophthalmic Plastic Surgery and Ocular Oncology Services, Advanced Eye Hospital and Institute, Navi Mumbai, India

D. Fell • S. Raouf
Stony Brook School of Medicine, Stony Brook University, New York, NY, USA

S. Kaliki (✉)
The Operation Eyesight Universal Institute for Eye Cancer, L V Prasad Eye Institute, Hyderabad, India
e-mail: swathikaliki@lvpei.org

J. Chhablani et al. (eds.), *Retinal and Choroidal Imaging in Systemic Diseases*,
https://doi.org/10.1007/978-981-10-5461-7_10

10.1 Epidemiology

10.1.1 Choroidal Metastases

Once considered a rare manifestation of systemic pathology, ocular metastatic lesions have for several decades been appreciated to be more prevalent than initially thought. The choroid is the most common site of metastatic lesions to the eye, and it is theorized that the highly perfused choroid vasculature is a source of hematogenous dissemination of tumors. In addition, the venous oxygen concentration of the choroid is only a few percent lower than that of pre-capillary arterioles, making the choroid particularly hospitable to metastatic lesion growth [1]. One large-scale study of known uveal metastases showed that the choroid was the site of metastases in 88% of the cases [2]. The majority of choroidal metastases are carcinomas, with metastatic melanomas and sarcomas being far less common [3].

It is difficult to accurately estimate the true incidence of choroidal metastases: asymptomatic cases may not always be detected and also the treatment of disseminated systemic metastases to vital organs may take precedence over ophthalmic complaints in advanced cases. The reported incidence of choroidal metastases has been estimated in several studies that examined large pools of patients with known systemic cancer. These reports taken together posit an incidence of choroidal metastasis between 2% and 12.6% [4–8]. Within this variation, these studies have established reliable trends in the most common primary sites of choroidal metastasis. For women, by far the most frequent primary cancer is of the breast (40–47%). In male patients, lung cancer (21–29%) is the most common primary malignancy resulting in choroidal metastasis. These top two causes of choroidal metastasis are followed by gastrointestinal (3–6%), renal (1–4%), and dermatologic (2–4%) malignancies [2, 9–11]. In three-fourths of metastatic ocular lesions, involvement was unilateral [12]. There is evidence to suggest that choroidal metastases from the breast are more likely to be multifocal and bilateral while lesions stemming from primary lung cancers were more frequently unifocal and unilateral [2, 10].

10.1.2 Retinal Metastases

Isolated retinal metastases are extremely uncommon and because of the infrequency of their occurrence, the incidence of retinal metastases is difficult to ascertain. Large-scale studies of ocular metastases have demonstrated retinal metastases to constitute less than 1% of all metastases to the eye [2]. As such, the study of retinal metastases has largely been the subject matter of case reports. It is believed that lesions travel to the eye by way of the internal carotid artery. Retinal metastases arise from cutaneous malignant melanomas and systemic carcinomas (including lung, breast, and gastrointestinal tissues) [13–16].

Due to the rare occurrence of ocular metastatic disease in general, it is critical to rule these lesions out when evaluating intraocular tumors. Using a wide variety of ophthalmic imaging techniques in conjunction with each other, it is possible to differentiate choroidal and retinal metastatic disease from primary ocular cancers. This approach gives ophthalmologists and oncologists the ability to provide their patients with quick and accurate diagnosis and the greatest chance for remission.

10.2 Fundoscopic Imaging

10.2.1 Choroidal Metastases

Of all the ocular structures, the choroid is the most commonly affected by metastases [2]. There exists significant variability in the appearance of metastatic lesions of the eye, depending on the location of the tumor [2]. However, there is a significant consistency of appearance in metastatic lesions to the choroid in particular. Multiple studies have demonstrated converging evidence for a classically appearing choroidal metastatic lesion: a yellow/orange subretinal mass, (98% of cases) (Figs. 10.1 and 10.2) in

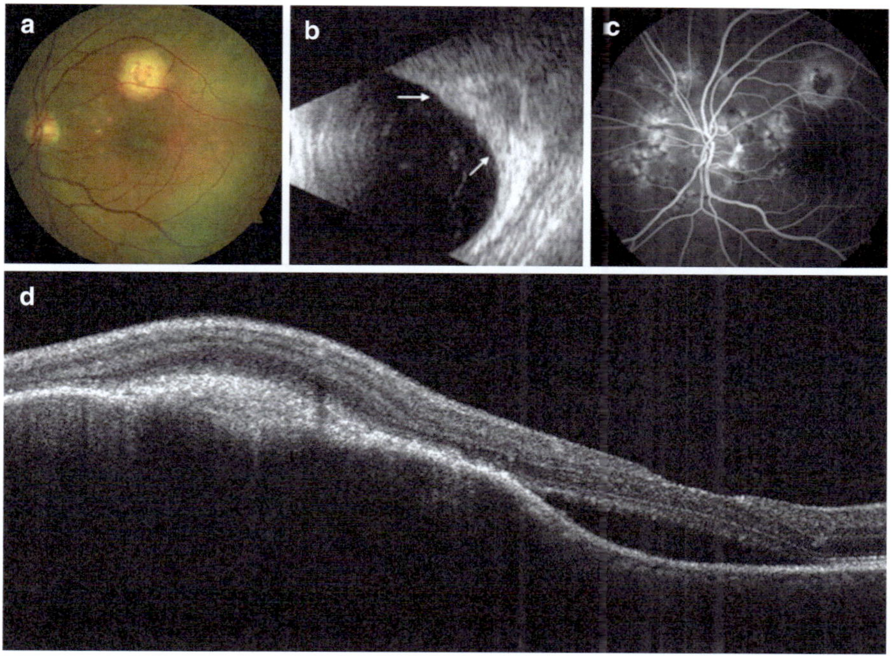

Fig. 10.1 (**a**) Color fundus photograph of a 78-year-old male with biopsy-proven adenocarcinoma of the lung showing yellowish subretinal deposits. Note the retinal vessels passing over the lesion indicating that the lesions are sub-retinal, i.e. choroidal in location. (**b**) Ultrasound B-scan showing acoustically solid thickening of choroid (*White arrows*) suggestive of choroidal metastases. (**c**) Fluorescein angiogram demonstrating the classical pinpoint leakage at the tumor border. The larger choroidal tumor is seen superior to the macula. Note the dilation of retinal capillaries at the edge of the lesion. (**d**) Enhanced depth optical coherence tomography image of the choroidal metastases. Note the irregular, undulating configuration of the choroidal lesion referred to as "lumpy-bumpy" appearance. Also note the adjacent subretinal fluid accumulation

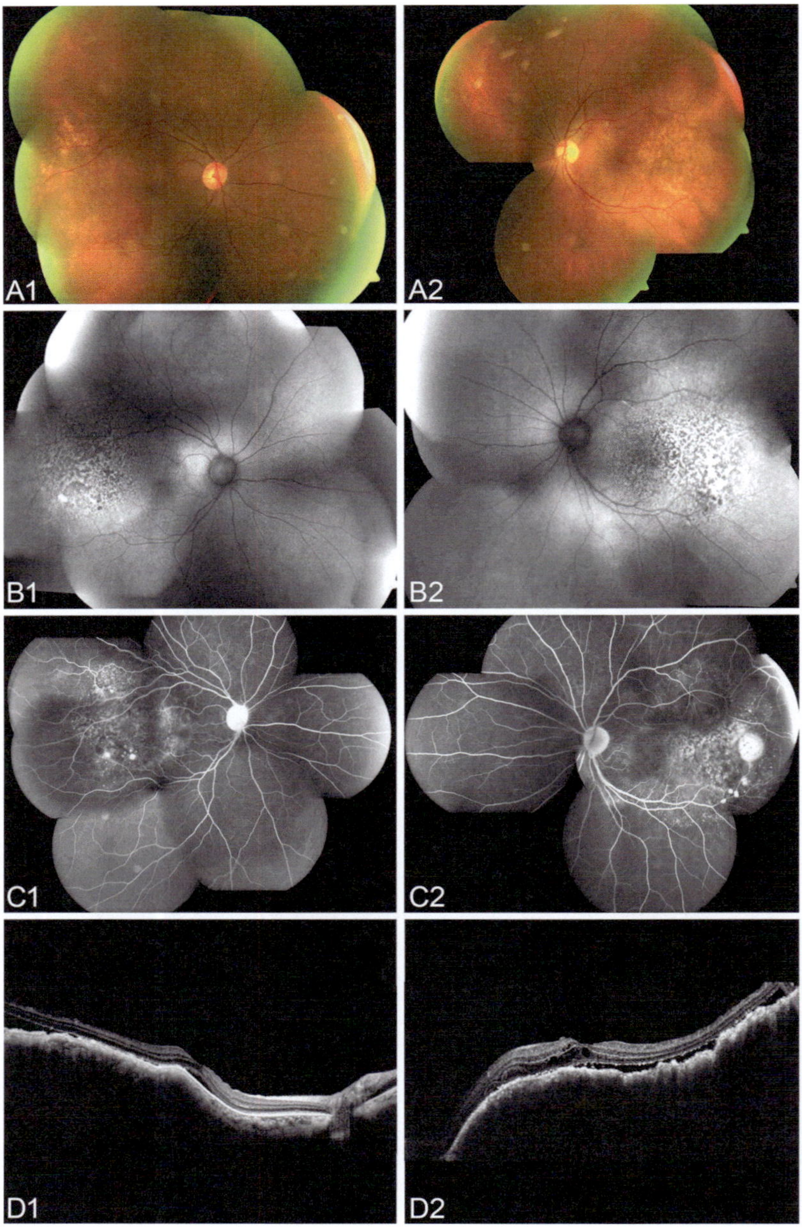

Fig. 10.2 A 57-year-old male with a history of lung adenocarcinoma with bilateral choroidal metastasis (**A1**) Color fundus photographs showing creamy yellow mass temporal to fovea in the right eye and (**A2**) in the macular region in the left eye (**B1**, **B2**) Fundus autofluorescence delineating the mass with hyper autofluorescence of the overlying lipofuscin pigment (**C1**, **C2**) Fluorescein angiography revealing hypoautofluorescence of the mass with overlying areas of staining and leakage (**D1**, **D2**) Enhanced depth imaging optical coherence tomography revealing lumpy bumpy appearance of anterior tumor surface

a plateau (61–77%) or dome configuration (23–38%) with accompanying subretinal fluid collection (64–85%) [2, 12, 17]. The average dimensions of choroidal metastatic lesions are measured to be a mean of 9 mm in basal diameter and 3 mm in thickness. The majority of the choroidal metastases were in the radial anatomical location between the macula and the equator (80%), with remaining lesions in the macula (12%) and in the radial space between the equator and the ora serrata (8%) [2].

10.2.2 Retinal Metastases

Because of the scarcity of documented metastatic disease of the retina, what is known of the fundoscopic appearance of these lesions has come from the accumulated case reports on this pathology. Difficulty in diagnosing retinal metastases comes from the fact that these lesions mimic retinitis in appearance. They are so rare that they are almost always originally misdiagnosed at first as inflammatory or infectious retinitis, or simply as a primary intraocular tumor [13]. There is some consensus that retinal lesions originating from primary carcinomas have a yellow-white appearance with perivascular infiltration [13, 18]. Associated changes that arise secondary to metastasis can include retinal hemorrhage, ischemia and even exudative detachment [13].

10.3 Ultrasonography

Ultrasound (B-scan) imaging has served an important role in intraocular imaging since its initial use in 1956 [19]. It gives practitioners a unique ability to visualize posterior structures in the eye in the presence of anterior opacities. There are specific ultrasonographic characteristics that can help to differentiate choroidal metastases from other tumors of the choroid, specifically choroidal melanoma. These differences are due to the patterns of growth that each of these lesions displays. While melanomas originate in a small area of choroid, grow outward toward and through Bruch's membrane, and assume a nodular, "mushroom-like" shape, metastases penetrate and diffusely replace a larger segment of the choroid. This results in a significantly lower height-to-base ratio observed in metastases (Fig. 10.1) as opposed to melanomas [20]. Because of the lack of detail in the layers of the retina, it is difficult to distinguish the exact location of the tumor whether the metastasis is in the choroid or superficial retina.

10.4 Optical Coherence Tomography (OCT)

10.4.1 Choroidal Metastases

Since its transition to a mainstay of ophthalmologic examination, OCT has given insight into the physiological details of conditions that are beyond the scope of external and funduscopic visualization. Though it is possible to diagnose choroidal and retinal metastases from history and funduscopic exam alone, OCT has given practitioners insight into qualities that separate metastases from other benign and malignant ocular lesions. Additionally, it has allowed for earlier diagnosis of metastatic lesions that may be too subtle for detection by conventional ultrasonography [21]. Though these tumors are often small and located parafoveally, the ability to evaluate choroidal metastases using OCT may be limited in the case of larger, more peripherally located tumors [22].

Early studies using time-domain OCT (TD-OCT) described thickening of the RPE and an undulating surface with clinically evident, overlying subretinal fluid, but failed to elaborate on characteristics of the tumor itself [23]. Studies since have used enhanced depth OCT (ED-OCT) imaging to evaluate the deeper layers of choroidal metastases. Choroidal metastases can be differentiated on OCT imaging by a "lumpy-bumpy" [22, 24, 25] appearance to their surface. In contrast, nevi and melanomas are usually described as having a "smooth, dome shaped topography" [22]. Metastatic choroidal lesions demonstrate compression and thinning of the choriocapillaris, a trait shared with choroidal nevi and melanoma, but which can help distinguish these lesions from choroidal hemangiomas [22, 24–27]. Subretinal lipofuscin deposition (in addition to subretinal fluid) and intraretinal edema were also common findings [22, 24–27]. Abnormalities of the RPE and the ellipsoid portion of photoreceptors have also been described, as well as "shaggy photoreceptors" and speckles within the previously established subretinal fluid (Figs. 10.1 and 10.2) [22, 26, 27]. The photoreceptor layer may also be anteriorly displaced [23]. Perhaps most importantly, OCT may be used to follow patients as they improve with treatment for their metastases. This includes resolution of subretinal fluid, restoration of choriocapillaris thickness, and smoothing of the photoreceptors [24].

10.4.2 Retinal Metastases

Though literature describing retinal metastases is few and far between, OCT has been used in rare cases to evaluate the fine characteristics of these tumors. Vertical OCT imaging of the lesion reveals "an inner retinal mass with outer retinal compression and contiguous edema." [18] Horizontal OCT imaging of the macula revealed exudative densities in the outer retina. The macula itself was spared in these lesions, but the presence of drusen was observed [18].

10.5 Fundus Fluorescein Angiography (FFA)

10.5.1 Choroidal Metastases

Intravenous FFA is the gold standard for evaluating retinal vasculature and plays a specific role in distinguishing choroidal metastases from choroidal melanoma. FFA of choroidal metastases demonstrates dilation of retinal capillaries with "pinpoint leakage at the tumor border," a trait less commonly seen in melanoma (Figs. 10.1 and 10.2) [28, 29]. Additionally, FFA demonstrates a hypoflurorescent arterial phase pattern with hyperfluorescence observed much later in the venous phase in metastases compared to melanoma [24, 28, 29]. This hyperfluorescence may vary from small irregular areas to bright, intrinsic vascularity seen in larger metastases [28]. The pinpoint leakages seen surrounding metastases on FA imaging holds an important role in differentiating metastatic lesions from primary melanomas as well. While a majority of choroidal metastases display this pattern of fluorescence, this observation is far less common in choroidal melanomas [28].

10.5.2 Retinal Metastases

FA imaging of retinal metastases reveals intrinsic vascularity and hemorrhage, resulting in hyperfluorescence [18].

10.6 Optical Coherence Tomography Angiography (OCTA)

Optical coherence tomography angiography is a novel imaging technique that utilizes the movement within vasculature in order to construct an angiogram of the retina. It has already been used to demonstrate choroidal neovascularization in age-related macular degeneration [30], as well as the vascular changes seen within the retina in diabetic retinopathy [31]. Though no research exists yet, examining the role that OCTA could play in diagnosing choroidal and retinal metastases, this will be an interesting area to explore given the changes in blood flow that occur in these tumors, as demonstrated by FFA.

10.7 Fundus Autofluorescence (FAF)

The technique of fundus autofluorescence (FAF) imaging relies on changes that occur within the RPE within a disease process. Choroidal metastases accumulate subretinal fluid as well as lipofuscin within the RPE leading to hyperfluorescent areas with hypofluorescent borders where there is RPE thickening [32–35]. These areas are not consistent throughout each lesion and there are varying direct correlations between the presence of both focal hyperpigmentation and subretinal fluid and the FAF patterns seen in these lesions [33, 34]. FAF patterns of choroidal metastases also show changes at their borders as these tumors grow [33].

Conclusion

Retinal and choroidal imaging plays a key role in the diagnosis of ocular diseases. Due to advances in different modes of imaging systems that highlight different facets of the disease process, clinicians can now take advantage of a combination of these imaging techniques that work together to ensure confidence in the diagnosis of choroidal and retinal metastases and allow patients to receive immediate and appropriate treatment, increasing overall survival.

References

1. Avram AM, Gielczyk R, Su L, Vine AK, Sisson JC. Choroidal and skin metastases from papillary thyroid cancer: case and a review of the literature. J Clin Endocrinol Metab. 2004;89(11):5303–7.
2. Shields CL, Shields JA, Gross NE, Schwartz GP, Lally SE. Survey of 520 eyes with uveal metastases. Ophthalmology. 1997;104(8):1265–76.
3. Shields CL. Plaque radiotherapy for the management of uveal metastasis. Curr Opin Ophthalmol. 1998;9(3):31–7.
4. Albert DM, Rubenstein RA, Scheie HG. Tumor metastasis to the eye. I. Incidence in 213 adult patients with generalized malignancy. Am J Ophthalmol. 1967;63(4):723–6.
5. Bloch RS, Gartner S. The incidence of ocular metastatic carcinoma. Arch Ophthalmol. 1971;85(6):673–5.
6. Eliassi-Rad B, Albert DM, Green WR. Frequency of ocular metastases in patients dying of cancer in eye bank populations. Br J Ophthalmol. 1996;80(2):125–8.
7. Kreusel K-M, Wiegel T, Stange M, Bornfeld N, Hinkelbein W, Foerster MH. Choroidal metastasis in disseminated lung cancer: frequency and risk factors. Am J Ophthalmol. 2002;134(3):445–7.
8. Shields JA, Shields CL, Scartozzi R. Survey of 1264 patients with orbital tumors and simulating lesions: the 2002 Montgomery lecture, part 1. Ophthalmology. 2004;111(5):997–1008.
9. Ferry AP, Font RL. Carcinoma metastatic to the eye and orbit. I. A clinicopathologic study of 227 cases. Arch Ophthalmol. 1974;92(4):276–86.
10. Freedman MI, Folk JC. Metastatic tumors to the eye and orbit. Patient survival and clinical characteristics. Arch Ophthalmol. 1987;105(9):1215–9.
11. Stephens RF, Shields JA. Diagnosis and management of cancer metastatic to the uvea: a study of 70 cases. Ophthalmology. 1979;86(7):1336–49.
12. Shah SU, Mashayekhi A, Shields CL, et al. Uveal metastasis from lung cancer: clinical features, treatment, and outcome in 194 patients. Ophthalmology. 2014;121(1):352–7.
13. Mack HG, Jakobiec FA. Isolated metastases to the retina or optic nerve. Int Ophthalmol Clin. 1997;37(4):251–60.
14. Klein R, Nicholson DH, Luxenberg MN. Retinal metastasis from squamous cell carcinoma of the lung. Am J Ophthalmol. 1977;83(3):358–61.
15. Letson AD, Davidorf FH. Bilateral retinal metastases from cutaneous malignant melanoma. Arch Ophthalmol. 1982;100(4):605–7.
16. Schmidt D, Ness T, Geissler M. Cotton-wool spots associated with pancreatic carcinoma. Eur J Med Res. 2001;6(3):101–4.
17. Demirci H, Shields CL, Chao A-N, Shields JA. Uveal metastasis from breast cancer in 264 patients. Am J Ophthalmol. 2003;136(2):264–71.
18. Shields CL, McMahon JF, Atalay HT, Hasanreisoglu M, Shields JA. Retinal metastasis from systemic cancer in 8 cases. JAMA Ophthalmol. 2014;132(11):1303–8.
19. Lizzi FL, Coleman DJ. History of ophthalmic ultrasound. J Ultrasound Med. 2004;23(10):1255–66.
20. Sobottka B, Schlote T, Krumpaszky HG, Kreissig I. Choroidal metastases and choroidal melanomas: comparison of ultrasonographic findings. Br J Ophthalmol. 1998;82:159–61.
21. Witkin AJ, Fischer DH, Shields CL, Reichstein D, Shields JA. Enhanced depth imaging spectral-domain optical coherence tomography of a subtle choroidal metastasis. Eye. 2012;26(12):1598–9.
22. Shields CL, Pellegrini M, Ferenczy S. Enhanced depth imaging optical coherence tomography of intraocular tumors: from placid to seasick to rock and rolling topography – the 2013 Francesco Orzalesi Lecture. Retina. 2014;34:1495–512.
23. Arevalo JF, Fernandez CF, Reinaldo GA. Optical coherence tomography characteristics of choroidal metastasis. Ophthalmology. 2005;112(9):1612–9.
24. Arepalli S, Kaliki S, Shields CL. Choroidal metastases: origin, features, and therapy. Indian J Ophthalmol. 2015;63(2):122–7.

25. Demirci H, Cullen A, Sundstrom JM. Enhanced depth imaging optical coherence tomography of choroidal metastasis. Retina. 2014;34(7):1354–9.
26. Shields CL, Manalac J, Chandana D, Saktanaste D. Review of spectral domain enhanced depth imaging optical coherence tomography of tumors of the choroid. Indian J Ophthalmol. 2015;63(2):117–22.
27. Al-Dahmash SA, Shields CL, Kaliki S, Johnson T, Shields JA. Enhanced depth imaging optical coherence tomography of choroidal metastasis in 14 eyes. Retina. 2014;34:1588–93.
28. Li L, Wang WJ, Chen RJ, Qian J, Luo CQ. Fundus fluorescein angiography in metastatic choroidal carcinomas and differentiating metastatic choroidal carcinomas from primary choroidal melanomas. Zhonghua Yan Ke Za Zhi. 2011;47(1):27–34.
29. Ditmar S, Holtz FG. Choroidal metastases. In: Fluorescence angiography in ophthalmology. Berlin: Springer; 2008. p. 214–5.
30. Jia Y, Bailey ST, Wilson DJ, Tan O. Quantitative optical coherence tomography angiography of choroidal neovascularization in age-related macular degeneration. Ophthalmology. 2014;121(7):1435–44.
31. Ishibazawa A, Nagaoka T, Takahashi A, Omae T. Optical coherence tomography angiography in diabetic retinopathy: a prospective pilot study. Am J Ophthalmol. 2015;160(1):35–44.
32. Singh P, Singh A. Choroidal melanoma. Oman J Ophthalmol. 2012;5(1):3–9.
33. Natesh S, Chin K, Finger PT. Choroidal metastases fundus autofluorescence imaging: correlation to clinical, OCT, and fluorescein angiographic findings. Ophthalmic Surg Lasers Imaging. 2010;41(4):406–12.
34. Collet LC, Pulido JS, Gunduz K, Diago T. Fundus autofluorescence in choroidal metastatic lesions: a pilot study. Retina. 2008;28(9):1251–6.
35. Almeida A, Kaliki S, Shields CL. Autofluorescence of intraocular tumors. Curr Opin Ophthalmol. 2013;24(3):222–32.

Phakomatosis

11

Nishant Radke, Carol L. Shields, J. Fernando Arevalo,
and Jay Chhablani

Abstract

Phakomatoses, also known as oculo-neuro-cutaneous syndromes, are multisystem disorders affecting the eye with varied manifestations. They are primarily either choristomas or hamartomas. Retinal astrocytoma primary or acquired is an ocular manifestation of tuberous sclerosis while neurofibromatosis 1 may manifest in a very diverse manner ranging from lid neurofibromas, iris nodules, choroidal naevi, astrocytomas and optic nerve gliomas. Neurofibromatosis 2 usually manifests as a combined hamartoma of the retina and retinal pigment epithelium along with an epiretinal membrane (ERM). Sturge–Weber syndrome manifests with choroidal haemangiomas and glaucoma. Racemose cavernous haemangioma, retinal capillary haemangioma are other types of vascular pathologies seen as a part of phakomatosis while the choroidal melanoma is a serious manifestation seen as a part of oculodermal melanocytosis. In this chapter we describe the findings and features of phakomatoses using imaging techniques like fundus fluorescein angiography (FFA), indocyanine angiography (ICG), fundus photography, spectral domain optical coherence tomography (OCT), wide field imaging, fundus autofluorescence and the newer techniques such as OCT-angiography and adaptive optics.

N. Radke
Shri Ganesh Vinayak Eye Hospital, Raipur, India

C.L. Shields
Ocular Oncology Service, Wills Eye Hospital, Thomas Jefferson University, Philadelphia, PA, USA

J.F. Arevalo
Department of Ophthalmology, Johns Hopkins Bayview Medical Center, Baltimore, MD, USA

Retina Division, Wilmer Eye Institute, The Johns Hopkins University School of Medicine, Baltimore, MD, USA

J. Chhablani (✉)
Smt.Kanuri Santhamma Retina Vitreous Centre, L. V. Prasad Eye Institute, Kallam Anji Reddy Campus, L.V. Prasad Marg, Banjara Hills, Hyderabad 500 034, Andhra Pradesh, India
e-mail: jay.chhablani@gmail.com

J. Chhablani et al. (eds.), *Retinal and Choroidal Imaging in Systemic Diseases*,
https://doi.org/10.1007/978-981-10-5461-7_11

Phakomatoses are basically a group of different syndrome complexes which are characterized by systemic hamartomas of different organs like eye, the brain, skin and sometimes also involve the bones and viscera [1–4]. Oculo-neuro-cutaneous syndrome is another name given to them because of the multiple system involvement in phakomatoses.

Van der Hoeve was the first person to use the term "Phakoma" in the year 1932 when he described a mother spot or birthmark in many such conditions [4]. Consequently several other entities like von Hippel–Lindau syndrome (retinal and cerebellar haemangiomatosis), Bourneville's syndrome (tuberous sclerosis), von Recklinghausen syndrome (neurofibromatosis), Sturge–Weber syndrome (encephalofacial haemangiomatosis), Wyburn-Mason syndrome (racemose angiomatosis), organoid naevus syndrome, oculocutaneous melanocytosis and cavernous haemangioma of the retina with coetaneous and central nervous system involvement have been categorized as well alongside these oculo-neuro-cutaneous syndromes.

Since most of these syndromes feature choristomas and hamartomas, we need to understand these two important terminologies. To simply put it a "Choristoma" is a tumour composed of normal elements in abnormal location whereas a "Hamartoma" is a tumour of normal elements in normal locations. Most of the phakomatosis are either hamartomas or choristomas.

11.1 Tuberous Sclerosis Complex

Also known as the Bourneville's syndrome, TSC is characterized by the presence of retinal astrocytic hamartomas, the so-called ashleaf macules (cutaneous depigmented lesions) or adenoma sebaceum and astrocytomas in the central nervous system. Other associations are tumours like cardiac rhabdomyoma and renal angiomyolipoma [5–13]. The classical manifestation is a triad of adenoma sebaceum, mental deficiency and seizures.

At times retinal tumour is the only manifestation of TSC. It is still unknown whether these tumours represent a separate entity or are a forme fruste lesion of the classical entity or simply a partial expression of TSC. Occasionally patients with neurofibromatosis 1 may show an identical tumour of the fundus.

TSC occurs with an incidence of about 1:10,000 population [9]. TSC has been identified in all races. There is no gender predilection identified. TSC appears to be transmitted in an autosomal dominant way with incomplete penetrance. Chromosome 9q34 and chromosome 16p13 are found to be linked with TSC [5].

Retinal Lesions

The characteristic retinal lesion of TSC is the retinal astrocytic hamartoma (Figs. 11.1 and 11.2) [5–7]. The variations are a non-calcified tumour, the calcified tumour or, more commonly, a combination of the two. A small non-calcified tumour may only appear as an ill-defined translucent thickening of the retinal nerve fibre layer whereas the larger tumours are more opaque and appear as sessile lesions at the level of the nerve fibre layer. The calcified variant shows the characteristic

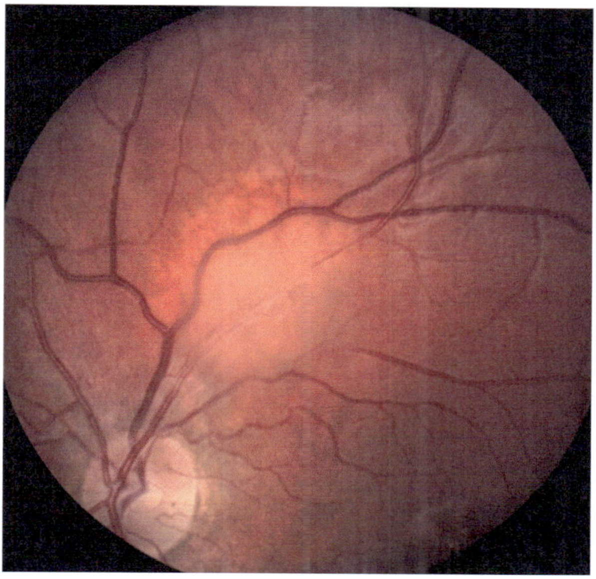

Fig. 11.1 A 10-year-old Caucasian female presented with seizures at 10 months of age. She was diagnosed with tuberous sclerosis based upon her history of seizures and the presence of ashleaf spots, adenoma sebaceum, angiomyolipomas and subependymal nodules. Genetic testing was positive for TSC2. Ocular examination of the left eye demonstrated a subtle, "gelatinous" appearing astrocytic hamartoma along the superotemporal arcade. (*Image courtesy of Mary Beth Aronow, MD*)

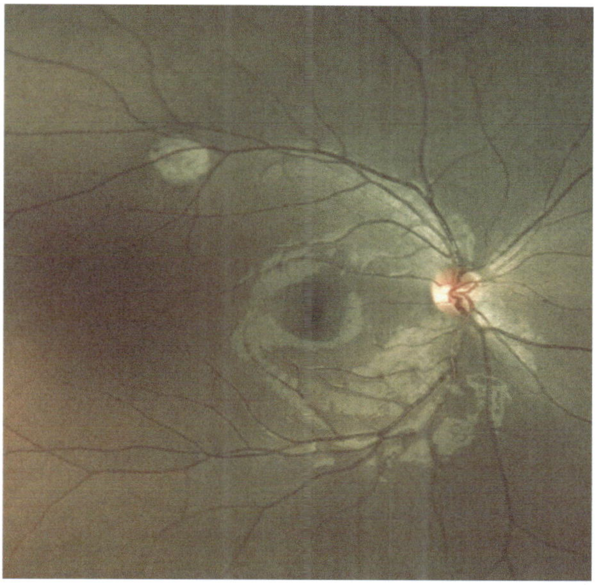

Fig. 11.2 A 23-year-old African American female with positive genetic testing for TSC had typical features including adenoma sebaceum, subependymal nodules, ashleaf spots and history of seizures. Dilated fundus examination revealed a flat, achromic patch along the superotemporal arcade of the right eye. (*Image courtesy of Mary Beth Aronow, MD*)

yellow, refractile structures resembling fish eggs or tapioca. The hamartoma is usually a small and stable innocuous lesion. However, occasionally it can cause retinal traction or vitreous haemorrhage. The rare aggressive variant can show progression to exudative detachment with or without neovascular glaucoma, and at times may need enucleation. Extraocular extension into the orbital and epibulbar tissues has been recognized in these cases [13].

Fundus Autofluorescence Retinal astrocytic hamartoma, particularly the calcified variant, usually shows autofluorescence.

Fundus Fluorescein Angiography FFA is an ancillary aid in the diagnosis of tuberous sclerosis retinal astrocytic hamartoma. The tumour is relatively hypo fluorescent in the arterial phase. Venous phase reveals a network of fine blood vessels. These vessels leak in the late phase during re-circulation and cause staining of the mass (Fig. 11.3).

Ultrasonography Ultrasonography is useful in large retinal astrocytic hamartomas. On A- and B-scan ultrasonography, the mass is seen as a sessile or dome-shaped lesion with acoustic solidity. The presence of calcification within the substance causes orbital shadow artefacts [5] (Fig. 11.3).

Optical Coherence Tomography Time domain OCT features of retinal astrocytic hamartoma were first published by Shields et al. [14] in 2006 and they found tumour involvement of the inner portion of the retina without identification of a specific

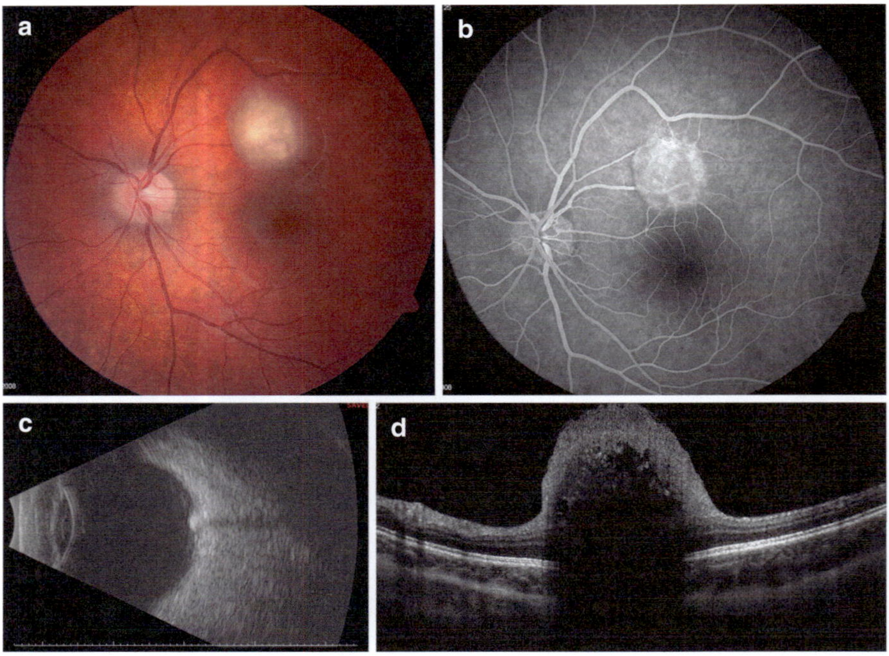

Fig. 11.3 Case of retinal astrocytoma: Fundus photograph (**a**) shows *yellowish* refracticle lesion. Fundus fluorescein angiography (**b**) shows network of blood vessels. Ultrasonography (**c**) shows hyperechoic lesion. Spectral domain optical coherence tomography (**d**) shows optical empty spaces with shadowing

layer because of lower TD OCT resolution. They also noted classic clear, so-called moth-eaten areas (or optically empty spaces [OESs]) which were attributed to intralesional calcification or cavitations that occasionally may be missed clinically. Pichi et al. [15] used spectral domain (SD) OCT in 43 patients with TSC which revealed more details about the intrinsic tumour features and led to a proposed classification based on SDOCT findings of tumour size, retinal traction and intralesional OESs.

Shields et al. [16] recently noted that the tumours were observed to originate from the inner retina, specifically the nerve fibre layer. All tumours show inward bowing and some degree of outward bowing with compression of the ganglion cell layer and the middle and the outer retinal layers, depending on tumour size. It was also found that in eyes with minimal posterior shadowing on SDOCT; the underlying choroid was unremarkable compared with the adjacent area. They noticed that macular tumours had a greater number of OESs compared with extramacular tumours ($P = 0.032$), but the OESs did not differ significantly in size (P = 0.824), whereas calcified tumours had larger OESs compared with non-calcified tumours ($P = 0.009$) but showed no statistically significant difference in OES number ($P = 0.189$). The SDOCT may also show adjacent retinal pathology like cystoid oedema and sub-retinal fluid. Shields et al. have also reported that in calcified tumours, the OESs likely represent intralesional calcification, whereas in the non-calcified tumours, they speculated that an OES could represent intralesional cavitation (Fig. 11.3). Veronese et al. documented the large, optically empty cavities on OCT, justifying the term cavitary retinal astrocytoma [17]. They further noted that the cavities evolved over time.

Pichi et al. [15] designed a classification of RAH in TSC based on SDOCT findings, identifying cavitation as type IV. Type I (flat without traction) was not associated with any systemic relationship, type II (thickness <500 mm and with traction) showed a relationship with cutaneous fibrous plaques, type III (calcified and thickness >500 mm) showed a relationship with subependymal astrocytoma and type IV (cavitary and thickness >500 mm) showed a relationship with pulmonary lymphangiomyomatosis [15].

11.1.1 Acquired Retinal Astrocytoma

Retinal astrocytic hamartoma is the commonest of the true glial tumours of the sensory retina and in most instances it is associated with other signs of TSC. The typical case that is unassociated with clinically evident TSC may represent a forme fruste of tuberous sclerosis in which only the ocular features are manifest. Occasionally, the retina can develop an acquired astrocytoma in somewhat older individuals without family history or clinical manifestations of TSC [18–22]. "Acquired retinal astrocytoma" was a term coined by Shields and Shields for such lesions, as opposed to the congenital astrocytic hamartoma of TSC [18]. It is typically yellow with abundant intrinsic vascularity which is best visualized with fluorescein angiography. Unlike the typical congenital astrocytic hamartoma, it generally lacks clinically evident calcification, is more likely to exhibit slowly progressive growth and is not associated with TSC. Intraretinal exudation and secondary retinal detachment are common as the tumour enlarges [18–22].

11.1.2 Fundus Fluorescein Angiography

Fluorescein angiography characteristically shows small, well-defined fine tumour blood vessels in the vascular filling phases with diffuse staining in late phase. Retinal feeder vessels can be apparent, but unlike in retinoblastoma and retinal haemangioblastoma they are not dilated or tortuous.

11.1.3 Ultrasonography

Ultrasonography usually discloses a non-calcified retinal mass with high internal reflectivity [18].

11.1.4 Infrared Imaging

Infrared imaging enhances visualization of the more minute lesions because it has a higher contrast in comparison to the background retina [23].

11.2 Neurofibromatosis

Neurofibromatosis is also known as oculo-neuro-cutaneous syndrome and involves multiple organ systems [24, 25]. It has an autosomal dominant inheritance and about 80% penetrance. Approximately half of the patients develop the lesions initially as spontaneous mutations and are without family history.

Neurofibromatosis is of two types: Type 1 and 2. Von Recklinghausen syndrome or the type 1 is also called as peripheral neurofibromatosis. Central neurofibromatosis is called as type 2 and presents as bilateral acoustic neurofibromatosis.

11.2.1 Neurofibromatosis 1

Neurofibromatosis type 1 has an incidence of 1:3000 persons. The frequency might actually be higher as some individuals will show only mild features and are thus undiagnosed. Decreased production of neurofibromin, a protein with tumour suppressor function, as a result of an autosomal dominant mutation in the NF1 gene has been found to be its cause. Deletion of even only one is sufficient to make it manifest. Out of seven prescribed diagnostic criteria for the diagnosis of NF1, two are ocular features, namely iris nodules also known as Lisch nodules and the second is the presence of optic nerve glioma.

11.2.2 Ophthalmologic Features

Amongst the different phakomatoses, NF has the most variegated manifestations (Fig. 11.4) [26–33]. This condition can involve various structures like eyelid, conjunctiva, aqueous outflow channels, uveal tract, retina, orbit and optic nerve. The lid involvement can be either nodular or plexiform. A diffuse thickening of the eyelid with a typical S-shaped curve of the eyelid is highly characteristic and suggestive of plexiform neurofibroma.

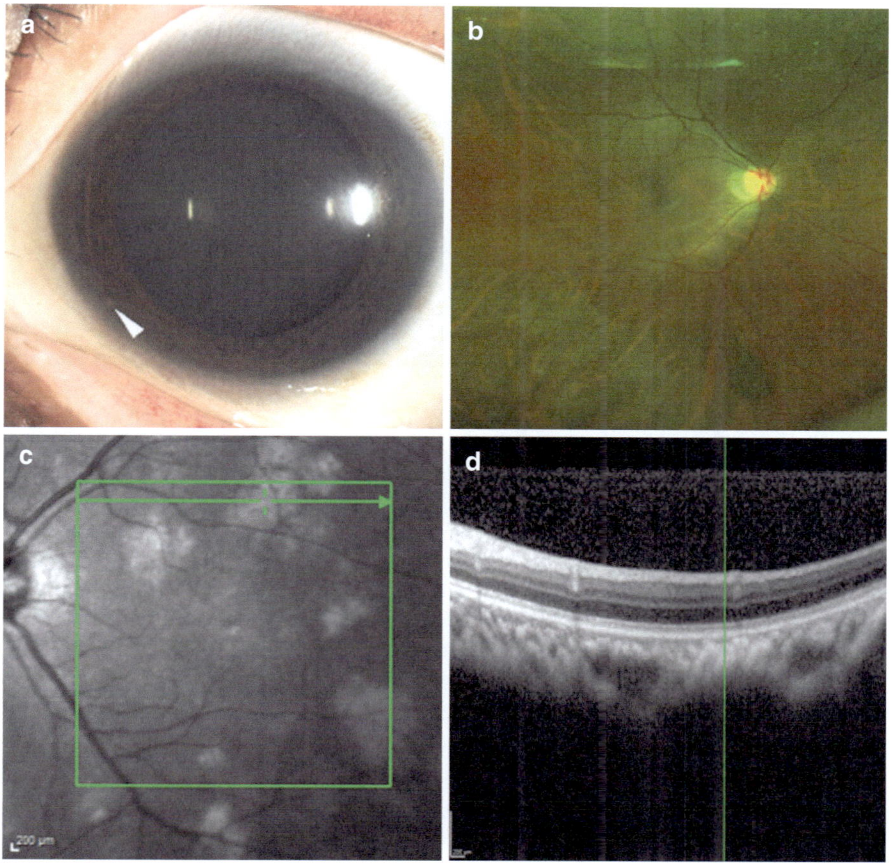

Fig. 11.4 A 31-year-old Caucasian male was diagnosed with NF1 based upon clinical criteria (multiple neurofibromas, cafe au lait spots and family history in multiple first degree relatives). Ophthalmic examination demonstrated typical ophthalmic features including Lisch nodules (**a**), an inferiorly located congenital hypertrophy of the RPE which has a possible association with NF1 (**b**) and choroidal patches apparent on SDOCT SLO reference images (**c**) which correspond to hyper-reflective lesions in the choroid (**d**) and have been associated with NF1. (*Images courtesy of Mary Beth Aronow, MD*). **Note, this OCT finding is not apparent on clinical examination and has been described in association with NF1 (Ishiko, BJO 2006; 90(8):1067–1068 and Kitaya, BJO 2002; 86:482–483)*

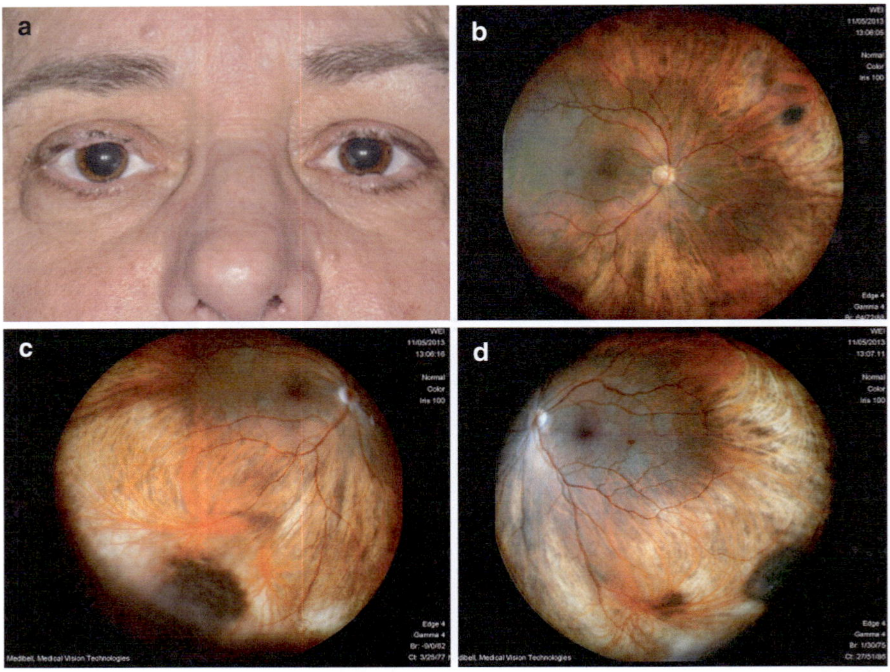

Fig. 11.5 A case of neurofibromatosis 1 shows S-shaped lids (**a**) with multiple bilateral choroidal naevi (**b–d**)

There is an increased incidence of congenital glaucoma in these patients and it may be secondary to several mechanisms [26]. Glioma of the optic nerve is highly associated with NF1 [28]. Multiple Lisch nodules (iris hamartomas) are the most common uveal and ophthalmic abnormality of NF1.

The choroidal involvement usually is in the form of an isolated choroidal naevus or multifocal choroidal naevi. Other manifestations in the choroid are in the form of a diffuse plexiform neurofibroma, neurilemmoma or sometimes a melanoma. The presence of multiple and bilateral choroidal naevi should raise the suspicion of neurofibromatosis type 1 (Fig. 11.5). The lesions appear as small, ill-defined naevi which have a random distribution. Choroidal neurofibroma usually presents in the form of diffusely thickened uveal tract from an increased number of neurofibromatous or melanocytic elements. Schwannoma also known as choroidal neurilemmoma, on the other hand, is rare and presents in the form of an elevated and circumscribed, amelanotic tumour [30]. The incidence of uveal melanoma is higher in patients with NF according to some studies [31, 32]. Retinal astrocytic hamartoma is more commonly seen in patients with TSC. However, patients with NF may also show the presence of retinal astrocytic hamartomas. Vasoproliferative retinal tumours may occur and if exudative in nature, the subsequent retinopathy may lead to blindness [33].

11.2.3 Infrared Imaging

Infrared imaging using the direct confocal mode in scanning laser ophthalmoscope (SLO) reveals patchy areas of brightness whereas indirect mode using SLO reveals dark patches [34, 35]. Infrared light travels through the retina better than visible spectrum thus imaging the choroid better [36]. Yasunari et al. found that when examined with Helium-Neon light, the bright patchy lesions seen on confocal IR imaging are choroidal in origin [34]. Yasunari et al. reported that choroidal abnormalities occurred in all patients (100%) as compared to plexiform neurofibroma (29%) or the Sakurai-Lisch nodules in the iris (76%) [34].

11.2.4 Optical Coherence Tomography

The choroid is one of the most commonly affected ocular structures in NF1. Infrared-fundus auto fluorescence (IR-FAF) is a common tool to identify choroidal pathologies like nodules in patients suffering from NF1 [37–41]. Despite normal routine ophthalmic examination, IR-FAF might reveal multiple patchy, bright choroidal lesions. Viola et al. found that 7% of normal individuals may show the presence of choroidal nodules when imaged with IR-FAF. This same number increased to 82% in their study on patients with NF1 [42]. Maximum accuracy was found with a cut-off value of 1.5 in their study on choroidal nodules. Ishiko et al. found that a collection and proliferation of neural crest-derived melanocytes and neural cells within the choroid of patients with NF1 causes an apparent thickening of the posterior fundus [38].

OCT reveals irregular hyper reflectivity which co-localizes with the choroidal lesions. Similar abnormalities were described on OCT by other investigators as well [40–42]. Makino and Tampo identified hypo reflective foci and speculated the long-standing nature of the nodules could result in focal atrophy of choriocapillaris thereby causing the hypo reflectivity seen on OCT images of the choroid [43]. The presence of normal integrity of the outer retinal structures seems to suggest that the changes are localized to the choroid alone and do not affect the retina. To summarize, patients with NF1 may have typical choroidal lesions visible on IR-FAF. OCT images help in confirming the extent and location of choroidal involvement. The quantum of choroidal involvement is likely to vary among patients and it increases with age [38].

11.2.5 Near-Infrared Fundus Autofluorescence

Bright and multiple patchy areas have been noted in all of the eyes examined by near-infrared monochromatic light reflectance (NIR-R) using a scanning laser ophthalmoscope [34]. Thus, NIR-R has become a commonly used tool to detect choroidal nodules in patients with NF1. One of the commonest ocular structures involved in NF1 is the choroid [34, 38, 42]. Melanosomes in the retinal pigment epithelium

(RPE) and the choroid have been located as the source for near-infrared autofluorescence (NIR-AF) [44]. NIR-AF also visualizes the melanin in age-related macular degeneration and some other retinal diseases [45, 46].

Tomoko Ueda-Consolvo et al. [41] noticed irregular hyper-reflective foci in the choroid on OCT which was found to coincide with the bright and patchy areas seen on NIR-R. However, they also notices some hypo reflective foci in the choroid on OCT scans in the same region which were found to be bright and patchy with NIR-R in a patient. The locations of the hypo fluorescent regions revealed on ICGA were found to correspond with those of the bright patchy regions revealed by NIR-R and NIR-AF. Focal choriocapillary atrophy as a result of the long-standing nature of the choroidal nodules is speculated to be the cause of hypocyanescence on ICGA. Similar to other studies they noted the presence of normal integrity of the outer retinal structures thereby suggesting that the changes are localized to the choroid alone and do not affect the retina.

11.2.6 Indo Cyanine Green Angiography

Fluorescein angiography shows areas of irregular and transmitted hyper fluorescence due to retinal pigmented epithelium (RPE) alterations. FA is, however, unable to identify any underlying choroidal pathologies. ICGA, on the other hand, shows diffuse hypo fluorescence which is unrelated to the lesion observed on clinical fundus examination or on FA. Deep choroidal vessels are seen in all phases of ICGA. The presence of this diffuse hypo fluorescence is believed to be due to the diffuse scattering effect of the neurofibromatous tissue. Byun et al. in their study using ICGA demonstrated multiple hypo fluorescent areas which persist till the late phase. They thought that these choroidal neurofibromas were not causing any overlying RPE abnormalities [47].

Retinal microvascular abnormalities in the form of corkscrew shaped vessels have also been demonstrated using FFA in NF1 patients [48].

11.2.7 Enhanced Depth Imaging Spectral Domain Optical Coherence Tomography

Rao et al. [49] studied choroidal neurofibromatosis using EDI-SDOCT and imaging through the NIR lesions revealed the presence of hyper-reflective choroidal nodules. The nodules were found to abut the overlying choroid and choriocapillaris with an associated loss of choroidal lucency. This was suggestive of compromise of the choroidal vasculature by compression. Despite the possible compression on the choroidal vasculature, no overlying retinal abnormalities were observed. Even they felt that in the presence of patchy NIR changes and corresponding ICG hypo fluorescence along with lack or reduced retinal findings on dilated examination, FA, FAF and red-free imaging are sensitive and specific modalities for diagnosing choroidal neurofibromatosis [49].

11.2.7.1 Neurofibromatosis Type 2

General Considerations

Central neurofibromatosis or the type 2 (NF2) is a multisystem disorder as well but has prominent features involving the central nervous system in the form of tumours like bilateral acoustic neuromas (vestibular schwannomas), schwannomas of the spinal cord, gliomas, meningiomas and a juvenile posterior subcapsular cataract (PSC). The constellation of multiple inherited schwannomas meningiomas and ependymomas is referred to as MISME syndrome [50]. Skin involvement is less common in NF2.

Ophthalmologic Features

NF2 has three important eye manifestations. Juvenile PSC, combined hamartoma of the retina and retinal pigment epithelium (CHRRPE), and epiretinal membranes (ERM) are these important features. Juvenile PSC (<50 years) is a criterion for diagnosis. Eighty percent of patients with advanced features of NF2 have been found to have an ERM [51]. CHRRPE lesions lead to prominent retinal and macular dragging with resultant corkscrew type retinal vessels. The hamartoma has a gray–green appearance and may lead to tumour formation [52, 53].

11.2.8 SDOCT of CHRRPE

Juvenile PSC, CHRRPE, ERM, optic nerve meningioma, optic disc glioma, intra-ocular schwannoma and neurotrophic keratopathy are the ocular manifestations in NF2 [54–59]. SDOCT in CHRRPE in patients with NF 2 reveals a hyper-reflective ERM with traction and retinal folds [60]. The inner layers of the underlying retina were found to be irregularly thickened, but outer photoreceptor layers were not grossly affected (Fig. 11.6).

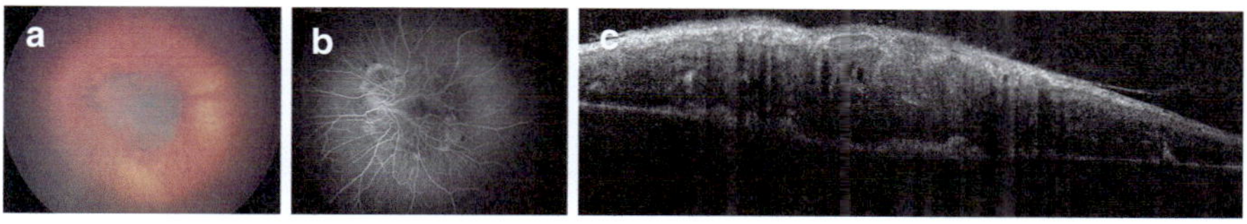

Fig. 11.6 A case of neurofibromatosis 2 shows a typical combined hamartoma of the retinal and retinal pigment epithelium on colour fundus photograph (**a**). Fluorescein angiography (**b**) shows tortuosity of the vessels and extent of the lesion. Spectral domain optical coherence tomography (**c**) shows hyper-reflective inner retina with few cystic spaces

11.2.9 Fundus Fluorescein Angiography

FFA shows tortuosity of the vessels and localized pinpoint leakages with late retinal vascular leakage. These findings correspond to the location of the lesion.

11.3 Sturge–Weber Syndrome (Encephalofacial Haemangiomatosis)

The Sturge–Weber (SW) syndrome is a syndrome complex characterized by the presence of congenital hamartomas in the eye, skin and brain which manifest at different times during life. Most common presentations are in childhood. The typical haemangiomas affect the choroid, face (port wine stain) and brain. Intra-cranial calcification is also noted [61–65].

The incidence is 1:50,000. Retinal vessels are tortuous and the presence of a diffuse choroidal haemangioma is noted in the posterior segment. In a study on SW syndrome 55% patients were found to have diffuse choroidal haemangioma which is indeed the most common pathology affecting the uveal tract in patients with SW syndrome [66, 67]. The fundus reflex seen through the pupil appears bright red in these patients when compared with the reflex in the fellow eye, the so-called the tomato catsup fundus.

11.3.1 Colour Fundus Photography

While imaging choroidal haemangiomas, it is important to remember the method of imaging. A scanning laser ophthalmoscope makes them look brown thereby leading to an erroneous conclusion of the more serious choroidal melanoma. In contrast when imaged with the panoret-1000 system, its true colour is recorded and displayed.

11.3.2 Fundus Fluorescein Angiography

FFA in the arteriovenous phase reveals prominent hyper fluorescence in the area of haemangioma demonstrating the tumour vessels. While the late phase shows marked leakage (Fig. 11.7).

Shields et al. reported that the intrinsic vasculature displays hyper fluorescence through all the phases of the angiography [68]. Schulenburg et al. have concluded that ICG angiography and wide-angle ICG angiography carry more diagnostic value than FFA [69]. Strong intra-tumoural hyper fluorescence of the vessels in arterial phase with a late phase significant washout and thus relative hypo fluorescence compared to the neighbouring choroid was observed by them [69].

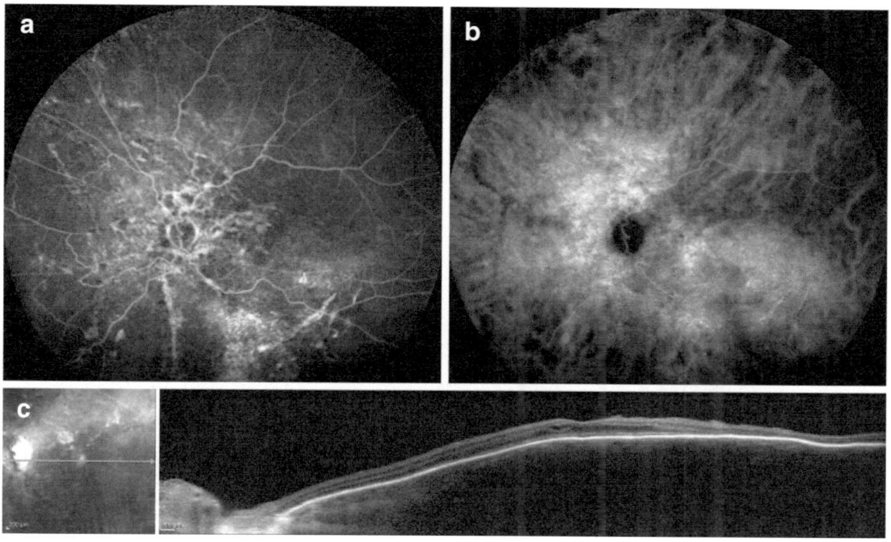

Fig. 11.7 Fluorescein angiography (**a**) and indocyanine green angiography (**b**) of a case of choroidal haemangioma show tumoural vessels. Spectral domain optical coherence tomography (**c**) shows choroidal elevation with few cystic changes of the retina

11.3.3 Spectral Domain Optical Coherence Tomography

The trend now a day is to monitor the secondary effects after treatment of choroidal haemangioma with SDOCT [70]. It is particularly useful for monitoring treatment response, like resolution of the exudative RD or macular oedema.

Sub-retinal and intra retinal fluid, schitic changes, loss of outer retina and retinal atrophy are some of the changes noted on OCT [71–74]. The overlying retina may be normal as well. The RPE layer usually shows a dome-shaped uninterrupted elevation over the haemangioma (Fig. 11.7) [72, 74]. Chronic cases lead to sub-retinal fibrosis and RPE alterations. CMO and sub-foveal fluid are changes which may be noted on SDOCT at the macula [75]. EDI of circumscribed choroidal haemangiomas reveals a low-to-medium reflective band with a homogenous signal and intrinsic spaces [76]. Posterior border of choroidal haemangiomas can be identified only if the tumour is <0.9 mm in thickness. The haemangioma itself may, however, be identified and distinguished from the neighbouring choroidal tissue on imaging [76].

11.3.4 Fundus Autofluorescence

Choroidal haemangioma appears hypo- or isofluorescent in comparison to the surrounding tissue [73]. The autofluorescence shows granularity. Overlying orange pigmentation is strongly hyperautofluorescent, while regions with fibrosis and

RPE atrophy appear hypoautofluorescent. Fresh sub-retinal fluid is hyper autofluorescent. By contrast, chronic sub-retinal fluid is hypoautofluorescent [73]. Following treatment, the relative hypoautofluorescence of the haemangiomas increases [73].

11.3.5 B Scan USG

B scan USG demonstrates scan ultrasonography and shows a diffuse, highly echoic thickened area of choroid (Fig. 11.8) with high internal reflectivity similar to that of the surrounding choroidal tissue. Usually a choroidal haemangioma is unilateral; however, bilateral cases have been noted particularly in patients with bilateral facial naevus flammeus. Exudative retinal detachment can be localized and at times total with extensive exudation in diffuse choroidal haemangiomas. Chronic cases of such exudative RD may lead to secondary neovascular glaucoma (Fig. 11.9).

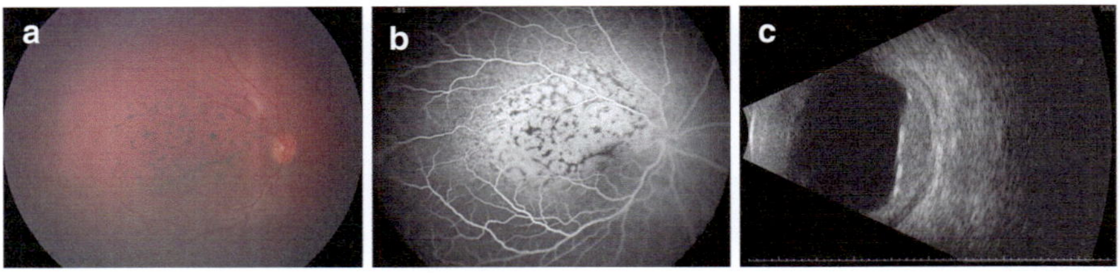

Fig. 11.8 (**a**) Case of choroidal haemangioma with pigmentary changes (**b**) shows vasculature changes on fluorescein angiography. Ultrasonography (**c**) shows high echogenic thickening of choroid

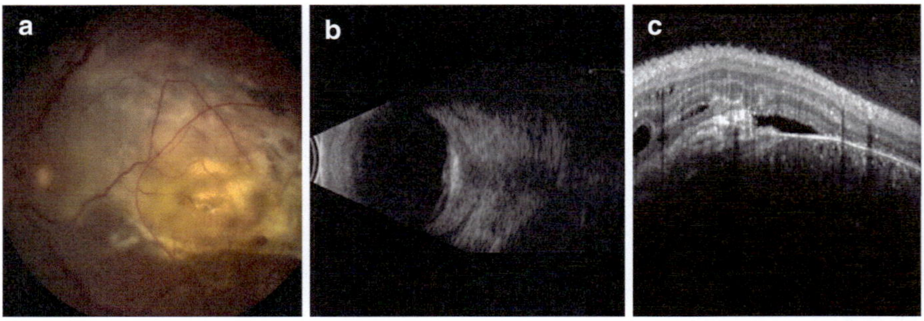

Fig. 11.9 A 10-year-old boy had cutaneous naevus flammeus (or port wine stain) typical of Sturge–Weber syndrome. Fundus examination of the left eye demonstrated extensive chorioretinal scarring in the macula and exudative retinal detachment secondary to chronic, diffuse choroidal haemangioma (**a**). B-scan ultrasonography demonstrated diffuse choroidal thickening (**b**). SDOCT revealed choroidal thickening with overlying intraretinal and sub-retinal fluid (**c**). (*Images courtesy of Adam Wenick, MD*)

Other changes seen in fundus include congenital retinal vascular tortuosity and retinal pigmentary alterations. Chronic exudative retinal detachment sometimes causes a "pseudo-retinitis pigmentosa" like picture.

11.3.5.1 Management

The management of a diffuse choroidal haemangioma depends on the size and expanse of the tumour along with the presence of any associated exudative retinal detachment. A minimally elevated tumour with no SRF can be observed. The necessary hyperopic refractive correction can be prescribed. Tumours with SRF or thicker lesions need PDT or external beam radiation. Paediatric patients with the presence of any lesion in macula or SRF need careful monitoring for amblyopia [77].

11.4 Racemose Haemangiomatosis (Wyburn-Mason Syndrome)

Retinoencephalofacial angiomatosis is a racemose haemangioma and is also called as the Wyburn-Mason syndrome or Bonnet–Dechaume–Blanc syndrome [78]. It is a rare congenital condition with no heredity and consists of arterio-venous malformations (AVM) that affect the mid-brain, ipsilateral retina, visual pathways and facial structures. Usually it is symptom free. Unlike other oculo-neuro-cutaneous syndromes, it shows minimal skin changes except for small haemangiomas. The characteristic AVM can be either subtle asymptomatic lesions or at times are more extensive forming tumour-like vascular masses, often referred to as racemose or cirsoid haemangiomas (Fig. 11.10). Racemose haemangioma may affect the retina,

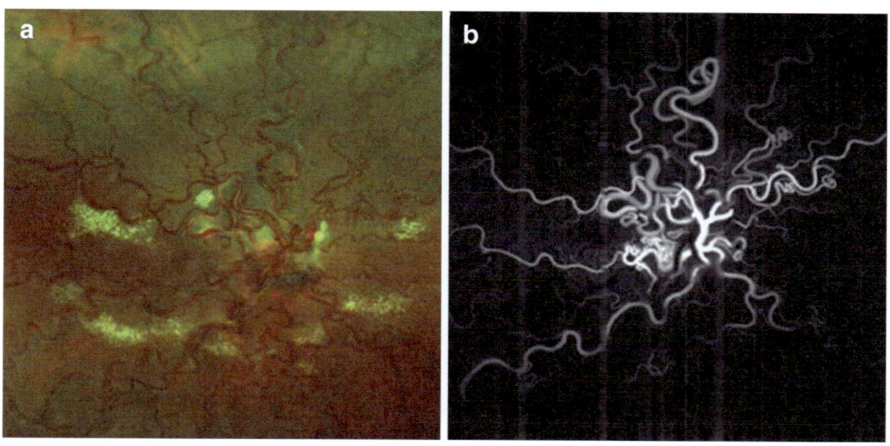

Fig. 11.10 A 13-year-old Caucasian female presented with unilateral dilated tortuous vessels and retinal arteriovenous malformation (**a**). Fluorescein angiography demonstrated rapid arteriovenous transit of blood through the anomalous anastomoses in the right eye (**b**). (*Images courtesy of Adam Wenick, MD*)

orbit or adjacent structures. However, the characteristic eye lesion is the retinal racemose haemangioma. Archers classification group III type is the most unmistakable variant characterized by an extensive complex AVM. This particular group III type is often associated with visual loss. One or more dilated and tortuous arteries run a variable distance from the optic nerve head (ONH) and culminate into the AVM. The dilated and tortuous veins then head back to the ONH for drainage.

11.4.1 Fundus Fluorescein Angiography

FFA notably shows no leakage (Fig. 11.10).

BRVO and vitreous haemorrhage with subsequent associated complications may occur which warrant treatment in the form of laser, intravitreal anti-VEGF injections or vitrectomy.

11.5 Retinal Cavernous Haemangiomatosis

There are two variants described. First is the sporadic variant which is not associated with syndrome and the second is associated with cutaneous and central nervous system vascular malformations. This second type is a part of the phakomatoses. Retinal cavernous haemangioma is its only ocular manifestation. Clinically, it manifests in the form of a dark grape-like cluster of venous intraretinal aneurysms located either at the ONH, macula or in the periphery [79–81]. The lesion usually lies along the path of a vein and feeder vessels are absent. These lesions do not leak any exudate or sub-retinal fluid. There is a risk of repetitive vitreous haemorrhages which may be mild thereby leading to whitish fibroglial membrane proliferation on the surface. The main complication is vitreous haemorrhage. Larger tumours may be associated with severe fibroglial membrane formation which may cause retinal dragging with macular ectopia.

11.5.1 Fundus Fluorescein Angiography

FFA is the most important diagnostic test. Clusters of hypo fluorescence which persist till late phase without leakage from the aneurysms are seen. Fluorescein accumulated in the venous aneurysms pools in the plasma component of the superior part of each vascular space, whereas the blood components sediment in the lower portion producing the characteristic hemispheres of hyper- and hypo fluorescence. This typical fluorescein–blood interface in the late angiograms characterizes the lesion complex (Fig. 11.11).

11.5.2 Optical Coherence Tomography

OCT shows lobulated, hyper-reflective masses located at the level of inner retina and anatomically correspond to the aneurysms. Optically empty cystic spaces

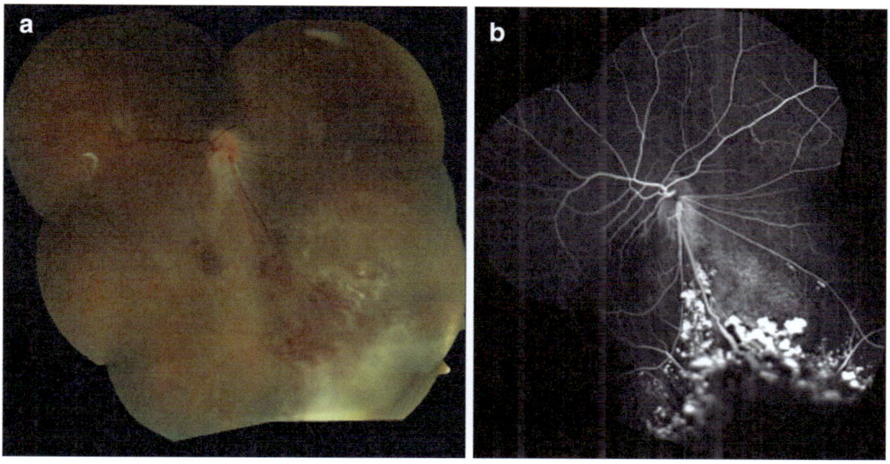

Fig. 11.11 (**a**) case of retinal cavernous haemangioma - Colour Montage (b) Fluorescein angiography showing hyper- and hypo-fluorescent hemispheres (*Images courtesy of SwathiKalki, MD*)

may be present within these hyper-reflective masses [82, 83]. Secondary features like epiretinal membrane may be noted with or without traction but SRF is absent.

11.6 Oculodermal Melanocytosis

Ocular or oculodermal melanocytosis is also known as congenital melanosis bulbi, naevus fuscoceruleus ophthalmomaxillaris or naevus of Ota and it is a congenital pigmentary condition affecting the periocular skin, sclera, uvea, orbit, palate, ear drum and meninges [80, 81, 84–87]. Important risk predisposed is that of a melanoma. Uveal Melanoma is the most common site although occasionally orbit or meninges may get involved as well [87–92].

11.6.1 Fundus Autofluorescence

FAF is based on the intrinsic property of certain molecules to show transient emission of light, or fluorescence, when illuminated by an external light source. In the eye, many tissues have autofluorescence properties such as the cornea, lens and the RPE. The main source of FAF is believed to be the fluorophore A2 E found in lipofuscin. Lipofuscin accumulates and gets deposited in the retinal tissue as a result of ageing. However, the deposits may also be noted in conditions leading to degeneration of the retinal pigment epithelium like Stargardt's dystrophy, astrocytoma, Bests disease, etc.

FAF depicts the intrinsic characteristics of melanoma along with the changes at the level of the RPE. It also highlights the presence of drusen and lipofuscin pigment accumulation. OCT is helpful to identify the presence of any fluid accumulation within the retina or at the level of neurosensory retina.

Shields et al. reported that [93] choroidal melanoma showed different types of AF. They reported hypoautofluorescence (39%), isoautofluorescence (6%) and hyperautofluorescence (55%) in their study. The autofluorescence was found to be more in larger, pigmented and tumours with disruption of the RPE. The autofluorescence pattern was granular in 92% and nongranular in 8% [93]. Near-infrared wavelengths (780–820 nm) penetrate deeper into the choroid as compared to the shorter wavelengths. These are also known to excite melanin-associated fluorophores [94]. These may have a role in future.

11.6.2 Optical Coherence Tomography

OCT shows three different types of findings, viz., serous retinal detachment, cystic changes within the overlying retina and loss of normal retinal architecture above the tumour.

EDI-OCT of small choroidal melanomas was studied by Shields et al. [95]. EDI-OCT allows in vivo quantification of tumour size and cross-sectional details of the tumour and the neighbouring choroidal tissue. On EDI, small choroidal melanomas appear as homogeneous and optically reflective lesions located along the anterior surface, with gradual shadowing noted more deeply. The internal characteristics of the tumour were found to be irresolvable. Optical shadowing can be either partial or complete. They concluded that the EDI-OCT features found more often with significance in choroidal melanoma compared with choroidal naevus are the presence of increased shaggy photoreceptors or structural abnormality at their level, loss of external limiting membrane (ELM), loss of inner segment–outer segment (IS-OS) junction, retinal oedema, irregular inner plexiform layer and irregularity of ganglion cell layer.

11.6.3 Von Hippel Lindau (VHL) Disease

Retinal capillary angiomas or haemangioblastomas may be seen in isolation or with the systemic association of VHL disease. VHL is a rare autosomal dominant disorder with a prevalence of 1:36,000 live births. It encompasses multiple benign or malignant tumours or cysts in the tissues of the brain, spinal cord, inner ear, retina, kidneys, pancreas, adrenal glands, epididymis and the broad ligament [96]. The retinal capillary haemangioblastomas are many times the first manifestation of VHL and can range from very small innocuous lesions to large leaky lesions resulting in visual morbidity. Initially they appear like a subtle red or gray dot. The lesion has a fibro-vascular component as it grows and the afferent and efferent blood vessels to and from the lesion become enlarged and tortuous with secondary changes which gives its characteristic nodular appearance. Secondary changes like exudative retinal detachment, perilesional retinal oedema, hard exudates and macular oedema may be noted. Fibrous component can lead to tractional detachment as well as haemorrhage and long-standing lesions with increasing chronicity may lead to neovascular glaucoma. Common location is in the retinal periphery and posterior pole lesions are rare. Spontaneous regression is rare and has been shown to occur as well [97]. Tumours involving the posterior pole or optic nerve tend to cause vision loss earlier and are thus identified early compared to peripheral retinal lesions which are incidentally discovered at times.

Diagnosis The diagnosis of retinal capillary haemangioblastomas is clinical. Tests are ancillary to monitor the disease progression or course and to plan treatment.

Fundus Photography Montage or wide-angled fundus photography is useful to monitor the changes in the tumour. The tumour usually appears like a well-circumscribed orange lesion usually in the periphery with feeder vessels.

Fundus Fluorescein Angiography Shows early leakage with marked hyper fluorescence in early phase. This increases in late phase but may decrease at times as well. Petalloid pooling is seen if macular oedema is concomitantly associated (Fig. 11.12).

Optical Coherence Tomography Has no role in diagnosis of the angiomas; however, it can be helpful for diagnosis and management of macular oedema because of the VHL. OCT features of peripapillary angiomas have been studied. Chin et al. reported that they appear like a round masses with dense shadowing which is in continuity of outer retina and extends into the sub-retinal space. Adjoining areas of sub-retinal fluid may be present with macular oedema [98].

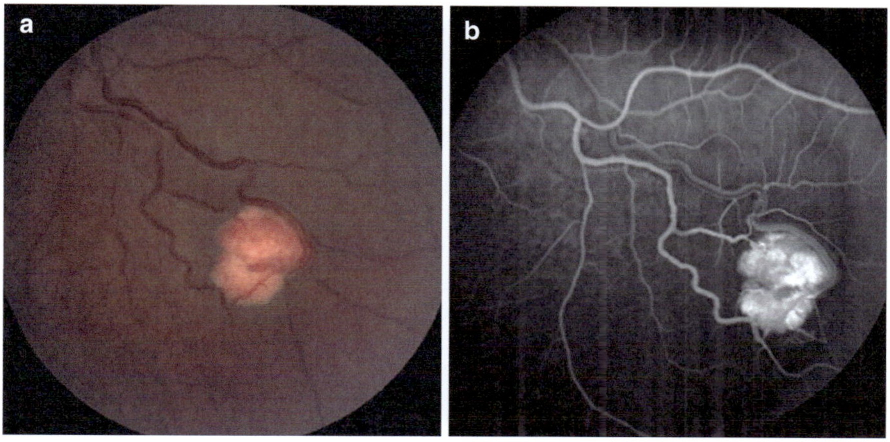

Fig. 11.12 A 23-year-old Caucasian female presented with a retinal capillary haemangioblastoma. A feeding arteriole and draining venule are apparent on colour fundus photography (**a**). Fluorescein angiography demonstrates rapid filling confirming the vascular nature of this lesion (**b**). (*Images courtesy of Adam Wenick, MD*)

Ultrasonography Shows the presence of a solid retinal lesion with smooth anterior edge but variable internal reflectivity. Orbital shadowing or choroidal excavation is not seen.

Peripheral treatment in the form of local laser for small laser or combination of cryotherapy and laser for larger tumours may lead to regression of the lesions. In the process "Ablatio Fugax" may develop; a term used to describe sudden drop in vision due to massive exudation and macular oedema post-laser or cryotherapy. Optic nerve lesions are difficult to treat and PDT has been tried with limited success. TRD may need vitrectomy. Anti-VEGF agents and steroid intravitreal injections are options worth considering along with combination of PDT but results are not always excellent.

References

1. Shields JA, Shields CL. Systemic hamartomatoses ("Phakomatoses"). In: Intraocular tumours. A text and atlas. Philadelphia: WB Saunders; 1992. p. 513–39.
2. Shields JA, Shields CL, editors. Intraocular tumours. An atlas and textbook. 2nd ed. Philadelphia: Lippincott Williams and Wilkins; 2008.
3. Shields JA, Shields CL. The systemic hamartomatoses ("Phakomatoses"). In: Mannis MJ, Macsai MS, Huntley AC, editors. Eye and skin disease. New York: Lippincott-Raven; 1996. p. 367–80.
4. Van der Hoeve J. The Doyne memorial lecture. Eye symptoms in phakomatoses. Trans Ophthalmol Soc UK. 1932;52:380–401.
5. Shields JA, Shields CL. Intraocular tumours. An atlas and textbook. 2nd ed. Philadelphia: Williams & Wilkins; 2008.
6. Shields JA, Shields CL. Eyelid, conjunctival and orbital tumours. An atlas and textbook. 2nd ed. Philadelphia: Williams & Wilkins; 2008.
7. Shields JA, Shields CL. The systemic hamartomatoses ("phakomatoses"). In: Nelson LA, Olitsky SE, editors. Harley's pediatric ophthalmology. 5th ed. Philadelphia: Williams & Wilkins; 2005. p. 436–47.
8. Bourneville D. Sclereusetubereuse des circonvolutioncerebrales. Idioteetepilepsiehemiphlegique. Arch Neurol (Paris). 1880;1:81–91.
9. Kwiatkowski DJ, Short MP. Tuberous sclerosis. Arch Dermatol. 1994;130:348–54.
10. Lucchese NJ, Goldberg MF. Iris and fundus pigmentary changes in tuberous sclerosis. J Pediatr Ophthalmol Strabismus. 1981;18:45–6.
11. Lagos JC, Gomez MR. Tuberous sclerosis. Reappraisal of a clinical entity. Mayo Clin Proc. 1967;42:26–49.
12. Reed WB, Nickel WR, Campion G. Internal manifestations of tuberous sclerosis. Arch Dermatol. 1963;87:715–28.
13. Shields JA, Eagle RC Jr, Shields CL, Marr BP. Aggressive retinal astrocytomas in 4 patients with tuberous sclerosis complex. The first John Dickerson lecture. Arch Ophthalmol. 2005;123:856–63.
14. Shields CL, Benavides R, Materin MA, Shields JA. Optical coherence tomography of retinal astrocytic hamartoma in 15 cases. Ophthalmology. 2006;113:1553–7.
15. Pichi F, Massaro D, Serafino M, et al. Retinal astrocytic hamartoma: optical coherence tomography classification and correlation with tuberous sclerosis complex. Retina. 2016;36(6):1199–208. DOI: 10.1097/IAE.0000000000000829.
16. Shields CL, Say EA, Fuller T, Arora S, Samara WA, Shields JA. Retinal astrocytic hamartoma arises in nerve fiber layer and shows "moth-eaten" optically empty spaces on optical coherence tomography. Ophthalmology. 2016;123:1809–16. DOI: 10.1016/j.ophtha.2016.04.011. pii: S0161-6420(16)30104-X. [Epub ahead of print].

17. Veronese C, Pichi F, Guidi SG, et al. Cystoid changes within astrocytic hamartomas of the retina in tuberous sclerosis. Retin Cases Brief Rep. 2011;5:113–6.
18. Shields JA, Shields CL. Glial tumours of the retina and optic disc. In: Shields JA, Shields CL, editors. Intraocular tumors an atlas and textbook. 2nd ed. Philadelphia: Lippincott Williams & Wilkins; 2009. p. 406–27.
19. Ramsay RC, Kinyoun JL, Hill CW, Aturaliya UP, Knobloch WH. Retinal astrocytoma. Am J Ophthalmol. 1979;88:32–3.
20. Reeser FH, Aaberg TM, Van Horn DL. Astrocytic hamartoma of the retina not associated with tuberous sclerosis. Am J Ophthalmol. 1978;86:688–98.
21. Bornfeld N, Messmer EP, Theodossiadis G, Meyer-Schwickerath G, Wessing A. Giant cell astrocytoma of the retina. Clinicopathologic report of a case not associated with Bourneville's disease. Retina. 1987;7:183–9.
22. Shields CL, Shields JA, Eagle RC Jr, Cangemi F. Progressive enlargement of acquired retinal astrocytoma in two cases. Ophthalmology. 2004;111:363–8.
23. Xu L, Burke TR, Greenberg JP, Mahajan VB, Tsang SH. Infrared imaging and optical coherence tomography reveal early-stage astrocytic hamartomas not detectable by fundoscopy. Am J Ophthalmol. 2012;153(5):883–889.e2. DOI: 10.1016/j.ajo.2011.10.033.
24. Von Recklinghausen FD. Uber die multiplenfibrome der haut und ihrebeziehungenzu den neurrommen. Festschr Feierfundfund-zwanzigjahrigen. Berlin Institute of Pathology. Berlin: Hirschwald; 1882.
25. Brasfield RD, Das Gupta TK. Von Recklinghausen's disease: a clinicopathological study. Ann Surg. 1972;175:86–104.
26. Grant WM, Walton DS. Distinctive gonioscopic findings in glaucoma due to neurofibromatosis. Arch Ophthalmol. 1968;79:127–34.
27. Lewis RA, Riccardi VM. von Recklinghausen neurofibromatosis. Incidence of iris hamartoma. Ophthalmology. 1981;88:348–54.
28. Lewis RA, Gerson LP, Axelson KA, et al. Von Recklinghausen neurofibromatosis II. Incidence of optic gliomata. Ophthalmology. 1984;91:929–35.
29. Kaiser-Kupfer MI, Freidlin V, Dariles MB, et al. The association of posterior capsular lens opacities with bilateral acoustic neuromas in patients with neurofibromatosis type 2. Arch Ophthalmol. 1989;107:541–4.
30. Shields JA, Sanborn GE, Kurz GH, et al. Benign peripheral nerve tumour of the choroid. Ophthalmology. 1981;88:1322–9.
31. Wiznia RA, Freedman JE, Mancini AD, et al. Malignant melanoma of the choroid in neurofibromatosis. Am J Ophthalmol. 1978;86:684–7.
32. Honavar S, Singh AD, et al. Iris melanoma in a patient with neurofibromatosis. Surv Ophthalmol. 2000;45:231–6.
33. Shields CL, Shields JA, Barrett J, et al. Vasoproliferativetumors of the ocular fundus. Classification and clinical manifestations in 103 patients. Arch Ophthalmol. 1995;113: 615–23.
34. Yasunari T, Shiraki K, Hattori H, et al. Frequency of choroidal abnormalities in neurofibromatosis type 1. Lancet. 2000;356:988–92.
35. Haynes RJ, Manivannan A, Walker S, et al. Imaging of optic nerve head drusen with the scanning laser ophthalmoscope. Br J Ophthalmol. 1997;81:654–7.
36. Shiraki K. Fundus examination using a scanning laser ophthalmoscope. Folia Ophthalmol Jpn. 1996;47:629–36.
37. Mori F, Kitaya N, Hikichi T, Yoshida A. Choroidal abnormalities in neurofibromatosis type 1 with non-invasive infrared imaging. Br J Ophthalmol. 2002;86(4):482–3.
38. Nakakura S, Shiraki K, Yasunari T, Hayashi Y, Ataka S, Kohno T. Quantification and anatomic distribution of choroidal abnormalities in patients with type I neurofibromatosis. Graefes Arch Clin Exp Ophthalmol. 2005;243(10):980–4.
39. Ishiko S, Yoshida A, Kato Y, Kagokawa H. Occult retinal and choroidal lesions in neurofibromatosis type 1. Br J Ophthalmol. 2006;90(8):1067–8.
40. Ayata A, Unal M, Ersanli D, Tatlipinar S. Near infrared fluorescence and OCT features of choroidal abnormalities in type 1 neurofibromatosis. Clin Exp Ophthalmol. 2008;36(4):390–2.

41. Ueda-Consolvo T, Miyakoshi A, Ozaki H, Houki S, Hayashi A. Near-infrared fundus autofluorescence-visualized melanin in the choroidal abnormalities of neurofibromatosis type 1. Clin Ophthalmol. 2012;6:1191–4.
42. Viola F, Villani E, Natacci F, et al. Choroidal abnormalities detected by near-infrared reflectance imaging as a new diagnostic criterion for neurofibromatosis 1. Ophthalmology. 2012;119(2):369–75.
43. Makino S, Tampo H. Optical Coherence Tomography Imaging of Choroidal Abnormalities in Neurofibromatosis Type 1. Case Rep Ophthalmol Med. 2013;2013:292981. DOI: 10.1155/2013/292981.
44. Gibbs D, Cideciyan AV, Jacobson SG, Williams DS. Retinal pigment epithelium defects in humans and mice with mutations in MYO7A: imaging melanosome-specific autofluorescence. Invest Ophthalmol Vis Sci. 2009;50(9):4386–93. DOI: 10.1167/iovs.09-3471.
45. Weinberger AWA, Lappas A, Kirschkamp T, et al. Fundus near infrared fluorescence correlates with fundus near infrared reflectance. Invest Ophthalmol Vis Sci. 2006;47:3098–108.
46. Kellner U, Kellner S, Weinitz S. Fundus autofluorescence (488 nm) and near-infrared autofluorescence (787 nm) visualize different retinal pigment epitjelium alterations in patients with age-related macular degeneration. Retina. 2010;30:6–15.
47. Byun YS, Park YH. Indocyanine green angiographic findings of obscure choroidal abnormalities in eurofibromatosis. Korean J Ophthalmol. 2012;26(3):230–4.
48. Muci-Mendoza R, Ramella M, Fuenmayor-Rivera D. Corkscrew retinal vessels in neurofibromatosis type 1: report of 12 cases. Br J Ophthalmol. 2002;86:282–4.
49. Rao RC, Choudhry N. Enhanced depth imaging spectral-domain optical coherence tomography findings in choroidal neurofibromatosis. Ophthalmic Surg Lasers Imaging Retina. 2014;45(5):466–8. DOI: 10.3928/23258160-20140818-01.
50. Evans DG. Neurofibromatosis 2 (Bilateral acoustic neurofibromatosis, central neurofibromatosis, NF2, neurofibromatosis type II). Genet Med. 2009;11:599–610.
51. Meyers SM, Gutman FA, Kaye LD, et al. Retinal changes associated with neurofibromatosis 2. Trans Am Ophthalmol Soc. 1995;93:245–57.
52. Shields CL, Mashayekhi A, Dai VV, et al. Optical coherence tomography findings of combined hamartoma of the retina and retinal pigment epithelium in 11 patients. Arch Ophthalmol. 2005;123:1746–50.
53. Shields CL, Thangappan A, Hartzell K, et al. Combined hamartoma of the retina and retinal pigment epithelium in 77 consecutive patients. Visual outcome based on macular versus extramacular tumour location. Ophthalmology. 2008;115:2246–52.
54. Pearson-Webb MA, Kaiser-Kupfer MI, Eldridge R. Eye findings in bilateral acoustic (central) neurofibromatosis: association with presenile lens opacities and cataracts but absence of Lisch nodules. N Engl J Med. 1986;315:1553–4.
55. Bouzas EA, Freidlin V, Parry DM, et al. Lens opacities in neurofibromatosis 2: further significant correlations. Br J Ophthalmol. 1993;77:354–7.
56. Landau K, Dossetor FM, Hoyt WF, Muci-Mendoza R. Retinal hamartoma in neurofibromatosis 2. Arch Ophthalmol. 1990;108:328–9.
57. Kaye LD, Rothner AD, Beauchamp GR, et al. Ocular findings associated with neurofibromatosis type II. Ophthalmology. 1992;99:1424–9.
58. Dossetor FM, Landau K, Hoyt WF. Optic disk glioma in neurofibromatosis type 2. Am J Ophthalmol. 1989;108:602–3.
59. Freedman SF, Elner VM, Donev I, et al. Intraocular neurilemmoma arising from the posterior ciliary nerve in neurofibromatosis: pathologic findings. Ophthalmology. 1988;95:1559–64.
60. Kang HM, Koh HJ, Chung EJ. Spectral-domain optical coherence tomography of combined hamartoma of the retina and retinal pigment epithelium in neurofibromatosis. Korean J Ophthalmol. 2013;27(1):68–71. DOI: 10.3341/kjo.2013.27.1.68.
61. Sturge WA. A case of partial epilepsy apparently due to a lesion of one of the vasomotor centers of the brain. Trans Clin Soc Lond. 1879;12:162–7.

62. Weber FP. Right-sided hemihypertrophy resulting from right-sided congenital spastic hemiplegia with a morbid condition of the left side of the brain revealed by radiogram. J Neurol Psycho-Pathol (London). 1922;37:301–11.
63. Stevenson RF, Morin JD. Ocular findings in nevus flammeus. Can J Ophthalmol. 1975;10:136–9.
64. Susac JO, Smith JL, Scelfo RJ. The "tomato catsup" fundus in Sturge–Weber syndrome. Arch Ophthalmol. 1974;92:69–70.
65. Lindsey P, Shields JA, Goldberg RE, et al. Bilateral nevus flammeus and bilateral choroidal hemangiomas. Retina. 1981;1:88–95.
66. Sullivan TJ, Clarke MP, Morin JD. The ocular manifestations of the Sturge–Weber syndrome. J Pediatr Ophthalmol Strabismus. 1992;29:349–56.
67. Witschel H, Font RL. Hemangioma of the choroid. A clinicopathologic study of 71 cases and a review of the literature. Surv Ophthalmol. 1976;20:415–31.
68. Shields CL, Honavar SG, Shields JA, Cater J, Demirci H. Circumscribed choroidal hemangioma: clinical manifestations and factors predictive of visual outcome in 200 consecutive cases. Ophthalmology. 2001;108(12):2237–48.
69. Schalenbourg A, Piguet B, Zografos L. Indocyanine green angiographic findings in choroidal hemangiomas: a study of 75 cases. Ophthalmologica. 2000;214(4):246–52.
70. Blasi MA, Tiberti AC, Scupola A, Balestrazzi A, Colangelo E, Valente P, et al. Photodynamic therapy with verteporfin for symptomatic circumscribed choroidal hemangioma: five-year outcomes. Ophthalmology. 2010;117(8):1630–7.
71. Say EAT, Shah SU, Ferenczy S, Shields CL. Optical coherence tomography of retinal and choroidal tumours. J Ophthalmol. 2012;2012:385058.
72. Sayanagi K, Pelayes DE, Kaiser PK, Singh AD. 3D Spectral domain optical coherence tomography findings in choroidal tumours. Eur J Ophthalmol. 2011;21(3):271–5.
73. Ramasubramanian A, Shields CL, Harmon SA, Shields JA. Autofluorescence of choroidal hemangioma in 34 consecutive eyes. Retina. 2010;30(1):16–22.
74. Liu W, Zhang Y, Xu G, Qian J, Jiang C, Li L. Optical coherence tomography for evaluation of photodynamic therapy in symptomatic circumscribed choroidal hemangioma. Retina. 2011;31(2):336–43.
75. Kwon HJ, Kim M, Lee CS, Lee SC. Treatment of serous macular detachment associated with circumscribed choroidal hemangioma. Am J Ophthalmol. 2012;154(1):137–45.
76. Torres VLL, Brugnoni N, Kaiser PK, Singh AD. Optical coherence tomography enhanced depth imaging of choroidal tumours. Am J Ophthalmol. 2011;151(4):586–93.
77. Ramasubramanian A, Shields CL. The current management of choroidal hemangioma. Retina Today. 2010;1:52–5.
78. Wyburn-Mason R. Arteriovenous aneurysm of midbrain and retina, facial naevi and mental changes. Brain. 1943;66:163–203.
79. Gass JDM. Cavernous hemangioma of the retina. A neuro-oculocutaneous syndrome. Am J Ophthalmol. 1971;71:799–814.
80. Lewis RA, Cohen MH, Wise GN. Cavernous hemangioma of the retina. A report of three cases and a review of the literature. Br J Ophthalmol. 1975;59:422–34.
81. Goldberg RE, Pheasant TR, Shields JA. Cavernous hemangioma of the retina. A four generation pedigree with neurocutaneous involvement. Arch Ophthalmol. 1979;97:2321–4.
82. Shields CL, Materin MA, Shields JA. Review of optical coherence tomography for intraocular tumours. Curr Opin Ophthalmol. 2005;16(3):141–54.
83. Andrade RE, Farah ME, Costa RA, Belfort R. Optical coherence tomography findings in macular cavernous haemangioma. Acta Ophthalmol Scand. 2005;83(2):267–9.
84. Shields CL, Shields JA. Tumors of the conjunctiva and cornea. Surv Ophthalmol. 2004;49:3–24.
85. Gonder JR, Nichol J, Augsburger JJ, Shields JA. Ocular and oculodermal melanocytosis. Can J Ophthalmol. 1985;20:176–8.
86. Gonder JR, Ezell PC, Shields JA, et al. Ocular melanocytosis: a study to determine the prevalence rate of ocular melanocytosis. Ophthalmology. 1982;89:950–2.

87. Velazquez N, Jones IS. Ocular and oculodermal melanocytosis associated with uveal melanoma. Ophthalmology. 1983;90:1472–6.
88. Gonder JR, Shields JA, Albert DM, et al. Uveal malignant melanoma associated with ocular and oculodermal melanocytosis. Ophthalmology. 1982;89:953–60.
89. Singh AD, De Potter P, Fijal BA, et al. Lifetime prevalence of uveal melanoma in Caucasian patients with ocular (dermal) melanocytosis. Ophthalmology. 1998;105:195–8.
90. Gunduz K, Shields JA, Shields CL, et al. Choroidal melanoma in a 14 year-old patient with ocular melanocytosis. Arch Ophthalmol. 1998;116:1112–4.
91. Shields JA, Shields CL, Eagle RC Jr, et al. Malignant melanoma arising from a large uveal melanocytoma in a patient with oculodermal melanocytosis. Arch Ophthalmol. 2000;118:990–3.
92. Honavar SG, Shields CL, Singh AD, et al. Two discrete choroidal melanomas in an eye with ocular melanocytosis. Ophthalmology. 2002;47:36–41.
93. Shields CL, Bianciotto C, Pirondini C, Materin MA, Harmon SA, Shields JA. Autofluorescence of choroidal melanoma in 51 cases. Br J Ophthalmol. 2008;92:617–22.
94. Elsner AE, Burns SA, Weiter JJ, Delori FC. Infrared imaging of sub-retinal structures in the human ocular fundus. Vis Res. 1996;36:191–205.
95. Shields CL, Kaliki S, Rojanaporn D, Ferenczy SR, Shields JA. Enhanced depth imaging optical coherence tomography of small choroidal melanoma: comparison with choroidal nevus. Arch Ophthalmol. 2012;130(7):850–6. DOI: 10.1001/archophthalmol.2012.1135.
96. Lonser RR, Glenn GM, Walther M, et al. Von Hippel–Lindau disease. Lancet. 2003;361:2059–67.
97. Whitson JT, Welch RB, Green WR. Von Hippel–Lindau disease: case report of a patient with spontaneous regression of a retinal angioma. Retina. 1986;6:253–9.
98. Chin EK, Trikha R, Morse LS, Zawadzki RJ, Werner JS, Park SS. Optical coherence tomography findings of exophytic retinal capillary hemangiomas of the posterior pole. Ophthalmic Surg Lasers Imaging. 2010. DOI: 10.3928/15428877-20100215-30.

12 Vogt–Koyanagi–Harada Disease

Hitesh Sharma, Parthopratim Dutta Majumder, and Manabu Mochizuki

Abstract

Vogt–Koyanagi–Harada disease is rare granulomatous inflammatory disease that affects pigmented structures, such as choroid, inner ear, meninges, hair, and skin. Ocular involvement is characterized by bilateral, diffuse, granulomatous panuveitis and exudative retinal detachment. Vogt–Koyanagi–Harada disease has usually a benign course if diagnosed early and adequately treated. Imaging remains an integral part of diagnosis of Vogt–Koyanagi–Harada disease and plays an important role in diagnosis, quantification of inflammation, and disease monitorization.

Vogt–Koyanagi–Harada (VKH) disease is an idiopathic bilateral chronic granulomatous panuveitis that may be associated with central nervous system (CNS), auditory, and integumentary manifestations.

Three researchers described separately the different spectrum of this single systemic inflammatory condition and hence the disease named so. Vogt [1] and Koyanagi [2] described bilateral anterior uveitis associated with vitiligo, alopecia, and poliosis and Harada [3] described five patients with posterior uveitis with exudative retinal detachment and cerebrospinal fluid (CSF) pleocytosis.

The prevalence of VKH disease is variable among different populations. In Japan, VKH disease represents 10.1% of all uveitis cases [4] whereas the disease

M. Mochizuki
Department of Ophthalmology and Visual Science, Tokyo Medical and Dental University Graduate School of Medicine, Tokyo, Japan

H. Sharma • P.D. Majumder (✉)
Department of Uvea and Intraocular Inflammation, Sankara Nethralaya, 18, College Road, Chennai, India
e-mail: drparthopratim@gmail.com

J. Chhablani et al. (eds.), *Retinal and Choroidal Imaging in Systemic Diseases*, https://doi.org/10.1007/978-981-10-5461-7_12

accounts only for 2% of all uveitis cases in India [5]. VKH disease is believed to affect people with certain genetic predispositions and pigmented races like Asians, Hispanics, Native Americans, and Asian Indians. However, the disease is less common in blacks from sub-Saharan countries [6]. The disease usually occurs in patients between the ages of 20 and 50 years, but any age group can be affected. Women are affected slightly more frequently than men. The etiology of VKH disease remains largely idiopathic. It is thought to be an autoimmune process directed against proteins related to stromal choroidal melanocytes [7].

VKH disease typically consists of four distinguished consecutive phases—prodromal, uveitic, convalescent, and chronic recurrent. The prodromal phase usually lasts 3–5 days and is characterized by neurologic and auditory manifestations, including headaches, tinnitus, neck stiffness, and hearing loss. In this stage, cerebrospinal fluid may reveal pleocytosis. Acute uveitis stage lasts for several weeks and is characterized bilateral posterior granulomatous uveitis. The underlying pathologic process primarily manifests as diffuse stromal choroiditis and exudative detachment of the neurosensory retina secondary to diffuse choroidal inflammation is common. As the inflammation extends anteriorly patients develop acute bilateral granulomatous iridocyclitis and often shallow anterior chamber secondary to ciliary body edema and suprachoroidal fluid collection. Convalescent stage is characterized by depigmentation of the integument and choroid and can manifest as depigmented fundus, vitiligo, alopecia, and poliosis. Approximately 17–73% of patients may progress to recurrence or chronicity, which is characterized by recurrent episodes of anterior uveitis. Ocular complications are common in convalescent and chronic stages (Table 12.1).

The diagnosis of VKH disease is usually clinical. Revised diagnostic criteria for VKH, created by a panel of experts convened at an international workshop in 1999, classifies the disease into three categories: complete, incomplete, and probable VKH [6] (Table 12.2).

Table 12.1 Ophthalmic manifestations of VKH

Clinical phase	Ophthalmic manifestations
Prodromal phase	Uncommon
	Optic nerve involvement can occur [8]
Acute uveitis phase	• Bilateral granulomatous uveitis, can be asymmetrical • Diffuse stromal choroiditis • Ciliochoroidal detachment, ciliary body edema • Serous retinal detachment • Optic disc edema
Chronic (convalescent) stage	• Depigmentation of choroid: "sunset glow fundus" • Dalen-Fuchs nodules • Sugiura sign: perilimbal vitiligo
Chronic recurrent stage	High chances of developing complications • Cataract • Glaucoma • Choroidal neovascular membranes (CNVM), and • Subretinal fibrosis

Table 12.2 Revised diagnostic criteria of Vogt–Koyanagi–Harada disease proposed by the International Nomenclature Committee [6]

1. *No history of penetrating ocular trauma or surgery preceding the initial onset of uveitis*
2. *No clinical or laboratory evidence suggestive of other ocular disease entities*
3. *Bilateral ocular involvement (a or b must be met, depending on the stage of disease when the patient is examined):* A. *Early manifestations of disease:* I. Evidence of diffuse choroiditis (with or without anterior uveitis, vitreous inflammatory reaction, or optic disc hyperemia), which may manifest as (A) focal areas of subretinal fluid, or (B) bullous exudative retinal detachments. II. If equivocal fundus findings, then both: A. Fluorescein angiography showing focal delayed choroidal perfusion, multiple areas of pinpoint leakage, large placoid areas of hyperfluorescence, pooling within subretinal fluid, and optic nerve staining; B. Ultrasonography showing diffuse choroidal thickening without evidence of posterior scleritis. B. *Late manifestations of disease:* I. History suggestive of prior presence of early findings noted in 3A and either (II) or (III) below, or multiple signs from (III) below: II. Ocular depigmentation: either (A) sunset glow fundus or (B) Sugiura sign. III. Other ocular signs including (A) nummular chorioretinal depigmented scars, or (B) retinal pigment epithelium clumping and/or migration, or (C) recurrent or chronic anterior uveitis. 4. *Neurological/auditory findings (may resolve by time of evaluation):* a. Meningismus (malaise, fever, headache, nausea, abdominal pain, stiffness of the neck and back, or a combination of these factors); note that headache alone is not sufficient to meet definition of meningismus. b. Tinnitus c. Cerebrospinal fluid pleocytosis 5. *Integumentary findings (not preceding onset of central nervous system or ocular disease):* a. Alopecia, or b. Poliosis, or c. Vitiligo.

Complete VKH: criteria 1–5 must be present
Incomplete VKH: criteria 1–3 and either 4 or 5 must be present
Probable VKHD (isolated ocular disease): criteria 1–3 must be present

12.1 Fundus Autofluorescence (FAF)

Fundus autofluorescence (FAF), based on excitation of inherent fluorophores like lipofuscin, which accumulate in retinal pigment epithelium (RPE) is a good indicator of RPE activity and metabolic stress. Being a non-invasive and rapid method, it has become very popular over the last decade.

RPE is extensively damaged in VKH, the posterior pole being involved in the acute phase and the periphery also involved in the convalescent and the chronic recurrent phase. FAF features in acute VKH were described by Koizumi et al. [9]. They described two distinct patterns; the first pattern was of mild hyperautofluorescence in patients who received early intense immunosuppression and the second pattern of widespread and more hyperautofluorescence seen in patients who did not receive treatment or received too late. Thus, FAF can help in monitoring and prognosticating acute phase of VKH.

In chronic VKH, hypoautofluorescence is mainly seen in areas of atrophy and scars, while hyperautofluorescence is mainly seen in areas of subretinal fluid in cases of recurrences [10, 11]. Vasconcelos-Santos et al. [10] have demonstrated the combined use of FAF and SD-OCT for evaluation of RPE and outer retinal changes and detecting subclinical recurrences in chronic VKH patients. Heussen et al. [11] have used wide field FAF to describe peripheral lesions in chronic VKH patients and includes multifocal hypofluorescent spots, focal hyperfluorescent spots, and a unique lattice-like hyperfluorescent streak. These changes may correlate with the proliferation of RPE leading to an increase in the total amount of fluorophores or their accumulation in the outer retina. Thus, FAF may be used as a supplement in monitoring RPE changes during the chronic phase as it is noninvasive and therefore can be repeated at closer intervals (Fig. 12.1).

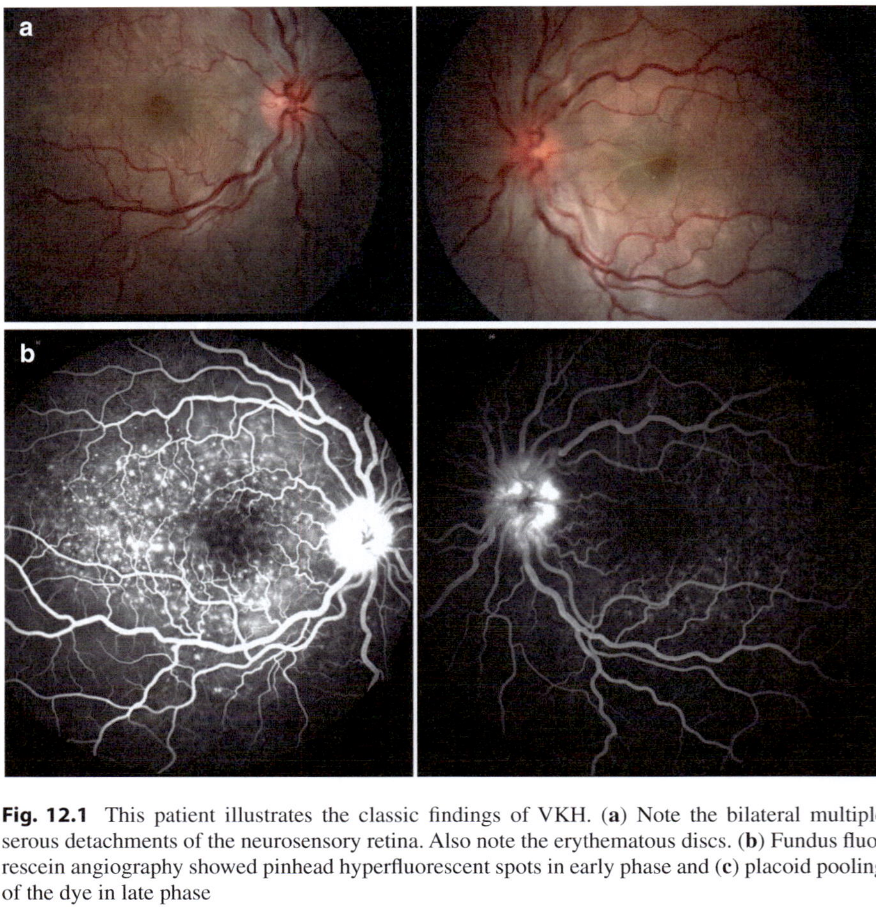

Fig. 12.1 This patient illustrates the classic findings of VKH. (**a**) Note the bilateral multiple serous detachments of the neurosensory retina. Also note the erythematous discs. (**b**) Fundus fluorescein angiography showed pinhead hyperfluorescent spots in early phase and (**c**) placoid pooling of the dye in late phase

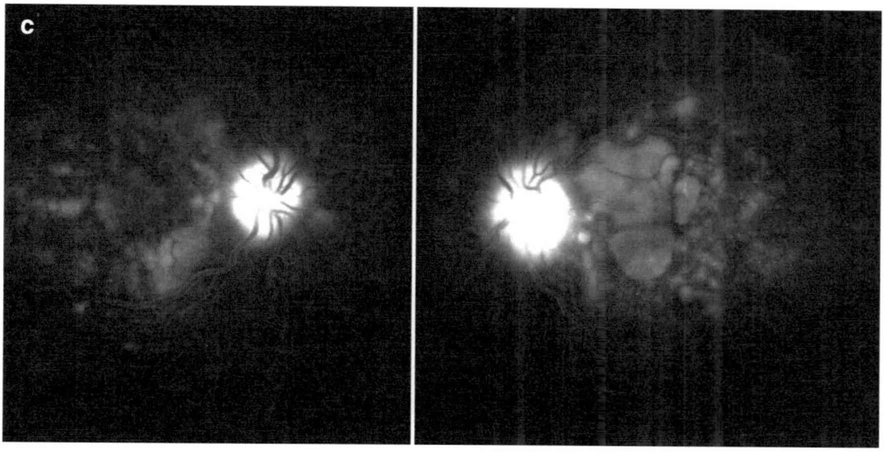

Fig. 12.1 (continued)

12.2 Fundus Fluorescein Angiography (FFA)

Fluorescein angiography is the most widely used ancillary investigation and helps to rule out similarly presenting conditions like central serous chorioretinopathy (CSCR), which is very important as the management of both the conditions is paradoxical.

In VKH, severe primary choroidal inflammation leads to spilling over of subretinal fluid to the retina, which in turn leaks profusely through the RPE causing an exudative retinal detachment. During the acute phase of VKH, the inflamed choroidal vessels become dilated and leak fluid, especially around the posterior pole. The choroidal inflammation usually spares the choriocapillaries but involves medium sized vessel. In majority of the patients, there is a delay in the choroidal filling, which is seen as spotted choroidal hyperfluorescence [12]. The RPE cells around the peripapillary region and macula are also inflamed during the acute phase of the disease. This is manifested as characteristic multiple punctate hyperfluorescent dots at the level of the RPE, often called as "stars at night" appearance. In subsequent phases of angiogram, the inflamed RPE allows the dye to leak and accumulate in the subretinal space over the posterior pole. This is manifested as placoid pooling of the dye and highlights the extent of exudative retinal detachment in the late phase of the angiogram. Optic disc hyperfluorescence is another important finding in angiogram and is seen in about 70% of patients in acute phase of the disease [13] (Fig. 12.2).

In the chronic recurrent stage, there are multiple hyperfluorescent RPE window defects and blocked fluorescence due to RPE hyperplasia. There can be alternating hyper- and hypofluorescence from RPE alterations, sometimes referred to as "moth-eaten" scars and "salt and pepper" pattern [14] (Fig. 12.3).

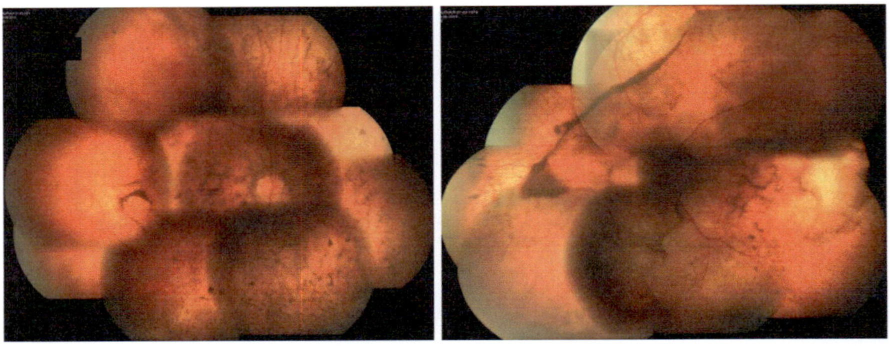

Fig. 12.2 Sunset glow fundus in VKH

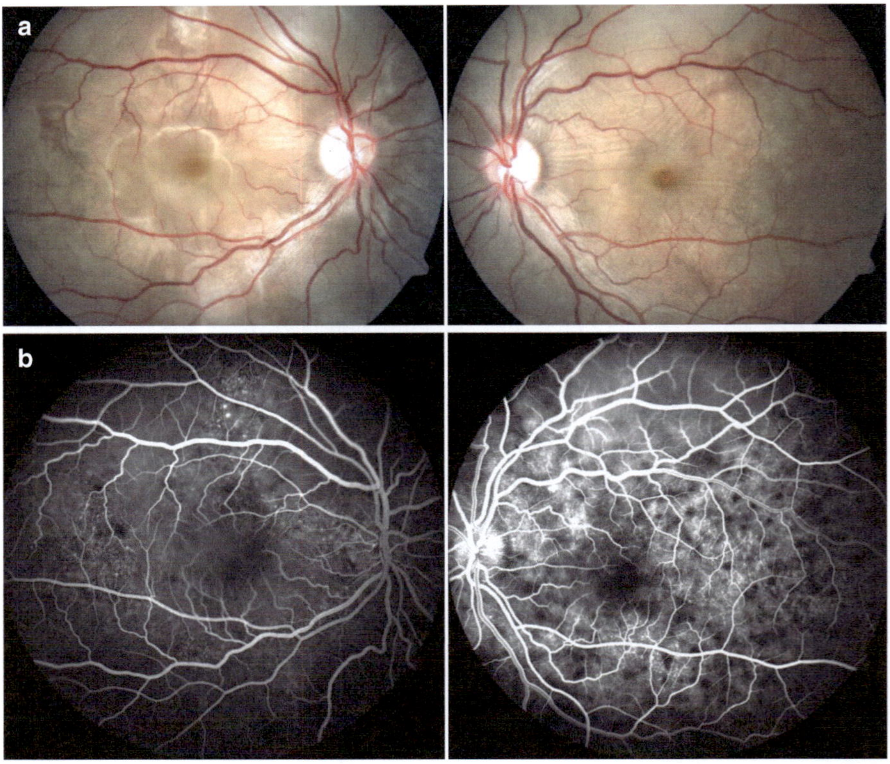

Fig. 12.3 This 54-year-old lady presented with headache, neck pain, and loss of vision in both eyes. Clinical examination revealed pockets of subretinal fluid and choroidal folds in both eyes (**a**). Early phase of the angiogram showed pin-head hyperfluorescent leaks (**b**) which increased and manifested as placoid pooling of the dye in late phase (**c**)

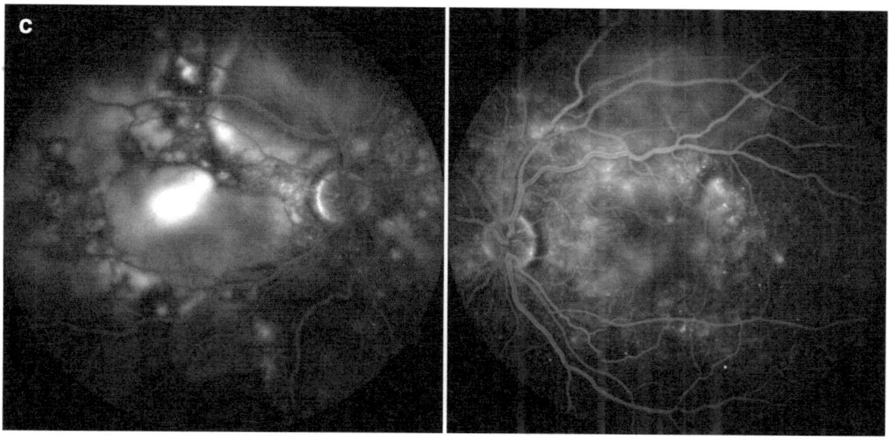

Fig. 12.3 (continued)

Table 12.3 FFA features in VKH and their clinical correlation

FFA features	Clinical correlation
Spotted choroidal hyperfluorescence	Choroidal inflammation
Early pinpoint hyperfluorescence	Breakdown of blood ocular barrier due to inflammation
Disc hyperfluorescence	Inflammation of the optic disc
Late placoid pooling of the dye	Subretinal fluid or exudative detachment
Spotted hyper and hypofluorescence (salt and pepper pattern)	RPE damage
Choroidal hypofluorescence	Delayed choroidal filling
Mixed band of hyper and hypofluorescence	Choroidal folds

Choroidal folds, undulations in the retinal pigment epithelium (RPE), the Bruch membrane, and inner aspects of the choroids are usually indiscernible on routine ophthalmoscopy in VKH. Recently this clinical manifestation was reported by several groups and thought to be a sign of severe choroidal inflammation. Wu et al. [15] observed choroidal folds in VKH to show hypofluorescence on FFA instead of alternating hypofluorescent and hyperfluorescent bands seen in choroidal folds in other clinical entities [16]. They postulated that compaction of RPE in the troughs decreases transmission of choroidal fluorescence and causes hypofluorescence, whereas the RPE in the peaks being normal do not show hyperfluorescence.

Chee et al. [17] have described the prognostic importance of FFA in VKH. They found that the absence of early pinpoint peripapillary hyperfluorescence on FA is a poor prognostic factor as it suggests that the disease is no longer in the hyperacute phase, and hence it may possibly need to be treated more aggressively and with a more prolonged course of immunosuppressive therapy (Table 12.3).

12.3 Indocyanine Green Angiography (ICG)

Indocyanine green (ICG) angiography is a very sensitive tool to show minimal and subclinical changes within the choroid and found to be an ideal ancillary test to investigate choroidal disorders. ICG can highlight the presence of small choroidal inflammatory foci and provide information on the choriocapillaris and choroidal stromal vessels (Fig. 12.4).

During acute phase, severe choroidal stromal inflammatory vasculopathy is manifested as early choroidal stromal vessel hyperfluorescence and leakage. Hypofluorescent dark spots, corresponding to choroidal foci or granuloma, are one of the most useful ICG sign for diagnosis and monitoring the activity of the

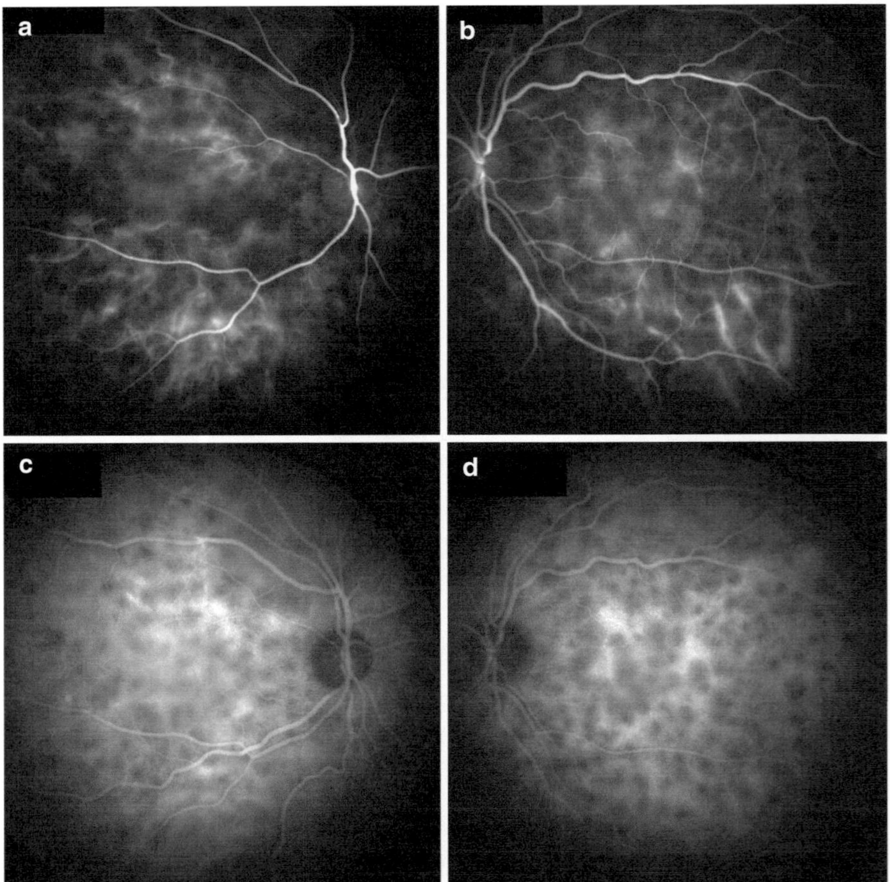

Fig. 12.4 ICG of a patient with VKH disease demonstrating choroidal stromal inflammatory vasculopathy as early choroidal stromal vessel hyperfluorescence and leakage (**a**, **b**). Note the hypofluorescent dark spots, corresponding to choroidal foci or granuloma (**c**, **d**)

Table 12.4 ICG features in VKH and their clinical correlation

ICG features	Clinical correlation
Early hyperfluorescence	Choroidal stromal inflammatory vasculopathy
Hypofluorescent dark spots	Choroidal granuloma
Disc hyperfluorescence	Severe disease
Small, irregular hyperfluorescent dots in periphery in chronic VKH	Dalen-Fuchs nodules

inflammation in VKH disease [18]. Serous retinal detachment usually appears hypofluorescence inside and around the detachment as highly protein-bound ICG molecule does not readily leak into the subneurosensory retinal space (Table 12.4).

12.4 Optical Coherence Tomography (OCT)

Optical coherence tomography is a non-invasive and a fast imaging modality which can pick up various features of vitreoretinal interface, retina and with newer machines the choroid in various phases of VKH.

OCT has been proven to be a better tool to visualize and understand the morphologic changes of the choroid in VKH patients. Cross-sectional images of multilobular serous retinal detachment in VKH disease have been studied in detail using OCT by various authors. Yamaguchi et al. observed that the subretinal fluid seen during the acute stage appeared to be divided into multiple compartments by inflammation-induced fibrous septa, creating the multilobular configuration of dye pooling sometimes demonstrated on FA in this disease [13].

Using a sequence of sectional images of the posterior pole obtained by OCT, cystoid structure within the retina in acute phase of VKH has been proposed by various authors [14, 19, 20]. Intraretinal fluid accumulation in the form of a cyst between the photoreceptor inner segment layers and the outer segment layers resolves earlier than subretinal fluid following treatment [20].

Choroid became significantly thicker during the active phase of VKH disease and choroidal thickness can be used as surrogate bio-marker to quantitatively evaluate the disease activity. EDI-OCT is an excellent method to directly visualize the choroid. It allows clear detection of the choroidal/retinal and choroidal/scleral interfaces, in vivo measurement of the total choroidal thickness. Choroidal thickness in active VKH disease is reported to exceed 800 μm compared with the normal choroid (379 μm) [21, 22]. The boundaries between the retina and the RPE and in turn between the RPE and the choroid are readily visible with the help of EDI-OCT. However, in case of choroidal thickening exceeding 1,000 μm, delineating the boundary between the choroid and the inner sclera may be difficult. EDI-OCT reveals a focal hyperreflectivity in the inner choroid, representing cross-sectional views of pericapillary arterioles and venules [23]. Reduction of focal hyperreflectivity in inner choroid is seen in both acute and convalescent stages of VKH. Fong et al. [23] attributed this feature due to compression and nonperfusion of small

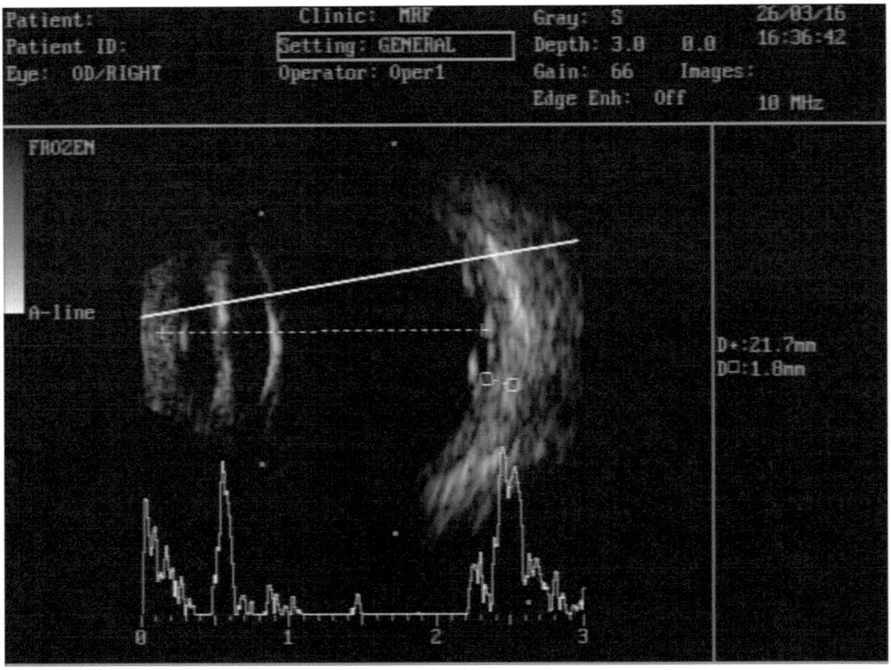

Fig. 12.5 Ultrasound B-scan of right eye of a patient with VKH showing multiple pockets of subretinal fluid with diffuse choroidal thickening

choroidal vessels from massive infiltration of inflammatory cells and granuloma in acute phase and shrinkage and dropout of small choroidal vessels caused by stromal scarring in convalescent stage of the disease (Fig. 12.5).

Choroidal folds are undulations or wrinkles in the retinal pigment epithelium (RPE), Bruch's membrane, and inner aspects choroid, and can be seen in various conditions like hypermetropia, hypotony, orbital diseases, choroidal tumors, ocular hypotony, scleritis, papilledema, choroidal detachment, etc. Choroidal folds are also observed in acute phase of VKH and are believed to be due to marked congestion and thickness of choroids which cause these folds to adapt the unchanged intraocular volume [24]. In VKH, choroidal folds are seen radiating from the optic disc to the periphery [15, 24].

Zhao et al. [24] concluded that the hypofluorescent lines on FFA are not always due to choroidal folds, but can be choroidal veins. According to them, choroidal veins can be differentiated from choroidal folds by discernibility on fundus photography, not straightly radiating from optic disc, irregular arrangement [24]. Gupta et al. [25] reported that changes in acute phase of the disease are seen mainly in the outer retinal segment like thickening or irregularity of the photoreceptor inner segment/outer segment (IS/OS) junction, with undulations and bumps on the surface of RPE on spectral domain OCT which resolved after systemic corticosteroids therapy.

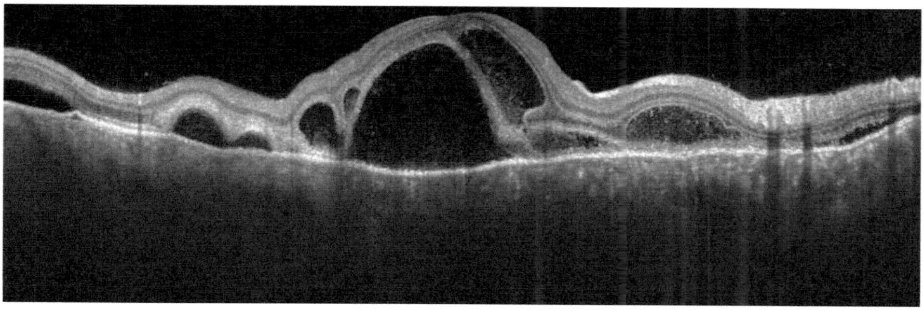

Fig. 12.6 Swept Source-OCT of right eye of the same patient showed multilobular serous retinal detachment

In a quantitative analysis for evaluating choroidal folds, Hosoda et al. [26] used RPE undulation index as a marker for choroidal folds in grading the disease severity of VKH. The RPE undulation index had a high value before steroid therapy, which was reduced after treatment and was strongly correlated with both retinal and choroidal thickness. Chee et al. [27] compared Swept Source-OCT and EDI-OCT in VKH patients and concluded that SS-OCT provides much better resolution images of the choroid than EDI-OCT resulting in accurate measurement of subfoveal choroidal thickness (Fig. 12.6).

12.5 Ultrasonography

Ultrasonography (USG) B scan is an important tool in diagnosis of VKH especially in cases where view of fundus is obscured by media opacity (e.g., extensive posterior synechiae preventing pupillary dilatation, cataract, or dense vitritis). It is also helpful in eyes where the amount of subretinal fluid is too extensive to be imaged by an OCT. USG B scan have been found to be useful in differentiating from posterior scleritis. In VKH, where sclera is secondarily involved, USG B scan shows diffuse, low to medium reflective choroidal thickening whereas in posterior scleritis the scleral thickening has high reflectivity and is frequently accompanied by retrobulbar edema in the peripapillary region resulting in the "T" sign [28]. USG B scan is also helpful in evaluation of choroidal detachment in VKH which, though rare, can occur in absence of prominent retinal detachment [29] (Fig. 12.7).

Various features seen on Ultrasonography B scan in VKH:

- Low to medium reflective thickening of the choroid
- Serous retinal detachments with shifting fluid
- Mild thickening of the sclera and/or episclera adjacent to areas of choroidal thickening
- Vitreous opacities.
- Extensive subretinal fibrosis in chronic cases.

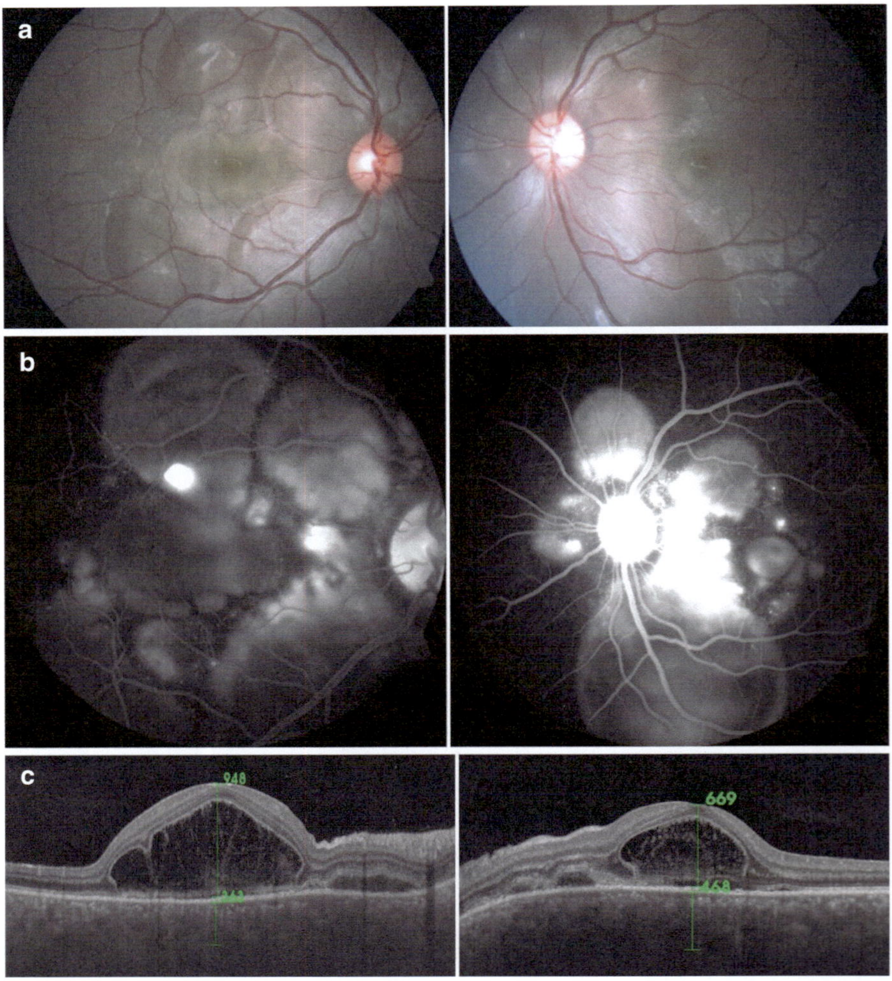

Fig. 12.7 A 14-year-old-girl presented with history of headache, ocular pain, redness followed by diminution of vision in both eyes. (**a**) Fundus examination of both eyes showed OU SRF pockets at posterior pole of both fundus. (**b**) Placoid pooling of the dye observed in late phases of angiogram. (**c**) OCT of the eyes showing multilobular serous retinal detachment with choroidal thickening

Ultrasound biomicroscopic (UBM) examination have demonstrated that ciliochoroidal detachment is a frequent finding in the acute stage of VKH disease and may be responsible for shallow anterior chamber encountered in the early stage of disease. The ciliary body is considered to be the most susceptible site for accumulation of suprachoroidal fluid. Ciliochoroidal detachment in VKH is usually depends on the severity and duration of insult to the choroidal vascular barrier by the inflammatory process. Acute angle closure can be the presenting sign of the disease and can complicate the diagnosis [30–33]. Using UBM, swollen ciliary bodies with anterior rotation of the ciliary processes were found to be responsible for anterior displacement of the peripheral iris and subsequent appositional closure of the anterior chamber angle [34]. Most of the published literature have shown resolution of ciliochoroidal detachment, ciliary body swelling, and deepening of anterior chamber depth significantly following steroid or immunosuppressive therapy.

12.6 Therapeutic Considerations

The aim of treatment in VKH is to suppress the active intraocular inflammation and prevent potential visual impairment. Early and aggressive treatment with systemic corticosteroids remains the mainstay of the initial therapy. Systemic steroid is administered either orally (1–1.5 mg/kg/day) or through a short course of intravenous methylprednisolone 1000 mg/day, for 3 days and slow tapering of oral corticosteroid. Rapid tapering or discontinuation of corticosteroid may incur in recurrences and the treatment should be continued for at least 6–9 months [35, 36]. Immunosuppressive agents are usually required to achieve long-term remission of the disease. However, these agents are also indicated in conditions inadequately controlled with corticosteroid alone or disease that warrants unacceptably high amount of corticosteroid. Use of immunosuppressive agents in VKH has been reported to have beneficiary effect and associated with reduced risk of vision loss [37].

References

1. Vogt A. Fruhzeitiges ergaruen der zilien und bemerkungen uber den sogenaten plotzlichen eintreitt dieser Veranderung. Klin Monatsbl Augenheilkd. 1906;44:228–42.
2. Koyanagi Y. Dysakusis, alopecia und poliosis bei schwerer uveitis nicht traumatischen Ursprugs. Klin Monatsbl Augenheilkd. 1929;82:194–211.
3. Harada E. Acute diffuse choroiditis. Acta Soc Ophthalmol Jpn. 1926;30:356–78.
4. Wakabayashi T, Morimura Y, Miyamoto Y, Okada AA. Changing patterns of intraocular inflammatory disease in Japan. Ocul Immunol Inflamm. 2003;11:277–86.
5. Mondkar SV, Biswas J, Ganesh SK. Analysis of 87 cases with Vogt-Koyanagi-Harada disease. Jpn J Ophthalmol. 2000;44:296–301.
6. Read RW, et al. Revised diagnostic criteria for Vogt-Koyanagi-Harada disease: report of an international committee on nomenclature. Am J Ophthalmol. 2001;131:647–52.
7. Sugita S, et al. Ocular infiltrating CD4+ T cells from patients with Vogt-Koyanagi-Harada disease recognize human melanocyte antigens. Invest Ophthalmol Vis Sci. 2006;47:2547–54.
8. Rajendram R, Evans M, Khurana RN, Tsai JH, Rao NA. Vogt-Koyanagi-Harada disease presenting as optic neuritis. Int Ophthalmol. 2007;27:217–20.
9. Koizumi H, Maruyama K, Kinoshita S. Blue light and near-infrared fundus autofluorescence in acute Vogt-Koyanagi-Harada disease. Br J Ophthalmol. 2010;94:1499–505.
10. Vasconcelos-Santos DV, Sohn EH, Sadda S, Rao NA. Retinal pigment epithelial changes in chronic Vogt-Koyanagi-Harada disease: fundus autofluorescence and spectral domain-optical coherence tomography findings. Retina Phila PA. 2010;30:33–41.
11. Heussen FM, et al. Ultra-wide-field green-light (532-nm) autofluorescence imaging in chronic Vogt-Koyanagi-Harada disease. Ophthalmic Surg Lasers Imaging Off J Int Soc Imaging Eye. 2011;42:272–7.

12. Arellanes-García L, Hernández-Barrios M, Fromow-Guerra J, Cervantes-Fanning P. Fluorescein fundus angiographic findings in Vogt-Koyanagi-Harada syndrome. Int Ophthalmol. 2007;27:155–61.
13. Yamaguchi Y, Otani T, Kishi S. Tomographic features of serous retinal detachment with multilobular dye pooling in acute Vogt-Koyanagi-Harada disease. Am J Ophthalmol. 2007;144:260–5.
14. Tsujikawa A, et al. Retinal cystoid spaces in acute Vogt-Koyanagi-Harada syndrome. Am J Ophthalmol. 2005;139:670–7.
15. Wu W, Wen F, Huang S, Luo G, Wu D. Choroidal folds in Vogt-Koyanagi-Harada disease. Am J Ophthalmol. 2007;143:900–1.
16. Newell FW. Choroidal folds. The seventh Harry Searls Gradle Memorial lecture. Am J Ophthalmol. 1973;75:930–42.
17. Chee S-P, Jap A, Cheung CMG. The prognostic value of angiography in Vogt-Koyanagi-Harada disease. Am J Ophthalmol. 2010;150:888–93.
18. Miyanaga M, et al. Indocyanine green angiography findings in initial acute pretreatment Vogt-Koyanagi-Harada disease in Japanese patients. Jpn J Ophthalmol. 2010;54:377–82.
19. Maruyama Y, Kishi S. Tomographic features of serous retinal detachment in Vogt-Koyanagi-Harada syndrome. Ophthalmic Surg Lasers Imaging Off J Int Soc Imaging Eye. 2004;35:239–42.
20. Lee JE, et al. Edema of the photoreceptor layer in Vogt-Koyanagi-Harada disease observed using high-resolution optical coherence tomography. Korean J Ophthalmol. 2009;23:74–9.
21. Maruko I, et al. Subfoveal choroidal thickness after treatment of Vogt-Koyanagi-Harada disease. Retina Phila PA. 2011;31:510–7.
22. Nakai K, et al. Choroidal observations in Vogt-Koyanagi-Harada disease using high-penetration optical coherence tomography. Graefes Arch Clin Exp Ophthalmol. 2012;250:1089–95.
23. Fong AHC, Li KKW, Wong D. Choroidal evaluation using enhanced depth imaging spectral-domain optical coherence tomography in Vogt-Koyanagi-Harada disease. Retina Phila PA. 2011;31:502–9.
24. Zhao C, et al. Choroidal folds in acute Vogt-Koyanagi-Harada disease. Ocul Immunol Inflamm. 2009;17:282–8.
25. Gupta V, Gupta A, Gupta P, Sharma A. Spectral-domain cirrus optical coherence tomography of choroidal striations seen in the acute stage of Vogt-Koyanagi-Harada disease. Am. J. Ophthalmol. 2009;147:148–153.e2.
26. Hosoda Y, et al. Relationship between retinal lesions and inward choroidal bulging in Vogt-Koyanagi-Harada disease. Am J Ophthalmol. 2014;157:1056–63.
27. Chee S-P, Chan S-WN, Jap A. Comparison of enhanced depth imaging and swept source optical coherence tomography in assessment of choroidal thickness in Vogt-Koyanagi-Harada disease. Ocul Immunol Inflamm. 2016:1–5. DOI: 10.3109/09273948.2016.1151896.
28. Forster DJ, Cano MR, Green RL, Rao NA. Echographic features of the Vogt-Koyanagi-Harada syndrome. Arch Ophthalmol Chic Ill. 1990;1960(108):1421–6.
29. Yamamoto N, Naito K. Annular choroidal detachment in a patient with Vogt-Koyanagi-Harada disease. Graefes Arch Clin Exp Ophthalmol. 2004;242:355–8.
30. Rathinam SR, Namperumalsamy P, Nozik RA, Cunningham ET. Angle closure glaucoma as a presenting sign of Vogt-Koyanagi-Harada syndrome. Br J Ophthalmol. 1997;81:608–9.
31. Forster DJ, Rao NA, Hill RA, Nguyen QH, Baerveldt G. Incidence and management of glaucoma in Vogt-Koyanagi-Harada syndrome. Ophthalmology. 1993;100:613–8.
32. Eibschitz-Tsimhoni M, Gelfand YA, Mezer E, Miller B. Bilateral angle closure glaucoma: an unusual presentation of Vogt-Koyanagi-Harada syndrome. Br J Ophthalmol. 1997;81:705–6.
33. Kimura R, Kasai M, Shoji K, Kanno C. Swollen ciliary processes as an initial symptom in Vogt-Koyanagi-Harada syndrome. Am J Ophthalmol. 1983;95:402–3.
34. Kishi A, Nao-i N, Sawada A. Ultrasound biomicroscopic findings of acute angle-closure glaucoma in Vogt-Koyanagi-Harada syndrome. Am J Ophthalmol. 1996;122:735–7.
35. Moorthy RS, Inomata H, Rao NA. Vogt-Koyanagi-Harada syndrome. Surv Ophthalmol. 1995;39:265–92.
36. Lai TYY, Chan RPS, Chan CKM, Lam DSC. Effects of the duration of initial oral corticosteroid treatment on the recurrence of inflammation in Vogt-Koyanagi-Harada disease. Eye Lond Engl. 2009;23:543–8.
37. Bykhovskaya I, Thorne JE, Kempen JH, Dunn JP, Jabs DA. Vogt-Koyanagi-Harada disease: clinical outcomes. Am J Ophthalmol. 2005;140:674–8.

Ocular Manifestations of Pregnancy 13

Michael T. Andreoli and William F. Mieler

Abstract

A variety of physiologic and pathologic changes may occur in the eye during pregnancy. Many of these variations are related to vascular and blood volume alterations in the mother. However, progression of various pre-existing conditions, such as diabetic retinopathy and intraocular tumors, may also occur. Ophthalmologists should be aware of these effects, as they may require modifications to screening or treatment patterns.

13.1 Introduction

Pregnancy may be associated with a wide array of ocular manifestations, many of which are vascular in etiology. These alterations may relate to pre-existing conditions or develop secondary to the pregnancy itself. Multiple retinal and choroidal pathologies are found at a higher rate in pregnant women. Additionally, common diseases such as diabetes mellitus, or uncommon intraocular tumors (uveal melanoma, choroidal hemangioma, and/or choroidal osteoma) may progress or grow during pregnancy as well.

M.T. Andreoli • W.F. Mieler (✉)
Department of Ophthalmology and Visual Sciences, University of Illinois at Chicago, Chicago, IL, USA
e-mail: wfmieler@gmail.com

J. Chhablani et al. (eds.), *Retinal and Choroidal Imaging in Systemic Diseases*,
https://doi.org/10.1007/978-981-10-5461-7_13

13.2 Physiologic Changes

13.2.1 Intraocular Pressure

Intraocular pressure may drop in the second half of pregnancy. The proposed mechanisms for this include increased uveoscleral outflow [1, 2] and decreased episcleral venous pressure [3]. The intraocular pressure generally returns to pre-pregnancy levels by two months postpartum [4].

13.2.2 Cornea

The cornea may exhibit several alterations during pregnancy, including decreased corneal sensitivity [5], increased thickness [6], and increased corneal curvature [7]. These factors may contribute to contact lens intolerance, which is common among pregnant women [8], and refractive shift [9]. Thus, new spectacle prescriptions should be delayed for several weeks postpartum.

13.3 Pathologic Conditions

13.3.1 Pregnancy-Induced Hypertension (Pre-Eclampsia, Eclampsia, HELLP Syndrome)

13.3.1.1 Pre-Eclampsia, and Eclampsia

Clinical Features

Pregnancy-induced hypertension (PIH), which includes pre-eclampsia and eclampsia, occurs in approximately 5% of pregnancies and may be associated with a variety of ocular abnormalities. Hypertension, peripheral edema, and proteinuria characterize pre-eclampsia. Eclampsia is pre-eclampsia accompanied by seizures.

Ocular Manifestations

The most common symptoms of PIH are blurred vision, photopsias, scotomata, and diplopia. Examination findings include retinal arteriolar abnormalities, serous retinal detachments, and ischemic optic neuropathy.

The most common retinal abnormality seen in pre-eclampsia is focal arteriolar spasm and narrowing, along with varying degrees of choroidal ischemia (Fig. 13.1) [10, 11]. This may also be associated with peripapillary or focal retinal edema, which may be mild (Fig. 13.2) or quite severe (Fig. 13.3). As vascular changes typically return to normal after delivery, permanent visual loss is rare, though retinal pigment epithelial mottling and/or varying degrees of optic atrophy may occur.

Serous retinal detachments occur in 1% of pre-eclamptic patients [12] and about 10% of eclamptic patients [13]. Choroidal ischemia is believed to play a role in the

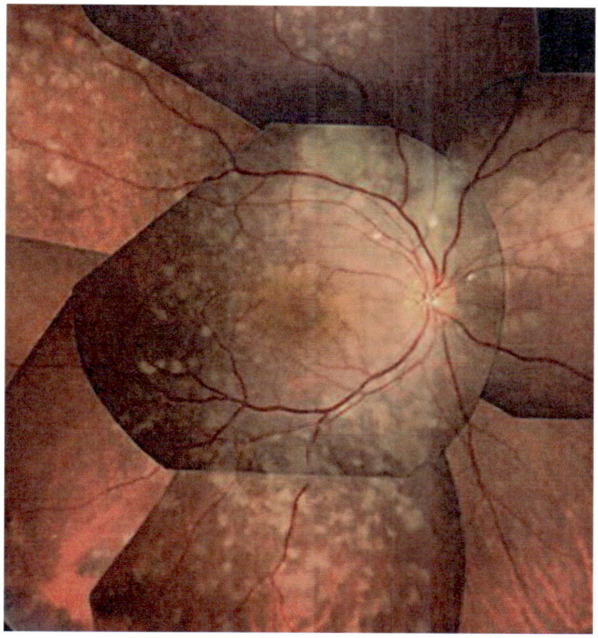

Fig. 13.1 Color photograph (right eye) in a patient with pre-eclampsia. The image reveals moderate retinal vascular attenuation and multiple areas of choroidal ischemia compatible with pre-eclampsia. The ischemic areas resolved post-partum, leaving mild retinal pigment epithelial mottling

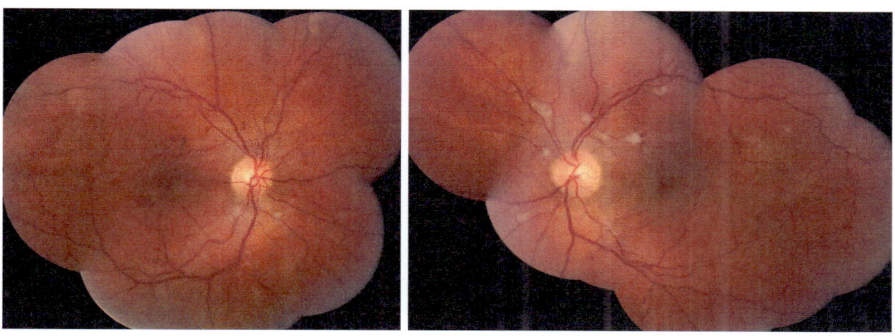

Fig. 13.2 Color photographs (both eyes) in a patient with pre-eclampsia. The photos reveal mild peripapillary edema compatible with the diagnosis

pathogenesis of these serous detachments [14]. The bullous serous elevations, which may be bilateral, occur in the absence of significant retinal vascular abnormalities. Most patients experience resolution of the detachments shortly after delivery. Although the visual prognosis is quite good, residual pigment epithelial alterations and optic atrophy may limit visual outcomes [15].

Acute ischemic optic neuropathy has been reported to occur in severe pre-eclampsia. The pathophysiology remains speculative [16].

Cortical blindness due to cerebral arteriolar vasospasm and cerebral edema may also be seen in PIH, although vision usually recovers completely [17, 18].

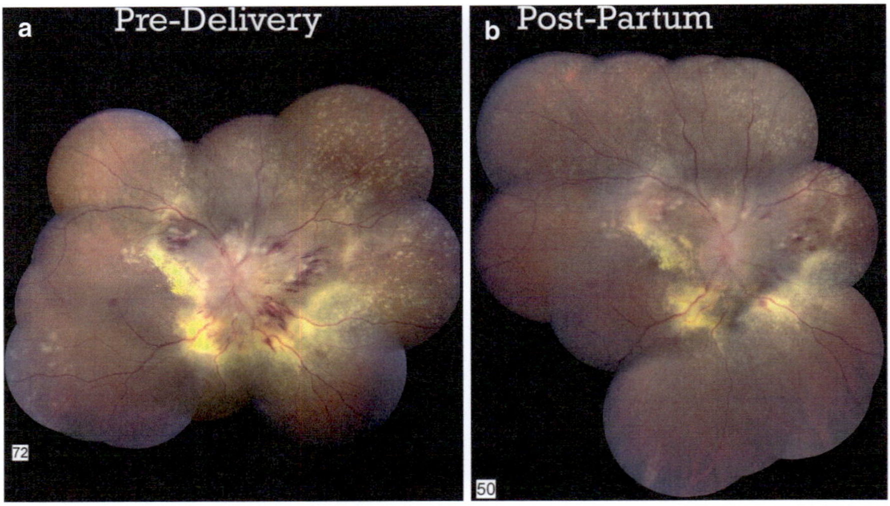

Fig. 13.3 Color photograph (right eye) in a patient with eclampsia (**a**) showing severe peripapillary retinal exudation with retinal edema and numerous intraretinal hemorrhages. These retinal changes improved significantly after delivery (**b**)

13.3.1.2 HELLP Syndrome

In approximately 10% of patients with severe PIH, the HELLP syndrome occurs. The HELLP syndrome, which is characterized by hemolysis, elevated liver enzymes, and low platelets, is associated with a poor maternal and fetal outcome. The ocular findings in this disorder include bilateral serous retinal detachments with yellow-white subretinal opacities (Fig. 13.4) [18], as well as possible vitreous hemorrhage [19].

Management of PIH

The management decisions for PIH are multifactorial, taking into account the maturity and health of the fetus. Medical treatment includes controlling the blood pressure and electrolyte imbalances.

Prognosis

Overall, the incidence of visual and retinal abnormalities has decreased due to improved medical management of PIH. The majority of the ocular abnormalities improve with medical management of PIH or with the delivery of the fetus.

13.3.2 Central Serous Chorioretinopathy

Central serous chorioretinopathy (CSCR) is characterized by a spontaneous, localized serous retinal detachment causing symptoms of decreased vision, metamorphopsia, and micropsia. The idiopathic form of disease primarily affects males in

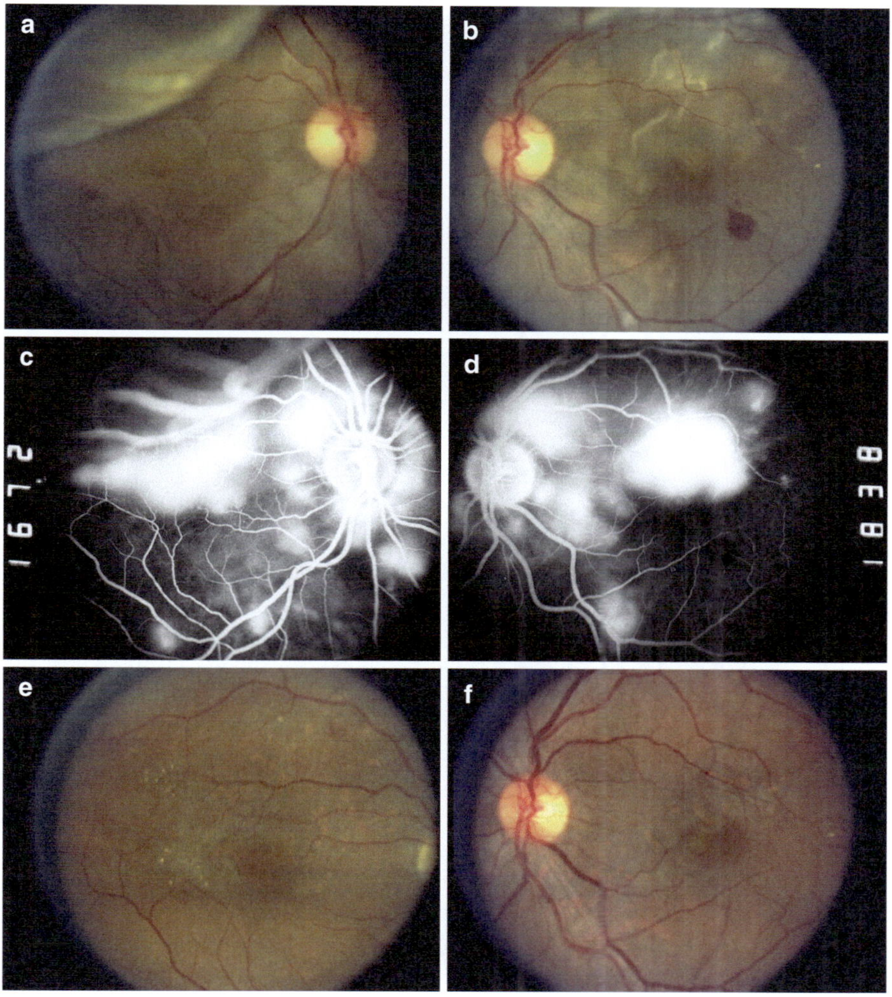

Fig. 13.4 Color photographs (both eyes) in a patient with HELLP syndrome (**a**, **b**) demonstrating extensive bilateral serous retinal detachments, with extensive leakage seen on fluorescein angiography (**c**, **d**). Following delivery, the retinal detachments resolved, leaving behind mild pigmentary changes to the retinal pigment epithelium (**e**, **f**)

the second to fourth decade of life. CSCR has been reported to occur in any trimester of pregnancy [20]. The etiology of CSCR in pregnancy is unknown, though hormonal [21], coagulation, and hemodynamic changes may play a role [22].

The presence of subretinal exudates with the serous retinal detachment is more often seen in CSCR associated with pregnancy (90%) than in non-pregnant patients (less than 20%) [23]. This exudate appears white or gray-white and represents fibrin in the subretinal space (Fig. 13.5) [23]. The diagnosis can generally be made by the clinical presentation, thus diagnostic fluorescein angiography is not necessary.

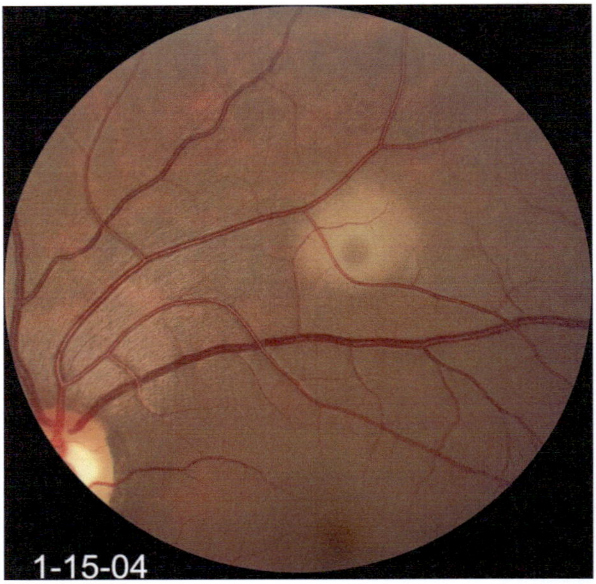

Fig. 13.5 Color photograph (left eye) showing a prominent serous retinal detachment of the macula with subretinal fibrin superiorly. This patient had just entered her second trimester of pregnancy. The findings were compatible with central serous chorioretinopathy

Both the serous detachment and the subretinal exudates tend to resolve near the end of pregnancy or in the postpartum period (Fig. 13.6). Patients who have experienced an episode of CSCR in pregnancy may have a recurrence outside of pregnancy or in a subsequent pregnancy [20].

13.3.3 Occlusive Vascular Disorders

A variety of occlusive vascular disorders may occur during pregnancy. These disorders include a Purtscher's-like retinopathy, or ocular changes associated with disseminated intravascular coagulation (DIC), thrombotic thrombocytopenic purpura (TTP), and/or amniotic fluid embolism.

13.3.3.1 Purtscher's-Like Retinopathy

A Purtscher's-like retinopathy has been reported, generally occurring within 24 h of childbirth [24]. It is usually associated with complications of the late stages of pregnancy, such as pre-eclampsia or pancreatitis. Patients experience severe, bilateral vision loss shortly after delivery. Funduscopic changes include widespread cotton wool spots with or without intraretinal hemorrhages (Fig. 13.7). Fluorescein angiography may demonstrate focal areas of arteriolar obstruction and varying degrees of retinal vascular leakage (Fig. 13.8). The retinal changes tend to resolve spontaneously, and vision recovers in most cases (Fig. 13.8). The etiology of this disorder is related to complement-induced granulocyte aggregation and vascular occlusion.

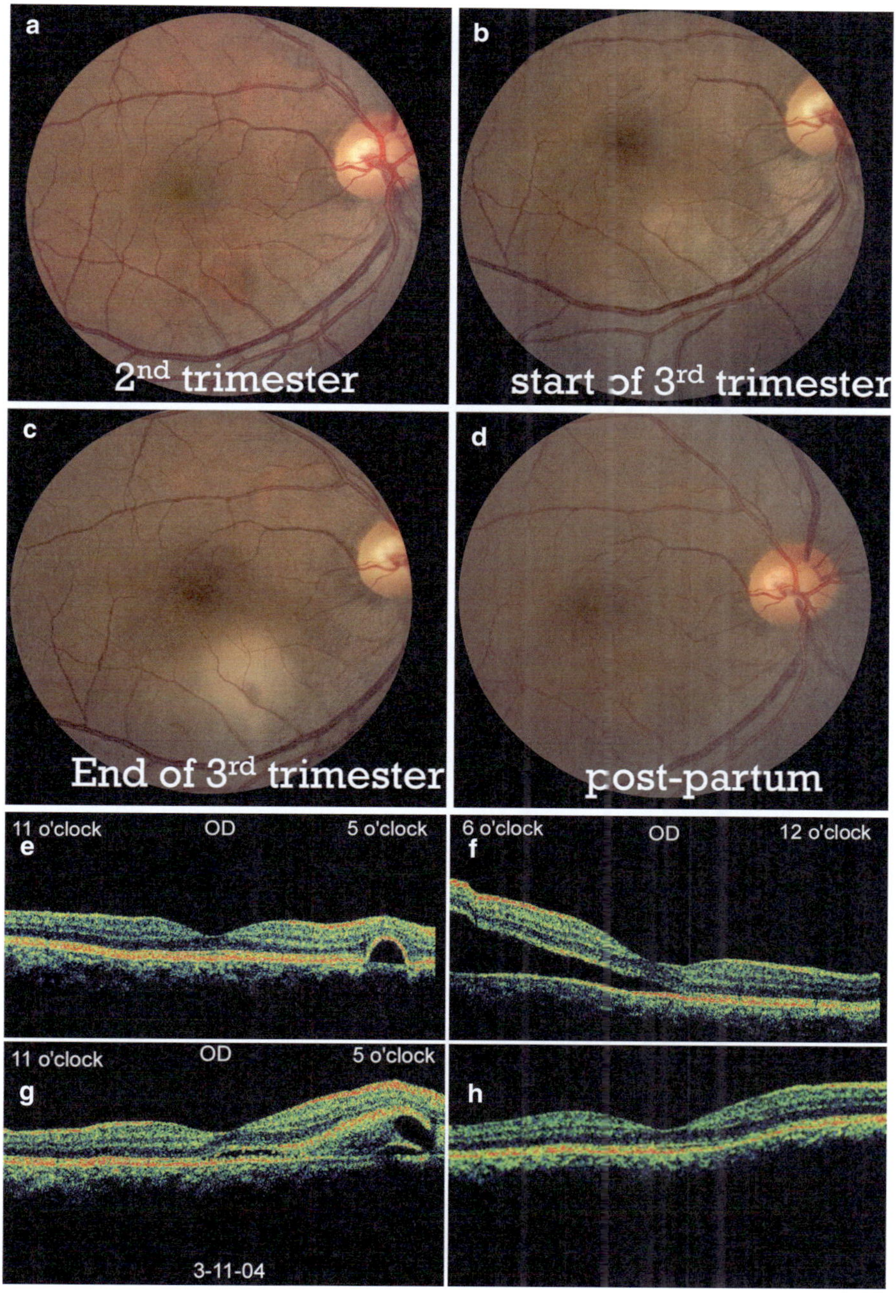

Fig. 13.6 Color photographs (right eye) (**a**–**d**) in a patient with bilateral CSCR at various stages during and post-pregnancy, with corresponding OCT images (**e**–**h**). The condition spontaneously improved without treatment

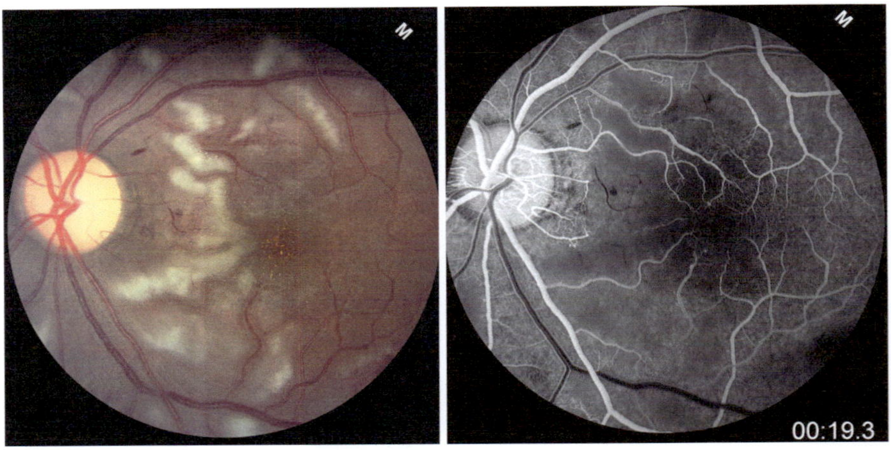

Fig. 13.7 Color photograph and fluorescein angiogram (right eye) in a patient immediately postpartum who experienced acute visual loss. The color photograph documents extensive temporal juxtapapillary retinal whitening while the fluorescein angiogram shows minimal capillary non-perfusion

13.3.3.2 Disseminated Intravascular Coagulation

Disseminated intravascular coagulation (DIC) may occur in complicated abortions, abruptio placenta, severe pre-eclampsia, and fetal compromise with retained tissue. DIC is characterized by widespread thrombus formation. The choroid is the most common intraocular structure involved [25, 26]. Occlusion of the choriocapillaris causes disruption of the overlying retinal pigment epithelium, leading to serous retinal detachment. With resolution of DIC, the serous detachment typically resolves. Retinal ischemia may also be seen (Fig. 13.9), along with residual retinal pigment epithelial alterations.

13.3.3.3 Thrombotic Thrombocytopenic Purpura

Thrombotic thrombocytopenic purpura (TTP) has been reported in the setting of pregnancy, and is characterized by thrombus deposition in vessels, hemolytic anemia, thrombocytopenia, neurologic changes, fever, and renal dysfunction. Ocular findings in this disorder include retinal vascular occlusions, retinal hemorrhages, serous retinal detachments, and optic disc neovascularization [27–29] (Fig. 13.10). The visual prognosis is generally very guarded. Purtscher's-like retinopathy has also been reported with TTP [30].

13.3.3.4 Amniotic Fluid Embolism

Amniotic fluid embolism is a serious complication of pregnancy, with an 80% mortality rate. It may occur during labor, delivery, or in the immediate postpartum period. Particulate matter from the amniotic fluid enters the maternal circulation, resulting in cardiopulmonary failure. Ophthalmic manifestations include retinal artery occlusions [31].

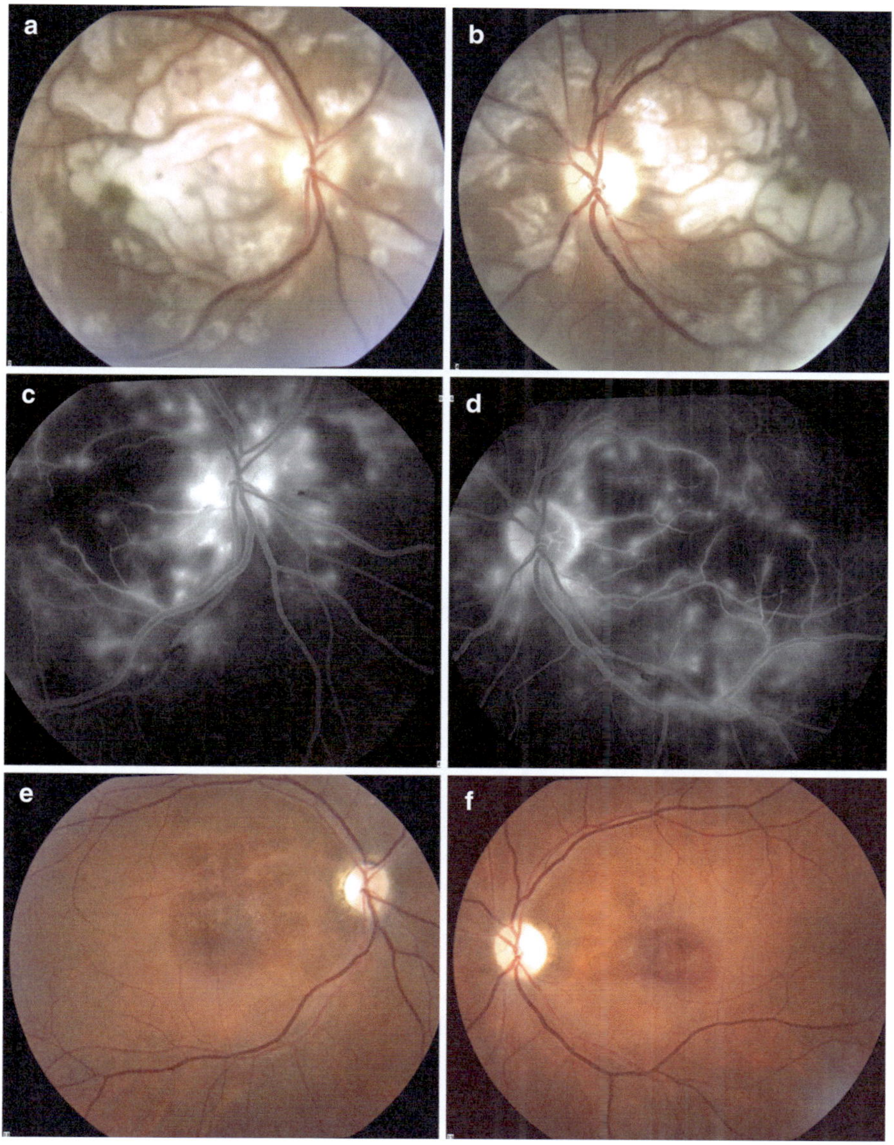

Fig. 13.8 Color photographs and fluorescein angiogram (both eyes) in a patient with Purtscher's-like retinopathy. (**a**, **b**) Color photographs document extensive peripapillary cotton-wool spots compatible with retinal ischemia, and this was documented on fluorescein angiography (**c**, **d**). Further in the post-delivery time frame (**e**, **f**), the cotton wool spots dissipated, though moderate retinal pigment epithelial mottling remained with mild visual impairment as well

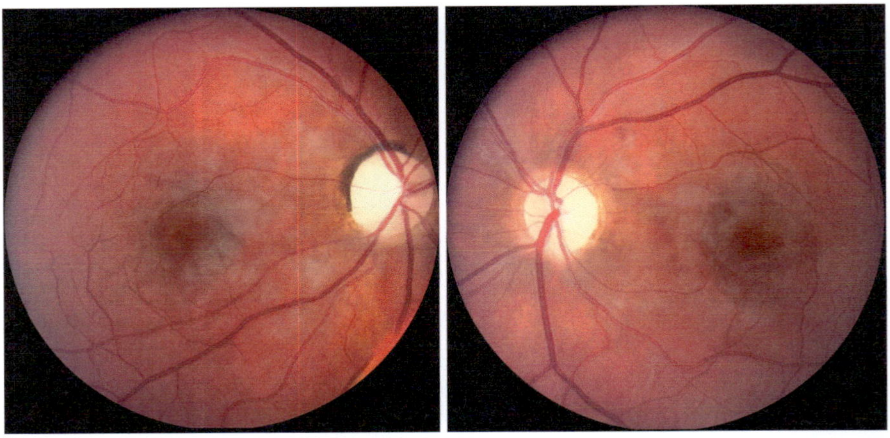

Fig. 13.9 Color photograph (both eyes) in a patient two months following a complicated abortion. Resolving cotton-wool spots are seen, and there was resultant retinal pigment epithelial mottling, though the vision was not adversely impacted

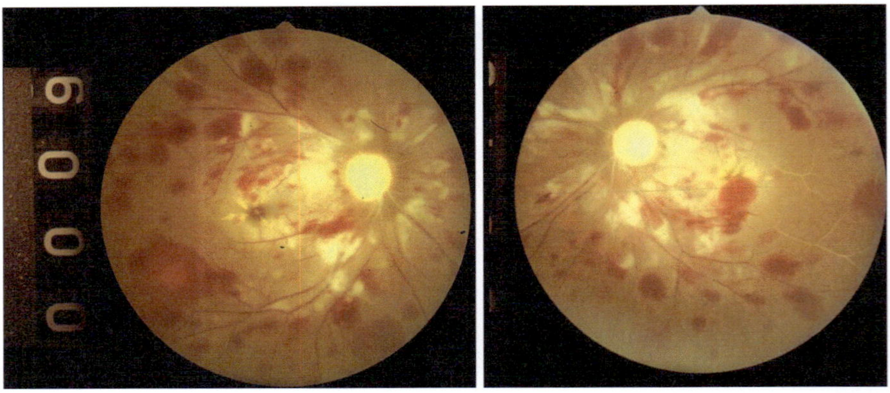

Fig. 13.10 Color photographs (both eye) in a pregnant patient who developed thrombotic thrombocytopenia purpura (TTP) and lost complete visual function

13.4 Pre-Existing Conditions

13.4.1 Diabetic Retinopathy

13.4.1.1 Progression

As reported by Klein and associates, pregnancy is a major risk factor for the progression of diabetic retinopathy (DR) [32]. Several studies have outlined the degree of the retinopathy progression during the course of pregnancy [33–35]. Axer-Siegel et al.

examined 65 patients with insulin dependent diabetes mellitus who became pregnant [36]. They reported that 26% of patients without DR at conception developed mild non-proliferative diabetic retinopathy (NPDR) during the course of pregnancy. Of the patients with initial NPDR, 55% had progression of their retinopathy. Twenty-two percent of patients with initial NPDR progressed to proliferative diabetic retinopathy (PDR) necessitating the need for pan-retinal photocoagulation (PRP).

Both NPDR and PDR occurring during the course of pregnancy have a high rate of spontaneous regression in the third trimester or in the post-partum time frame. In Axer-Siegel and coworkers' study, of the patients with no retinopathy at conception who then developed mild NPDR during pregnancy, 50% experienced total regression of their retinopathy and 30% had partial regression of their retinopathy after delivery [36]. The rate of total regression was not as high in patients with more advanced disease at the onset of pregnancy.

Diabetic macular edema (DME) may also occur during pregnancy [37]. As with the retinopathy, there is a high rate of spontaneous regression postpartum.

13.4.1.2 Factors Associated with Progression

The progression of DR is influenced by various factors including the duration of diabetes mellitus, metabolic control before and during pregnancy, severity of retinopathy at conception, and the presence of coexisting hypertension. Progression is more likely to occur in pregnant women who have had diabetes for a longer period of time, as is also the case for non-pregnant diabetics [36].

Several studies have also shown that both higher glycosylated hemoglobin levels at conception and rapid tightening of glycemic control during pregnancy have been associated with a higher risk of progression of retinopathy [33, 38]. In contrast, Lauszus and coworkers found no association between the progression of retinopathy and the glycosylated hemoglobin [39].

Another factor that influences the progression of DR during pregnancy is the degree of retinopathy at conception. Those patients with pre-existing DR are at a high risk of progression of their disease during pregnancy [36, 40]. Progression to PDR without the initial presence of NPDR in early pregnancy has been rarely described [41].

Finally, both high diastolic and systolic blood pressure have been reported to be associated independently with DR progression [32, 36].

13.4.1.3 Pathophysiology of Progression

The pathogenesis for the acceleration of DR during pregnancy is unclear. Several investigators have studied retinal circulatory changes in diabetic and control subjects during pregnancy. Chen and associates found an increase in retinal blood flow in pregnant women who had worsening of their DR [42]. In contrast, Schocket and coworkers noted that the retinal venous diameter and retinal blood flow decreased to a greater degree in diabetic mothers compared to non-diabetic mothers [43]. Thus, they proposed that the decrease in blood flow might exacerbate retinal ischemia and hypoxia, leading to the acceleration of DR.

13.4.1.4 Treatment Criteria for Diabetic Retinopathy

The treatment of PDR during pregnancy is based on the same criteria as in non-pregnant patients. DME is often observed without treatment due to the high rate of spontaneous regression in the post-partum period.

13.4.1.5 Follow-Up Guidelines

The American Academy of Ophthalmology has guidelines for the monitoring of pregnant diabetic patients in its Preferred Practice Patterns for diabetic retinopathy [44]. Ideally, pregnant diabetic women should receive an ophthalmologic examination prior to conception and then again in the first trimester. Subsequent exams should be at the discretion of the examiner, but at least every three months until delivery. Gestational diabetes does not carry the same risk of diabetic retinopathy and does not require fundus examination during pregnancy.

13.4.2 Intraocular Tumors

13.4.2.1 Uveal Melanoma

Uveal melanoma growth has been described during pregnancy [45–47]. Shields et al. reported a series of 16 pregnant patients with uveal melanoma [47]. Seven patients were diagnosed with active tumors at initial presentation and treated immediately. Of the remaining nine patients who had been followed for various lengths of time with suspicious lesions, seven patients demonstrated transformation into active melanoma during the course of pregnancy (Fig. 13.11). The histopathology

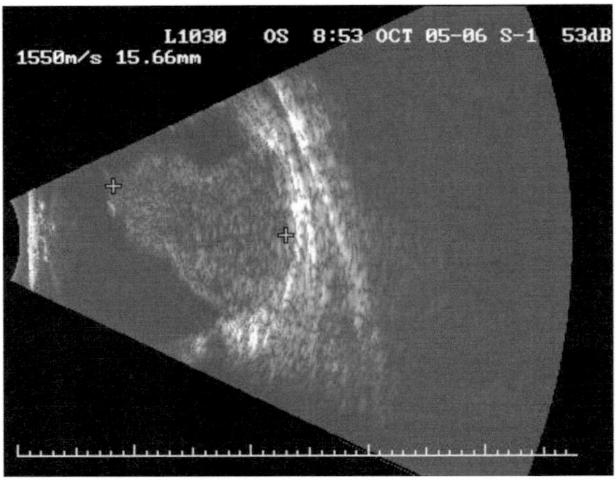

Fig. 13.11 Echogram (right eye) in a pregnant female who had been monitored with a pigmented lesion compatible with a medium-sized uveal melanoma. Initial plans were to wait until conclusion of the pregnancy to treat the lesion with brachytherapy, though with documented growth of the lesion (including a breakthrough Bruch's membrane), brachytherapy was carried out during the third trimester. The patient and child have done well

and survival rates of uveal melanoma in pregnant women were similar to non-pregnant patients. The etiology of transformation and growth during pregnancy is unknown.

13.4.2.2 Choroidal Osteoma

There have been several descriptions of choroidal osteomas presenting during pregnancy and/or changing in appearance [47]. The etiology for the exacerbation of the choroidal osteoma during pregnancy is unknown.

13.4.2.3 Choroidal Hemangioma

Choroidal hemangiomas have been documented to rapidly expand then spontaneously regress after delivery [48].

13.4.3 Diagnostic Agents

Fluorescein dye crosses the placenta and is present in breast milk for at least three days after administration [49]. No teratogenic or embryocidal effects have been reported in animals [50, 51]. Also, no adverse effects have been reported in humans.

Halperin and coworkers reviewed the use of fluorescein angiography in pregnant patients [52]. A retrospective study of neonatal outcomes in 105 pregnant patients who underwent fluorescein angiography revealed that there was not a high rate of birth anomalies or complications. Nonetheless, most vitreoretinal specialists likely would avoid obtaining an angiogram during pregnancy unless a sight-threatening lesion is suspected.

Indocyanine green (ICG) has been used in pregnant women for non-ophthalmic purposes, such as for measuring hepatic blood flow, without adverse effect on the mother or fetus. It does not cross the placenta, but it is not known whether it is present in breast milk [53]. Most retina specialists seem hesitant to order ICG angiography during pregnancy, despite its documented safety for non-ophthalmic purposes [54].

Conclusion

Pregnancy may be associated with a variety of ocular manifestations in the mother. Systemic hypertension may have a dramatic impact on the eye during pregnancy, inducing a variety of retinal, choroidal, and/or optic nerve abnormalities. Select vascular occlusive disorders such as Purtscher's-like retinopathy, DIC, or TTP also occur, though are extremely rare. Other conditions such as CSCR may occur with a greater frequency, though the visual changes generally stabilize post-partum.

Pre-existing conditions such as diabetes mellitus may be exacerbated during pregnancy. Finally, certain intraocular tumors such as uveal melanoma, choroidal osteoma, and choroidal hemangioma may grow or change during the course of pregnancy.

The majority of these conditions resolves or stabilizes during the post-partum time frame, though occasionally they may lead to permanent visual impairment. An understanding of these changes will aid in establishing the appropriate diagnosis and management of ocular conditions during pregnancy.

Acknowledgements A special thank you to David Sarraf, MD, Jules Stein Eye Institute, Los Angeles, CA, for use of several fundus photographs and fluorescein angiograms.

References

1. Hormonal influences in glaucoma. Br Med J. 1963;2(5354):404.
2. Phillips CI, Gore SM. Ocular hypotensive effect of late pregnancy with and without high blood pressure. Br J Ophthalmol. 1985;69(2):117–9.
3. Wilke K. Episcleral venous pressure and pregnancy [proceedings]. Acta Ophthalmol Suppl. 1975;125:40–1.
4. Horven I, Gjonnaess H. Corneal indentation pulse and intraocular pressure in pregnancy. Arch Ophthalmol. 1974;91(2):92–8.
5. Riss B, Riss P. Corneal sensitivity in pregnancy. Ophthalmologica. 1981;183(2):57–62.
6. Weinreb RN, Lu A, Beeson C. Maternal corneal thickness during pregnancy. Am J Ophthalmol. 1988;105(3):258–60.
7. Park SB, Lindahl KJ, Temnycky GO, Aquavella JV. The effect of pregnancy on corneal curvature. CLAO J. 1992;18(4):256–9.
8. Millodot M. The influence of pregnancy on the sensitivity of the cornea. Br J Ophthalmol. 1977;61(10):646–9.
9. Fatt IHM. Refractive index of the cornea as a function of its thickness. Am J Optom Physiol Optic. 1973;50:383–6.
10. Schreyer P, Tzadok J, Sherman DJ, Herman A, Bar-Itzhak R, Caspi E. Fluorescein angiography in hypertensive pregnancies. Int J Gynaecol Obstet. 1991;34(2):127–32.
11. Jaffe G, Schatz H. Ocular manifestations of preeclampsia. Am J Ophthalmol. 1987;103(3 Pt 1):309–15.
12. Dornan KJ, Mallek DR, Wittmann BK. The sequelae of serous retinal detachment in preeclampsia. Obstet Gynecol. 1982;60(5):657–63.
13. Hallum AV. Eye changes in hypertensive toxemia of pregnancy. JAMA. 1936;106:1649–51.
14. Valluri S, Adelberg DA, Curtis RS, Olk RJ. Diagnostic indocyanine green angiography in preeclampsia. Am J Ophthalmol. 1996;122(5):672–7.
15. Saito Y, Tano Y. Retinal pigment epithelial lesions associated with choroidal ischemia in preeclampsia. Retina. 1998;18(2):103–8.
16. Beck RW, Gamel JW, Willcourt RJ, Berman G. Acute ischemic optic neuropathy in severe preeclampsia. Am J Ophthalmol. 1980;90(3):342–6.
17. Grimes DA, Ekbladh LE, McCartney WH. Cortical blindness in preeclampsia. Int J Gynaecol Obstet. 1980;17(6):601–3.
18. Beeson JH, Duda EE. Computed axial tomography scan demonstration of cerebral edema in eclampsia preceded by blindness. Obstet Gynecol. 1982;60(4):529–32.
19. Leff SR, Yarian DL, Masciulli L, Green SN, Baldomero RE. Vitreous haemorrhage as a complication of HELLP syndrome. Br J Ophthalmol. 1990;74(8):498.
20. Sunness JS, Haller JA, Fine SL. Central serous chorioretinopathy and pregnancy. Arch Ophthalmol. 1993;111(3):360–4.
21. Chumbley LC, Frank RN. Central serous retinopathy and pregnancy. Am J Ophthalmol. 1974;77(2):158–60.
22. Fastenberg DM, Ober RR. Central serous choroidopathy in pregnancy. Arch Ophthalmol. 1983;101(7):1055–8.

23. Gass JD. Central serous chorioretinopathy and white subretinal exudation during pregnancy. Arch Ophthalmol. 1991;109(5):677–81.
24. Blodi BA, Johnson MW, Gass JD, Fine SL, Joffe LM. Purtscher's-like retinopathy after childbirth. Ophthalmology. 1990;97(12):1654–9.
25. Cogan DG. Ocular involvement in disseminated intravascular coagulopathy. Arch Ophthalmol. 1975;93(1):1–8.
26. Hoines J, Buettner H. Ocular complications of disseminated intravascular coagulation (DIC) in abruptio placentae. Retina. 1989;9(2):105–9.
27. Percival SP. The eye and Moschcowitz's disease (thrombotic thrombocytopenic purpura). Trans Ophthalmol Soc U K. 1970;90:375–82.
28. Lewellen DR Jr, Singerman LJ. Thrombotic thrombocytopenic purpura with optic disk neovascularization, vitreous hemorrhage, retinal detachment, and optic atrophy. Am J Ophthalmol. 1980;89(6):840–4.
29. Gum KB, Carter KD, Vine AK. Massive bilateral retinal vascular occlusion secondary to thrombotic thrombocytopenic purpura. Retina. 1988;8(3):185–7.
30. Power MH, Regillo MC, Custis PH. Thrombotic thrombocytopenic purpura associated with Purtscher retinopathy. Arch Ophthalmol. 1997;115(1):128–9.
31. Chang M, Herbert WN. Retinal arteriolar occlusions following amniotic fluid embolism. Ophthalmology. 1984;91(12):1634–7.
32. Klein BE, Moss SE, Klein R. Effect of pregnancy on progression of diabetic retinopathy. Diabetes Care. 1990;13(1):34–40.
33. Phelps RL, Sakol P, Metzger BE, Jampol LM, Freinkel N. Changes in diabetic retinopathy during pregnancy. Correlations with regulation of hyperglycemia. Arch Ophthalmol. 1986;104(12):1806–10.
34. Moloney JB, Drury MI. The effect of pregnancy on the natural course of diabetic retinopathy. Am J Ophthalmol. 1982;93(6):745–56.
35. Best RM, Chakravarthy U. Diabetic retinopathy in pregnancy. Br J Ophthalmol. 1997;81(3):249–51.
36. Axer-Siegel R, Hod M, Fink-Cohen S, et al. Diabetic retinopathy during pregnancy. Ophthalmology. 1996;103(11):1815–9.
37. Sinclair SH, Nesler C, Foxman B, Nichols CW, Gabbe S. Macular edema and pregnancy in insulin-dependent diabetes. Am J Ophthalmol. 1984;97(2):154–67.
38. Chew EY, Mills JL, Metzger BE, et al. Metabolic control and progression of retinopathy. The Diabetes in Early Pregnancy Study. National Institute of Child Health and Human Development Diabetes in Early Pregnancy Study. Diabetes Care. 1995;18(5):631–7.
39. Lauszus F, Klebe JG, Bek T. Diabetic retinopathy in pregnancy during tight metabolic control. Acta Obstet Gynecol Scand. 2000;79(5):367–70.
40. Sinclair SH, Nesler CL, Schwartz SS. Retinopathy in the pregnant diabetic. Clin Obstet Gynecol. 1985;28(3):536–52.
41. Kitzmiller JL, Main E, Ward B, Theiss T, Peterson DL. Insulin lispro and the development of proliferative diabetic retinopathy during pregnancy. Diabetes Care. 1999;22(5):874–6.
42. Chen HC, Newsom RS, Patel V, Cassar J, Mather H, Kohner EM. Retinal blood flow changes during pregnancy in women with diabetes. Invest Ophthalmol Vis Sci. 1994;35(8): 3199–208.
43. Schocket LS, Grunwald JE, Tsang AF, DuPont J. The effect of pregnancy on retinal hemodynamics in diabetic versus nondiabetic mothers. Am J Ophthalmol. 1999;128(4):477–84.
44. American Academy of Ophthalmology. San Francisco, CA: AAO; 2016. American academy of ophthalmology retina panel. Preferred practice pattern guidelines: Diabetic Retinopathy.
45. Siegel R, Ainslie WH. Malignant ocular melanoma during pregnancy. JAMA. 1963;185:542–3.
46. Seddon JM, MacLaughlin DT, Albert DM, Gragoudas ES, Ference M 3rd. Uveal melanomas presenting during pregnancy and the investigation of oestrogen receptors in melanomas. Br J Ophthalmol. 1982;66(11):695–704.
47. Shields CL, Shields JA, Eagle RC Jr, De Potter P, Menduke H. Uveal melanoma and pregnancy. A report of 16 cases. Ophthalmology. 1991;98(11):1667–73.

48. Pitta C, Bergen R, Littwin S. Spontaneous regression of a choroidal hemangioma following pregnancy. Ann Ophthalmol. 1979;11(5):772–4.
49. Mattern J, Mayer PR. Excretion of fluorescein into breast milk. Am J Ophthalmol. 1990;109(5):598–9.
50. McEnerney JK, Wong WP, Peyman GA. Evaluation of the teratogenicity of fluorescein sodium. Am J Ophthalmol. 1977;84(6):847–50.
51. Salem H, Loux JJ, Smith S, Nichols CW. Evaluation of the toxicologic and teratogenic potentials of sodium fluorescein in the rat. Toxicology. 1979;12(2):143–50.
52. Halperin LS, Olk RJ, Soubrane G, Coscas G. Safety of fluorescein angiography during pregnancy. Am J Ophthalmol. 1990;109(5):563–6.
53. Rudolf H, Goretzlehner G, Brugmann E, Towe J, Rudolf K. Assessment of liver function using indocyanine green (Ujoviridin) during normal pregnancy, during labor and in puerperium. Zentralbl Gynakol. 1977;99(25):1548–53.
54. Fineman MS, Maguire JI, Fineman SW, Benson WE. Safety of indocyanine green angiography during pregnancy: a survey of the retina, macula, and vitreous societies. Arch Ophthalmol. 2001;119(3):353–5.

Systemic Hypertension

14

Giuseppe Querques, Maria Vittoria Cicinelli, Lea Querques, Ilaria Zucchiatti, Lucia Benatti, Andrea Mazzaferro, Fatemeh Darvizeh, and Francesco Bandello

Abstract

Hypertensive retinopathy refers to a spectrum of ophthalmic changes secondary to elevated systemic blood pressure. Retinal arterioles can be visualized easily and non-invasively and share similar anatomical and physiological properties with cerebral and coronary microcirculation. Therefore, the retina provides a window to study the human circulation in hypertensive patients.

Both acute hypertensive peaks and chronically elevated blood pressure may have ocular involvement: arteriovenous nicking is the hallmark of long-standing disease. Retinopathy has been graded in mild, moderate, and severe according to ocular findings and systemic risk. Accurate diagnosis of hypertensive retinopathy, especially that associated with malignant hypertension, is necessary to avoid visual and systemic morbidity and to address prompt treatment.

In the United States, an estimated 25% of all adults and 60% of individuals over 60 years suffer from hypertension, corresponding to about 50 million people. Blacks have a higher prevalence than whites, and men are affected more than women until 50 years of age when women have a higher prevalence [1].

High blood pressure is classified into different classes:

- Essential hypertension, of unknown etiology and diagnosed when the average blood pressure measures >140 mmHg systolic or >90 mmHg diastolic.

G. Querques (✉) • M.V. Cicinelli • L. Querques • I. Zucchiatti • L. Benatti • A. Mazzaferro
F. Darvizeh • F. Bandello
Department of Ophthalmology, Scientific Institute San Raffaele, University Vita-Salute, via Olgettina 60, 20132 Milan, Italy
e-mail: giuseppe.querques@hotmail.it; cicinelli.mariavittoria@hsr.it; lea_querques@hotmail.com; ilaria.zucchiatti@gmail.com; l.benatti@studenti.unisr.it; andrea.mazzaferro@alice.it; fdarvizeh@gmail.com; bandello.francesco@hsr.it

J. Chhablani et al. (eds.), *Retinal and Choroidal Imaging in Systemic Diseases*, https://doi.org/10.1007/978-981-10-5461-7_14

- Secondary hypertension, when caused by medical o iatrogenic condition and can be cured with correction of the underlying disease.
- Malignant hypertension: affects 1% of the hypertensive population, occurring when the systolic blood pressure is ≥200 mmHg and the diastolic is ≥130 mmHg. Life-threatening complications are headache, proteinuria, stroke, kidney failure, and encephalopathy. Ocular symptoms include scotoma, diplopia, blurred vision, and photopsias.

Hypertension is often underdiagnosed or inadequately treated despite the relative ease of detection [2]. Untreated or inadequately treated hypertension carries significant cardiovascular and renal mortality. In patients with borderline hypertension, the relative risk of cardiovascular disease and end-stage renal disease is nearly double that of patients with optimal blood pressure [3].

Hypertensive retinopathy is nowadays evaluated as an indicator for organ damage along with left ventricular hypertrophy and chronic renal failure and is accepted as a prognosis-influencing factor in hypertensive patients [4]. However, most current guidelines for the management of arterial hypertension do not recommend fundoscopy as a routine screening test, as the presence of retinal lesions does not require changes in therapeutic management of these patients [5].

Over the past decade, large population-based studies have evaluated hypertensive retinopathy relying on retinal photography [6]. Data from these epidemiological studies indicate that hypertensive retinopathy signs occur in 3–14% of non-diabetic adults aged 40 years or older. Among the different retinal signs, focal arteriolar narrowing and arteriovenous (AV) nicking occur in 7–12% of hypertensive people, respectively, and the most common retinopathy lesions observed are isolated retinal hemorrhages or microaneurysms (3–17%), with cotton wool spots being relatively uncommon (0.3%).

14.1 Ocular Manifestations

Although the name hypertensive retinopathy implies exclusive retinal involvement, changes at different ocular structures are observed, depending on the chronicity and severity of the disease. In fact, the retina, the retinal pigment epithelium (RPE), the choroid, and the optic nerve may be affected, with variable associations. Subconjunctival hemorrhages, while usually secondary to a Valsalva maneuver, can also occur in conjunction with acute blood pressure elevation.

Retinal arterioles and capillaries are similar in anatomy to cerebral vessels in that they exhibit autoregulatory mechanisms to maintain a constant ocular perfusion pressure; moreover, tight junctions at endothelial level form the internal blood-retinal barrier, ensuring retinal isolation from systemic circulation. Choroidal arterioles and capillaries have fenestrations (no blood-ocular barrier) and do not exhibit autoregulation. Optic nerve head vessels feature intermediary characteristics with autoregulation but an incompetent blood-ocular barrier as a result of the peripapillary choroidal vessels [7].

Table 14.1 Clinical features of acute (on the left) and chronic (on the right) hypertensive retinopathy

Acute hypertensive retinopathy	Chronic hypertensive retinopathy
Cystoid macular edema/neurosensory retinal detachment	Arteriolosclerosis
Hypertensive choroidopathy	AV nicking
FIPTs	Stellate maculopathy
Cotton-wool spots	Collateral shunts, microaneurysms
Optic disc edema	Optic disc pallor
Systemic symptoms (proteinuria, stroke, kidney failure, encephalopathy)	RVO, macroaneurysm

AV arteriovenous, *FIPTs* focal intraretinal periarteriolar transudates, *RVO* retinal vein occlusion

These differences between the retina, the choroid, and the optic nerve explain why each of these anatomic regions responds differently to hypertension. In fact, acute hypertensive peaks, such as those reached in malignant hypertension or gravidic eclampsia, generally correspond to more striking clinical signs, with disc edema, choroidal infarction, and evident retinopathy. These events are related to diffuse vasoconstriction of arterial vascular beds secondary to the systemic release of catecholamines. Chronic hypertension leads to more subtle changes, affecting primarily the retinal vasculature, and patients are usually asymptomatic (Table 14.1).

14.2 Hypertensive Vasculopathy

First signs of hypertension-related ocular damage involve the retinal vasculature. Primary injury takes place at the microvascular level, where the physiological response of healthy retinal arterioles to high pressure is vasoconstriction (retinal circulatory system autoregulation) [8]. Arterial narrowing can be focal or generalized, when involves different arteriolar branches.

When this condition is sustained, vascular histological structure is diffusely affected. In detail, the tunica media of retinal vessel made of thin smooth muscle becomes hypertrophic, as a consequence of its prolonged state of contraction. Nutritional blood supply is likely to be insufficient to satisfy the increased metabolic demand of thickened muscular cells, and the fibers become ischemic and are replaced by hyaline scar. The outermost elastic layer of retinal arterioles gradually leaves place to thicker unelastic fibrotic coat; the thin endothelial monolayer that represents the internal blood-retinal barrier gets damaged by persistently high intraluminal blood pressure. This phenomenon is globally known as arteriolosclerosis and leads to increased optical density of retinal blood vessel walls; this is visible on ophthalmoscopy as sheathing of the vessels, or copper-wire appearance. When sheathing encircles the entire wall, it produces a silver-wire vessel (Fig. 14.1).

Morphological changes are more evident at AV crossing, where the pathologic rigid arteriole crosses, compresses, and dislocates the vein, as the vessels share a common adventitial sheath (Fig. 14.2).

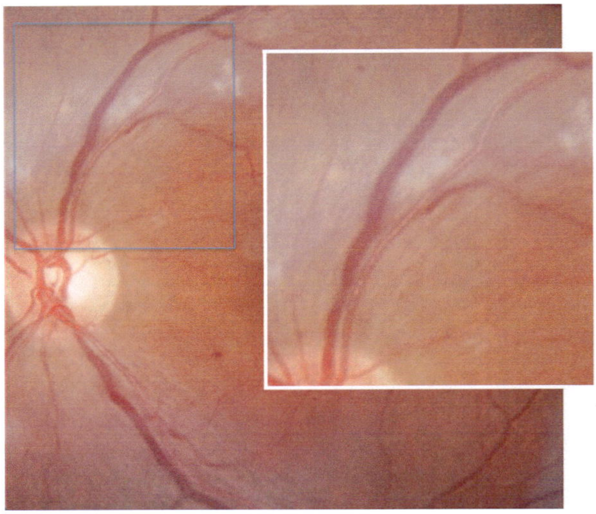

Fig. 14.1 Copper-wire arterioles. On the right magnification centered on the bright metallic reflex of the supero-temporal retinal arterioles

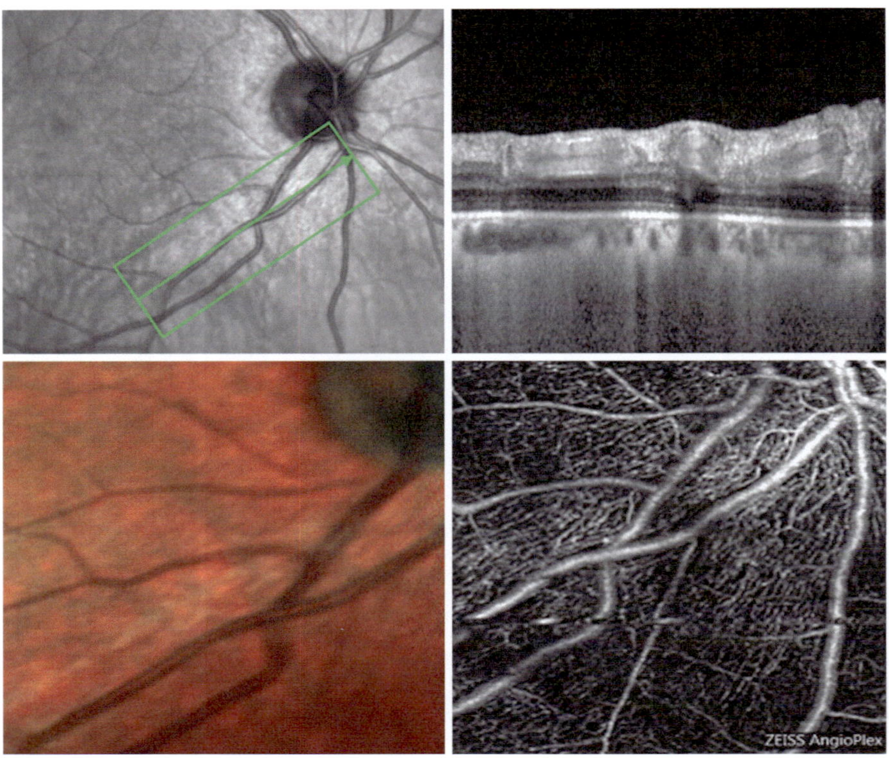

Fig. 14.2 Arteriovenous nicking. *Top*: infrared fundus image (*left*) and optical coherence tomography (OCT) (*right*) showing the anatomic relationship between the artery and the vein at arteriovenous crossing. *Bottom*: color fundus image (*left*) and OCT angiography (*right*) showing Gunn sign (see the text for explanation)

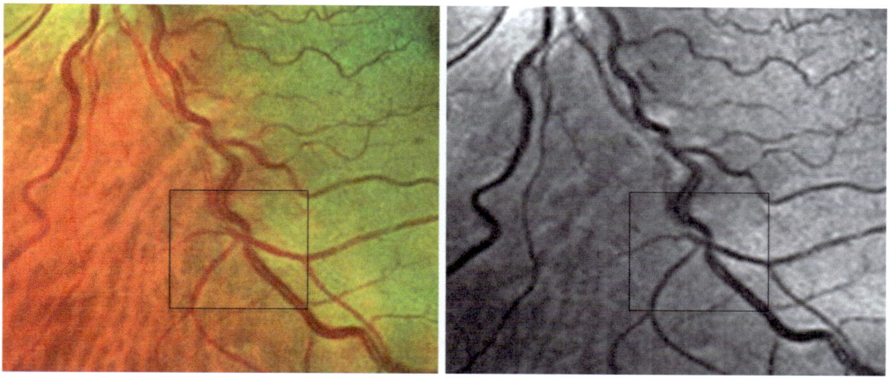

Fig. 14.3 Salus sign. Vein deviation under the enlarged arterioles at right-angle crossing points, where the venule crosses the arteriole in a horseshoe shape

Table 14.2 Clinical classification of hypertensive vasculopathy

Grade 1	Broadening of arteriolar light reflex, mild arteriolar attenuation, narrowing, and tortuosity, and vein concealment at the level of AV nicking
Grade 2	More evident broadening of arteriolar light reflex, higher arteriolar attenuation, and venous displacement at points where arterioles and venules cross over (Salus sign)
Grade 3	Bright arteriolar reflex (copper-wire), dilatation of veins distally to arteriovenous cross (Bonnet sign) and tapering of veins at both sides of AV cross (Gunn sign)
Grade 4	Brighter arteriolar reflex (silver-wire), associated with signs of grade 3 vasculopathy

AV arteriovenous

Since blood flow is impeded from AV nicking, the vein distal to compression shows hourglass constrictions (Gunn sign), aneurysmal-like dilatation (Bonnet sign), and increased tortuosity on both sides of the crossing. Moreover, sclerosis may alter the original length of retinal arterioles, and changes the orientation of the branches coming off, creating right angles between the main vessel and its minor branches. This change in length deflects the veins at the common sheath and changes their course in a horseshoe shape (Salus sign) (Fig. 14.3).

These features have been divided into four progressive stages (Scheie classification), not necessarily indicative for severity of the condition (Table 14.2) [9].

14.3 Hypertensive Retinopathy

Once vascular changes take place, the integrity of inner blood-retinal barrier is disrupted, endothelial permeability increases, and focal intraretinal periarteriolar transudates (FIPTs) accumulates in extracellular spaces. FIPTs are small, white, focal, oval lesions deep in the retina, associated with major arteriolar vessels and are among the earliest retinal lesions caused by malignant hypertension. Chronic retinal leakage, instead, results in lipid precipitation in the form of hard exudates with a peculiar speckled configuration that follows the radial orientation of Henle fiber layer, known as macular star (Fig. 14.4).

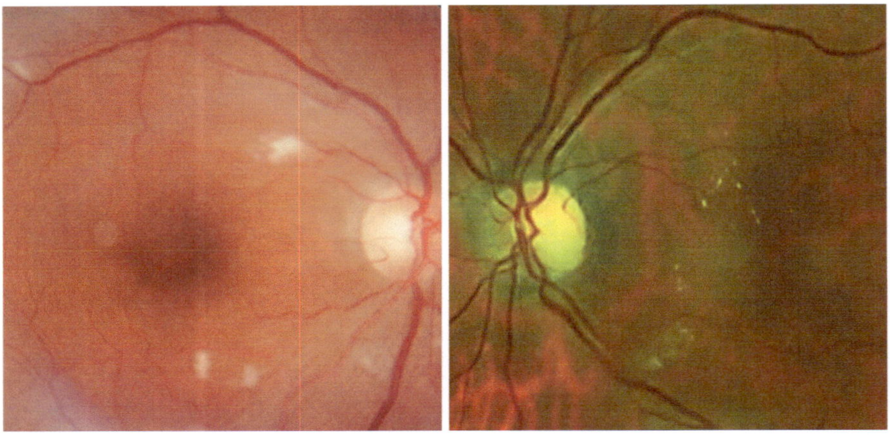

Fig. 14.4 *Left*: Intraretinal periarteriolar transudates, appearing as small, white, focal, oval lesions associated with arteriolar vessels, among the earliest lesions suggestive of malignant hypertension. *Right*: radial orientation of perimacular hard exudates

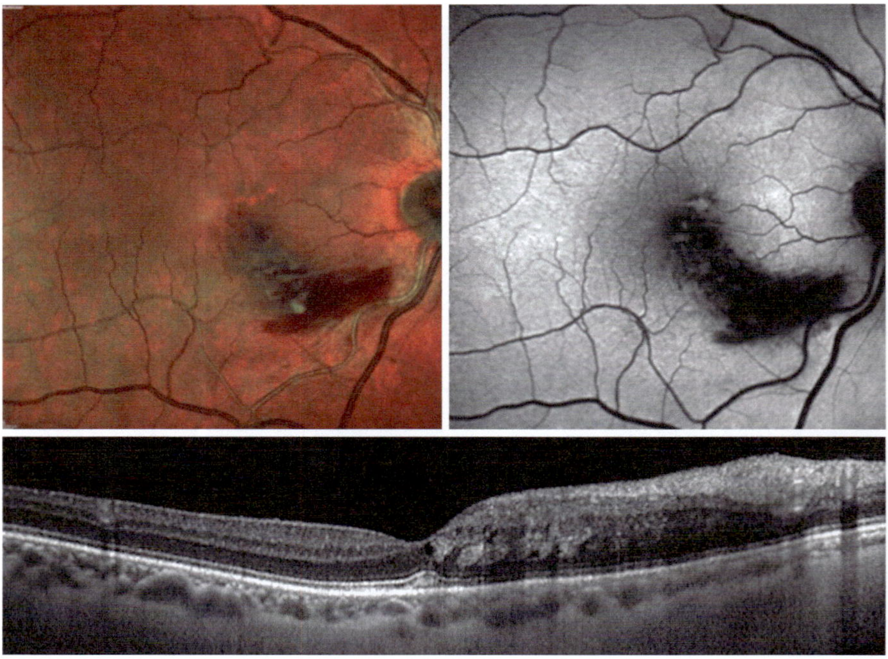

Fig. 14.5 Cotton-wool spots and flame-shaped hemorrhages in the nerve fiber layer imaged through color fundus (*top left*), posterior pole blue-light (588 nm) fundus autofluorescence (*top right*), and optical coherence tomography (*bottom*)

In severe cases, signs of retinal ischemia and venous stasis become detectable on fundus, including cotton-wool spots and flame-shaped hemorrhages in the nerve fiber layer (Fig. 14.5).

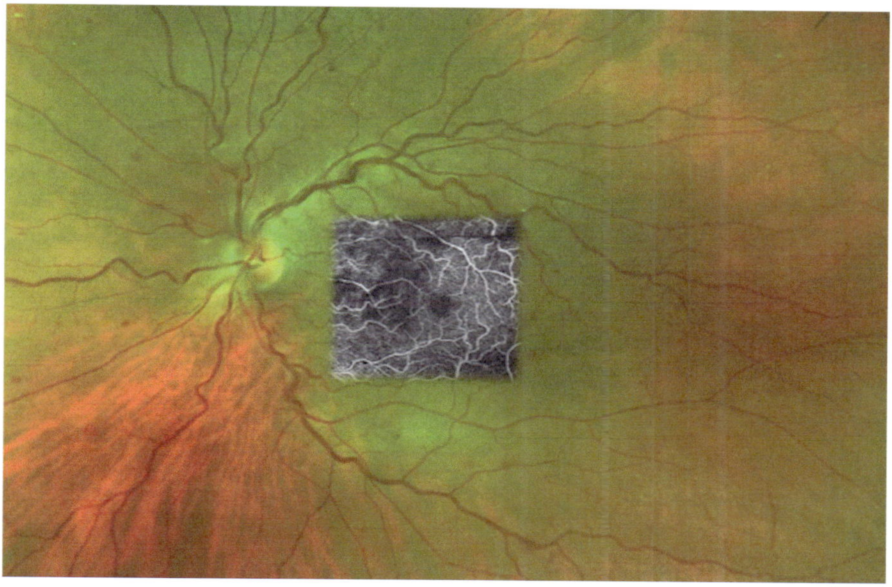

Fig. 14.6 Incipient retinal vein occlusion in highly hypertensive woman presenting with central scotoma: note marked vascular tortuosity, dot retinal hemorrhages, and initial macular hypoperfusion on superimposed optical coherence tomography angiography of the same eye

Compensatory changes to chronic capillary obliteration result in the development of microaneurysms, shunts, and collateral vessels. Possible vascular complications of untreated hypertensive retinopathy are vein occlusion and macroaneurysm (Fig. 14.6).

14.4 Hypertensive Choroidopathy

Choroid is rarely damaged in chronic hypertensive retinopathy; choroidal involvement is more common in accelerate setting, such as hypertensive crisis or toxemia of pregnancy [10]. Choroidal vascular involvement is typically more severe than retinal changes, and more closely resembles systemic arterial narrowing. Features of choroidopathy are often bilateral, share an acute ischemic pathogenesis, and represent microinfarcts of the terminal branches of the short posterior ciliary arteries (Fig. 14.7).

They include:

- Elschnig spots: small, confluent, pigmented lesions in correspondence to focal choroidal necrosis.
- Siegrist's streaks: linear flecks along vessel, indicative of fibrinoid necrosis.
- Neurosensory retinal detachment and intraretinal cystoid edema secondary to external blood-retinal barrier damage (Fig. 14.8).

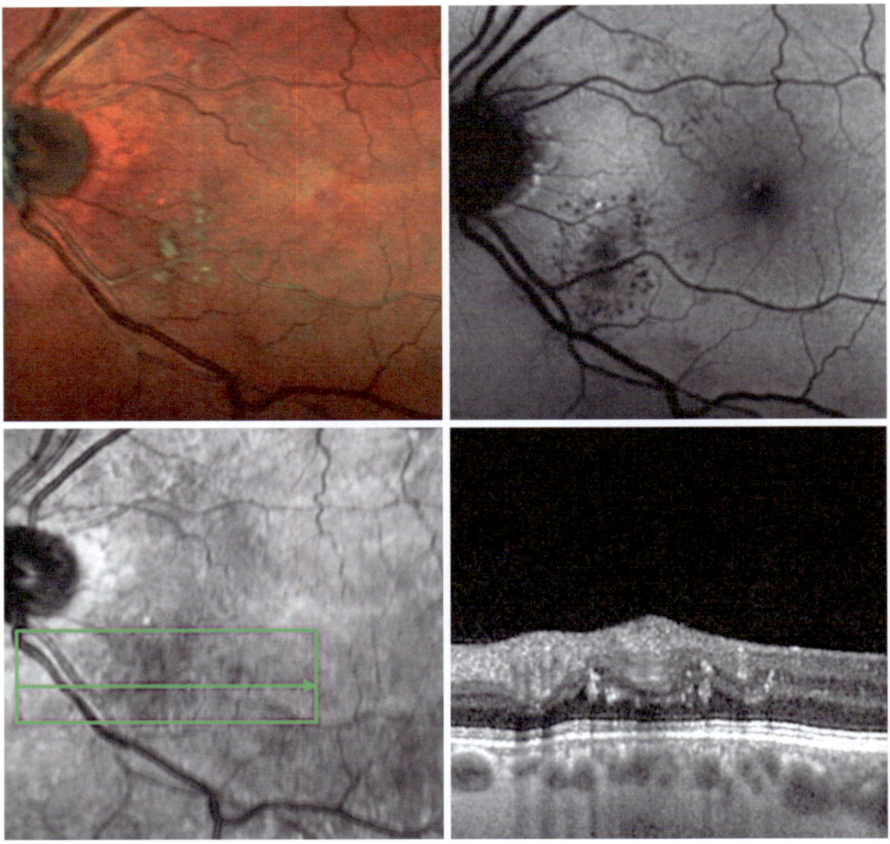

Fig. 14.7 Multimodal imaging of focal chorioretinal ischemia: color fundus image showing hard exudates and small hemorrhages (*top left*); fundus autofluorescence showing multiple focal hypo-autofluorescent dots, related to small choroidal infarctions (*top right*); infrared image and optical coherence tomography scan passing through the lesion, showing a circular three-dimensional disposition of the exudates around the occluded vessel (*bottom*)

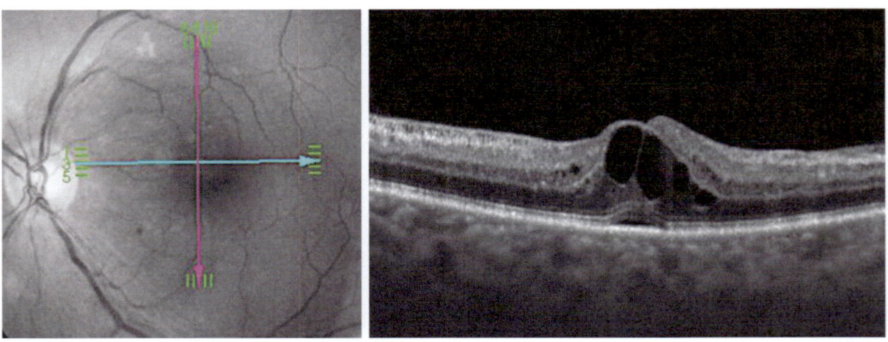

Fig. 14.8 Swept-source optical coherence tomography of a chronically hypertensive patient, showing intraretinal edema and foveal neurosensory detachment

14.5 Hypertensive Opticopathy

In hyper-acute cases, optic disc swelling takes place (Fig. 14.4). This is a form of non-arteritic anterior ischemic optic neuropathy (NAION), secondary to hormone-related vasoconstriction of the posterior ciliary arteries supplying the optic nerve head. Ischemia occurring in the optic nerve leads to stasis of axoplasmic flow, with peripapillary hemorrhages and cotton-wool spots. Optic disc pallor develops in chronic hypertension. Diabetic papillopathy and central retinal vein occlusion must be considered in the differential diagnosis of this clinical picture.

14.6 Instrumental Diagnosis

Hypertensive retinopathy is a clinical diagnosis, as visualized on slit-lamp biomicroscopy or indirect ophthalmoscopy. Diagnosis is confirmed by measurement of blood pressure and exclusion of all possible confounding factors. Fundus fluorescein angiography is not crucial for diagnosis, but helps in visualization of capillary nonperfusion, blockage from retinal hemorrhages and leakage where blood-retinal barrier is disrupted, at level of FIPTs. FIPTs are angiographically distinguishable from cotton-wool spots, as they appear hypofluorescent due to nonperfusion and capillary dropout. There may be delayed, patchy choroidal filling defects followed by late leakage when hypertensive choroidopathy is present. In case of optic neuropathy, leakage from a swollen optic nerve is detectable in late frames.

Optical coherence tomography (OCT) helps in diagnosis of macular edema and serous neuroretinal detachment; its utility is higher in the follow-up as it is noninvasive, dye-less, and no-time consuming (Fig. 14.8).

The development of specific computer-assisted imaging software has made it possible to objectively measure the retinal arteriolar caliber and the arteriole-to-venule ratio (AVR) in hypertensive patients [11]. Additional software exists for assessment of microvascular remodeling, branching angles, bifurcation, fractal dimension, tortuosity, vascular length-to-diameter ratio, and wall-to-lumen ratio (Fig. 14.9).

Further technological advancements in retinal imaging allowing dynamic evaluation of retinal vascular flow and remodeling, such as the dynamic vessel analyzer (DVA) and scanning laser Doppler flowmetry, have shown that venules may represent a dynamic component in response to hypertension [12] (Fig. 14.10).

Innovative retinal imaging tools, such as ultrawide-field retinal imaging (Fig. 14.10), adaptive optics, retinal oximetry, and Doppler optical coherence tomography, have emerged recently to evaluate in advance the link between the eye and hypertension. These tools have limited use in current clinical practice yet, and have been used mainly for research purpose; however, implementation of these methods would become a precious resource in primary screening of population at risk.

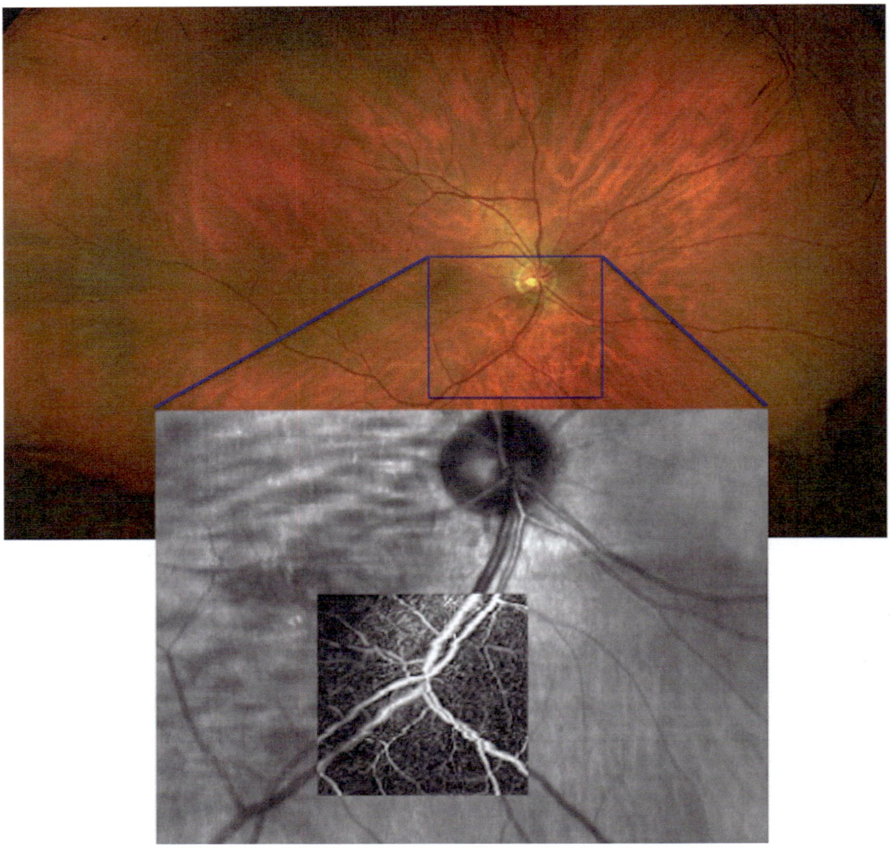

Fig. 14.9 Ultrawide-field retinal imaging and optical coherence tomography angiography showing arteriovenous nicking

14.7 Staging

The original classification system for hypertensive retinopathy was proposed in 1939 (Keith-Wagener-Barker classification) (Table 14.3). Since that time, other classification schemes have been proposed. However, there have been several criticisms of grading systems concerning the reproducibility and the relevance to clinical practice. In detail, the poor correlation of retinal signs with severity of hypertension; the presence of retinal signs in normotensives; a lack of predictable progression in clinical signs; the recognition of choroidopathy and optic neuropathy as separate manifestations; and poor inter-observer reliability have all led to disuse of these grading systems [13].

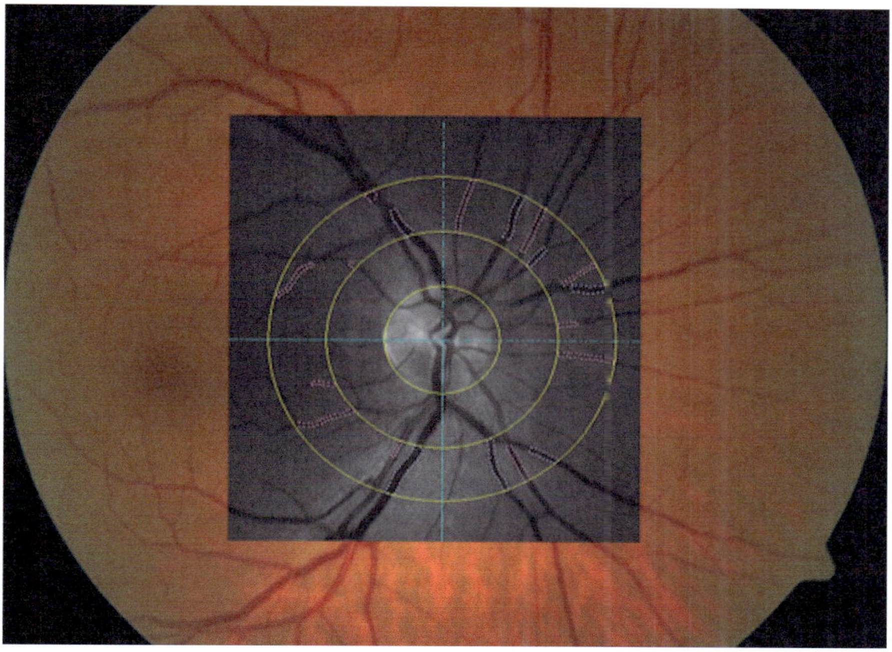

Fig. 14.10 Dynamic vessel analyzer (DVA) and analysis of retinal vascular caliber to calculate the arteriole-to-venule ratio (AVR)

Table 14.3 Keith-Wagener-Barker clinical classification of hypertensive retinopathy (1939)

Group 1	Mild generalized arteriolar narrowing, sclerosis and tortuosity, slight arterial light reflex
Group 2	Definite arteriolosclerosis, AV nicking, exaggerated arterial light reflex
Group 3	Cotton-wool sports, retinal hemorrhages, retinal exudates
Group 4	Choroidopathy, macular star, papilledema

14.8 Differential Diagnosis

In general, the degree and the duration of systemic hypertension are the primary determinants of hypertensive retinopathy grade. However, the changes described in the above sections are not unique for hypertension. Main differential diagnosis comprehends diabetic retinopathy, retinal venous occlusion, hyperviscosity syndromes, congenital hereditary retinal arterial tortuosity, ocular ischemic syndrome, infectious retinopathy (especially HIV-related), and radiation retinopathy. The retinopathy may also be more severe and more progressive when associated with other ocular or general medical conditions (i.e. diabetic retinopathy). Other factors, such as hyperlipidemia, may make the retinopathy worse as well.

14.9 Treatment

Chronic hypertensive retinopathy rarely results in significant vision loss. Urgency of treatment is related to presumed cerebral damages, including ischemic or hemorrhagic stroke, that may cause severe irreversible morbidity. Antihypertensive medication may reverse hypertensive retinopathy signs; newer studies, based on digital retinal photography and computerized analysis, have revealed that blood pressure reduction is associated with a reduction in arteriolar narrowing, widening of arteriolar branch angle, and an increase in arteriolar density among untreated hypertensive patients [14]. Treatment of chronic hypertension requires a detailed medical evaluation of the patient, to recognize the underlying cause and tailor the right treatment. In addition, appropriate patient education regarding low-sodium diet, exercise, and medication compliance is crucial.

Management of malignant hypertension (and therefore retinopathy, choroidopathy, and optic neuropathy) should require a primary care setting, with the goal of gradual lowering of the blood pressure to a level that minimizes end-organ damage. Too rapid decline can lead to ischemia of the optic nerve, brain, and other vital organs, resulting in permanent damage. Most patients resume normal vision after acute hypertensive events. If vision loss occurs, this may result from RPE changes secondary to retinal detachment or from optic atrophy due to prolonged optic disc swelling [15]. In patients with macular edema, in addition to systemic management of blood pressure, ocular adjuvant treatments that target vascular endothelial growth factor (VEGF) reduction have come to the forefront. These anti-VEGF agents presumably act by reducing vascular permeability, and they reduce macular edema in eyes with malignant hypertension. Although a few anecdotal reports available in the literature have shown good visual outcomes, the routine use of such therapies warrants further research [16, 17].

Key Learning Points

- Retina provides a window to cerebral circulation in hypertensive patients.
- Hypertensive retinopathy is evaluated as indicator for organ damage.
- Malignant hypertension is a life-threatening medical emergency
- Arterial narrowing and arteriovenous (AV) nicking are the hallmark of long-standing disease.
- New imaging software will provide non-invasive assessment of hypertensive retinopathy.

References

1. Joint National Committee on Prevention, Detection, Evaluation, and Treatment of High Blood Pressure. Sixth report of the Joint National Committee on prevention, detection, evaluation, and treatment of high blood pressure (JNC VI). Arch Intern Med. 1997;157:2413.
2. Burt VL, Cutler JA, Higgins M. Trends in the prevalence, awareness, treatment and control of hypertension in the adult US population: data from the Health Examination Surveys 1960–1991. Hypertension. 1995;26:60.

3. National High Blood Pressure Education Program Working Group. Report on primary prevention of hypertension. Arch Intern Med. 1993;153:186.
4. Chobanian AV, Bakris GL, Black HR, et al. The seventh report of the Joint National Committee on prevention, detection, evaluation, and treatment of high blood pressure: the JNC7 report. JAMA. 2003;289:2560–72.
5. Mancia G, De Backer G, Dominiczak A, et al. Guidelines for the management of arterial hypertension: the Task Force for the Management of Arterial Hypertension of the European Society of Hypertension (ESH) and of the European Society of Cardiology (ESC). J Hypertens. 2007;25:1105–87.
6. Ojaimi E, Nguyen TT, Klein R, et al. Retinopathy signs in people without diabetes. The multi-ethnic study of atherosclerosis. Ophthalmology. 2011;118:656–62.
7. Bill A, Sperber GO. Control of retinal and choroidal blood flow. Eye (Lond). 1990;4(Pt 2):319–25.
8. Robinson F, Riva CE, Grunwald JE, Petrig BL, Sinclair SH. Retinal blood flow autoregulation in response to an acute increase in blood pressure. Invest Ophthalmol Vis Sci. 1986;27(5):722–6.
9. Scheie HG. Evaluation of ophthalmoscopic changes of hypertension and arteriolar sclerosis. AMA Arch Ophthalmol. 1953;49(2):117–38.
10. Fastenberg DM, Fetkenhour CL, Choromolos E, et al. Choroidal vascular changes in toxemia of pregnancy. Am J Ophthalmol. 1980;89:362–8.
11. Hubbard L, Brothers RJ, King WL, et al. Methods for evaluation of retinal microvascular abnormalities associated with hypertension/sclerosis in the Atherosclerosis Risk in Communities Study. Ophthalmology. 1999;106:2269–80.
12. Cheung CY, Tay WT, Mitchell P, et al. Quantitative and qualitative retinal microvascular characteristics and blood pressure. J Hypertens. 2011;29:1380–91.
13. Hyman B. The eye as a target organ: an updated classification of hypertensive retinopathy. J Clin Hypertens. 2000;2:194–7.
14. Hughes AD, Stanton AV, Jabbar AS, et al. Effect of antihypertensive treatment on retinal microvascular changes in hypertension. J Hypertens. 2008;26: 703–7.
15. Kincaid-Smith P, McMichael J, Murphy EA. The clinical course and pathology of hypertension with papilloedema (malignant hypertension). Q J Med. 1958;27:117–53.
16. Zucchiatti I, Iacono P, Battaglia PM, et al. Intravitreal bevacizumab in a patient with a macular star in malignant hypertension. Eur J Ophthalmol. 2011;21:336–9.
17. Salman AG. Intravitreal bevacizumab in persistent retinopathy secondary to malignant hypertension. Saudi J Ophthalmol. 2013;27:25–9.

Intraocular Lymphoma

15

Mary E. Aronow

Abstract

Intraocular lymphoma encompasses a heterogeneous spectrum of lymphoid neoplasms. These are extranodal, non-Hodgkin's lymphomas, and the majority are of B-cell origin. Historically, there have been several nomenclature and classification systems used to describe these intraocular neoplasms. At present, most experts classify these entities based upon site of involvement and whether the lymphoma is primary or secondary. Intraocular lymphoma can therefore be subdivided into: primary vitreoretinal lymphoma (PVRL), primary uveal lymphoma, and secondary intraocular manifestations of systemic lymphoma. PVRL is a high-grade, aggressive malignancy associated with central nervous system involvement and poor survival rates despite treatment. Primary uveal lymphoma is predominantly a low-grade, indolent lymphoma which may cause significant ocular morbidity, but carries an overall favorable prognosis for survival. As all forms of intraocular lymphoma can masquerade as infectious and inflammatory conditions, establishing the diagnosis can be challenging. Clinical features alone can be non-specific at times, therefore ancillary ophthalmic imaging and systemic imaging studies are invaluable in facilitating the diagnostic work-up for individuals with suspected intraocular lymphoma. Familiarity with the clinical features as well as a comprehensive understanding of the unique patterns of systemic involvement for each form of intraocular lymphoma is important in the management of these diseases.

M.E. Aronow
Department of Ophthalmology, Retina Division, Wilmer Eye Institute, Johns Hopkins University School of Medicine, 600 North Wolfe Street, Maumenee 744, Baltimore, MD 21287-9277, USA
e-mail: maronow1@jhmi.edu

J. Chhablani et al. (eds.), *Retinal and Choroidal Imaging in Systemic Diseases*, https://doi.org/10.1007/978-981-10-5461-7_15

15.1 Introduction

Intraocular lymphoma can be broadly classified based upon site of involvement and whether the disease is primary or secondary. Intraocular lymphoma can be further subdivided into: primary vitreoretinal lymphoma, primary uveal lymphoma, and secondary intraocular manifestations of systemic lymphoma (Table 15.1). The vast majority are non-Hodgkin's B-cell lymphomas (rare T-cell variants exist). The distinction between forms of intraocular lymphoma is important, as the differential diagnosis, patterns of systemic involvement, and treatment strategies vary for each entity. Intraocular lymphoma frequently masquerades as inflammatory and infectious processes, resulting in delay in diagnosis and initiation of treatment. In the

Table 15.1 Clinical and imaging features of intraocular lymphoma

Lymphoma	Clinical features	Subtype	Imaging findings
Primary vitreoretinal lymphoma	Frequently bilateral vitreous cells retinal, sub-RPE infiltrates CNS involvement	High-grade DLBCL (majority)	FA: granular "leopard-spot" appearance
			ICG: hypofluorescent lesions in late phase
			OCT: sub-RPE infiltration, absence of macular edema
			FAF: autofluorescence in some cases
			MRI brain: potential CNS involvement
Primary uveal lymphoma	M>F usually unilateral clear vitreous diffuse choroidal thickening exudative retinal detachment	Low-grade EMZL (majority)	FA: foci of hyperfluorescence, staining in the late phase
			ICG: hypofluorescence corresponding to observed infiltrates
			OCT: choroidal thickening, "sea-sick" appearance
			USG: choroidal thickening, low internal reflectivity, extrascleral extension in some cases
			Systemic imaging: excludes potential systemic involvement
Secondary intraocular lymphoma	Variable: choroidal thickening iris infiltrates pseudohypopyon vitreous cells	Dependent upon systemic NHL	Majority demonstrate choroidal involvement with imaging findings similar to uveal lymphoma

RPE retinal pigment epithelium, *CNS* central nervous system, *DLBCL* diffuse large B-cell lymphoma, *FA* fluorescein angiography, *ICG* indocyanine green angiography, *OCT* optical coherence tomography, *FAF* fundus autofluorescence, *MRI* magnetic resonance imaging, *M* males, *F* females, *EMZL* extranodal marginal zone lymphoma, *USG* ultrasonography, *NHL* non-Hodgkin's lymphoma following chapter, a discussion follows regarding each of the major forms of intraocular lymphoma, including a description of the typical clinical features, recommended examination and ancillary imaging investigations, patterns of systemic involvement, treatment strategies, and prognosis.

15.2 Primary Vitreoretinal Lymphoma

Primary vitreoretinal lymphoma (PVRL) is considered a variant of primary central nervous system lymphoma (PCNSL), with predominantly vitreoretinal involvement. PVRL has previously been termed primary intraocular lymphoma (PIOL or PCNSL-O), "reticulum cell sarcoma" and "microgliomatosis" [1, 2]. As the vitreous and retina are the major site of involvement, PVRL is the preferred name for this entity, particularly as earlier descriptors misleadingly suggest that the disease arises from reticulum or microglial cells.

PCNSL is an aggressive diffuse large B-cell lymphoma associated with poor survival (ranging from 1 to 8 years) depending upon factors such as Karnofsky performance status and age [3]. PCNSL originates in the brain parenchyma, leptomeninges, spinal cord, and the eyes [4]. In the United States, the age-adjusted incidence of PCNSL is 4.8 per million population [5]. As PVRL occurs as a subset of PCNSL, the exact incidence is unknown due to the small number of cases. In the United States, between 1999 and 2002, there were approximately 100 reported cases of PVRL which illustrates the rare nature of this disease [5]. Co-existence of PVRL with PCNSL is variable, with CNS disease manifesting prior to, at the same time of ocular presentation, or following ocular diagnosis. Of those with PCNSL, approximately 25% will have PVRL at the time of CNS diagnosis [7]. In contrast, 56–90% of individuals initially diagnosed PVRL will subsequently develop central nervous system within 8–29 months of follow-up [8–13]. The peak incidence of PVRL is in the fifth to seventh decades in immunocompetent individuals. In immunocompromised patients, such as those with autoimmune deficiency syndrome (AIDS), PVRL may occur at a younger age. The most common presenting symptoms are painless decrease in vision and floaters [10]. Those who are asymptomatic may be diagnosed during routine ophthalmic screening in the setting of known PCNSL. For PCNSL, common presenting symptoms may include personality changes or cognitive decline. Seizures are an unusual feature of this form of lymphoma.

15.2.1 Clinical Features

The hallmark clinical feature of PVRL is vitreous cells (Fig. 15.1a). Unlike more typical cases of posterior uveitis, lymphoma cells within the vitreous cavity may appear larger, and form sheets and/or clusters resulting in an "aurora borealis" appearance [12]. Vitreous haze may be present. Yellow-to white retinal, and particularly sub-retinal pigment epithelium (sub-RPE) infiltrates are characteristic. Bilateral disease is present in 80% of cases, and is typically asymmetric [8]. Anterior

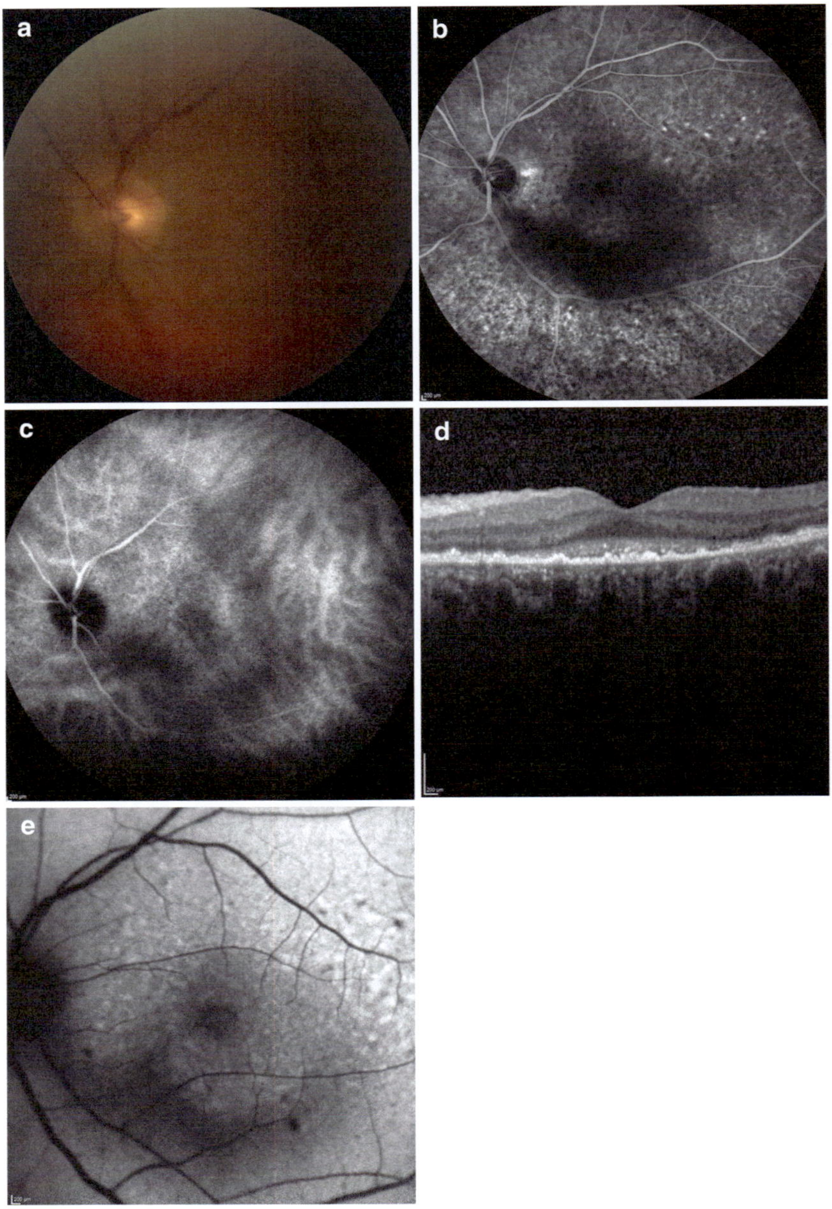

Fig. 15.1 A 64-year-old male presented with vitritis and decreased vision unresponsive to steroids. Soon after ocular presentation, he developed central nervous systemic lesions. Biopsy confirmed diffuse large B-cell lymphoma. Fundus photograph of the left eye demonstrates vitreous haze and mild vitreous cells (**a**). Fluorescein angiogram demonstrates a "leopard spot" appearance of the fundus (**b**). Indocyanine green angiography reveals hypofluorescent spots in the late phase of the angiogram (**c**). Optical coherent tomography (OCT) shows hyperreflective, nodular, infiltrate beneath the retinal pigment epithelium (**d**). Fundus autofluorescence demonstrates subtle autofluorescence corresponding to these infiltrates (**e**)

segment manifestations such as aqueous cells, keratic precipitates, and iris nodules have been reported, however these findings are non-specific [14]. Other less frequently reported features include perivasculitis [10], retinal artery occlusion [15], exudative retinal detachment [16], multifocal "punched-out" lesions of the retinal pigment epithelium (RPE) [17], disc edema, and optic atrophy [18]. Fundus photography is helpful to document the initial clinical findings and response to therapy.

15.2.2 Differential Diagnosis

Delayed diagnosis is common in PVRL due to the non-specific ophthalmic manifestations, many of which masquerade as inflammatory, infectious, and other neoplastic entities. In a series of 32 individuals with histologically confirmed PVRL, the average time between ocular symptoms and establishment of the diagnosis was 21 months [11]. The differential diagnosis includes such entities as sarcoidosis, syphilis, tuberculosis, birdshot retinochoroidopathy, multifocal chorioretinitis, acute posterior multifocal placoid pigmentary epitheliopathy (APMPPE), punctate inner choroidopathy, and serpiginous choroiditis [19]. When subretinal or choroidal involvement is present, other neoplastic entities such as metastases and potentially amelanotic melanoma should be considered. In immunocompromised patients, infections such as cytomegalovirus, toxoplasmosis, and pneumocystis choroiditis should be included in the differential diagnosis.

15.2.3 Fluorescein Angiography (FA)

The FA features of PVRL are typical and include: granularity giving rise to a "leopard spot" appearance to the fundus (Fig. 15.1b), blocked fluorescence, and late staining [20]. These features correlate histopathologically with clinically observed lymphoma cells located between the RPE and Bruch's membrane [20]. In contrast, fluorescein angiographic features which are common in posterior uveitis such as perivascular staining, vascular leakage, and petaloid leakage (cystoid macular edema) rarely occur in PVRL [20]. In a series of 53 patients with histopathologically confirmed PVRL, the fluorescein angiographic features were compared to 133 individuals with simulating conditions (infectious uveitis, autoimmune-mediated uveitis, and choroidal metastases) [21]. Small, round, hypofluorescent lesions (50–250 μm in diameter) were observed in the posterior pole in the early to late phase of the FA in 45% of PVRL patients, however these findings were observed in only 2% of non-lymphoma cases ($p < 0.001$) [21]. The FA features correlated with the clinically observed small, subtle, white punctuate lesions scattered throughout the fundus.

15.2.4 Indocyanine Green (ICG) Angiography

In PVRL, the lymphoma cells are typically confined to the vitreous cavity and sub-RPE space, rather than the choroid. ICG angiography is particularly useful in characterizing the choroidal circulation, however this modality still demonstrates distinct features when compared to ICG angiograms obtained from individuals with simulating posterior uveitis. Small, round hypofluorescent lesions (Fig. 15.1c) that disappear in the later phase were observed in 26% of individuals with PVRL, but only 9% of non-lymphoma cases ($p = 0.014$) [21]. It has been suggested that this finding represents a reactive lymphocytic response within the choroid [22, 23].

15.2.5 Optical Coherence Tomography (OCT)

OCT findings are not diagnostic for PVRL, however they may be useful as an ancillary imaging technique in differentiating PVRL from other simulating forms of posterior uveitis. OCT has demonstrated that central foveal thickness is near normal in individuals with PVRL (mean: 231 μm, standard deviation: 45 μm), in contrast to the central foveal thickness in eyes with posterior uveitis in which foveal thickness is frequently increased due to the presence of macular edema (mean: 327 μm, standard deviation: 114 μm) ($p < 0.001$) [21]. In this same series, hyperreflective, nodular RPE lesions (Fig. 15.1d) were observed on the OCT in 42% of patients with PVRL compared to 15% of eyes with non-lymphoma diagnoses ($p = 0.076$) [21].

15.2.6 Fundus Autofluorescence (FAF)

While FAF is not routinely used in the work-up of PVRL, it may potentially highlight some unique features. In one series of five eyes, sub-RPE infiltrates exhibited weak autofluorescence (Fig. 15.1e) by FAF [24]. Brownish clumps on the surface of these lesions revealed bright autofluorescence. In contrast, diffuse retinal infiltrates or retinal whitening showed hypoautofluorescence. This method is useful in characterizing regions of RPE atrophy that appear hypoautofluorescent following therapy [24].

15.2.7 Additional Diagnostic Testing

As clinical findings are often non-specific, biopsy is the gold standard for definitive diagnosis of PVRL [25–29]. An exception is in setting of established PCNSL, with classic ocular findings. In these cases, the diagnosis of PVRL is straightforward, and most experts would concur that ocular biopsy is unnecessary for initiation of treatment. Collaboration with a cytopathologist with experience in diagnosing lymphoma is ideal. The majority of cases of PVRL are aggressive, diffuse large B-cell lymphoma (DLBCL). In a multi-center retrospective review of 221 patients with histologically confirmed PCNSL with ocular involvement, the subtype was determined to be DLBCL in 73%, T-cell in 2%, and type not specified in the remaining 25% [30]. Cytology demonstrates typical features. The cells in PVRL are 2–4 times larger than normal lymphocytes, demonstrate pleomorphism, and contain scant cytoplasm [28]. The nuclei are large and may be round or oval-shaped, with conspicuous nuclear membranes, finger-like protrusions, and multiple, prominent, eccentrically located nucleoli. Mitotic figures are characteristic [28]. Electron microscopy demonstrates intranuclear inclusions, cytoplasmic crystalloids, pseudopodal cytoplasmic extensions, cytosomes, and autophagic vacuoles [31].

Several biopsy techniques can be employed to confirm diagnosis: vitreous biopsy, retinal biopsy, and sub-retinal biopsy. A common approach is to perform diagnostic 23-Gauge pars plana vitrectomy. Alternatively, 25-Gauge sutureless vitrectomy may be used for improved patient comfort and shorter operative times [27]. Proper surgical technique and handling of vitreous biopsy specimens are essential for optimizing diagnostic accuracy. Vitreous aspirates are typically have low cellularity and lymphoma cells are inherently fragile, making them prone to lysis at the time of sample collection. Biopsy techniques vary by treatment center. A frequently described approach is to procure an undiluted vitreous biopsy (approximately 1–2 mL) before the start of the saline infusion [25, 32]. Next, the saline infusion is initiated, and a second, dilute vitreous sample is procured in a separate syringe [33]. The vitreous cassette can also be submitted as an additional sample [27]. If fresh (unfixed) samples will be analyzed, the biopsy material should be sent to the laboratory within one hour of collection [25]. It is common for multiple vitreous biopsies to be performed to establish the correct diagnosis.

When sub-retinal infiltrates are the predominant clinical feature, a retinal or subretinal biopsy may be preferred. Subretinal biopsy techniques have been previously described in detail [34]. Briefly, a core vitrectomy is performed to allow entry into the subretinal space. Vitreous separation is induced and a thorough vitrectomy is then performed overlying the optimal biopsy site. The retina is incised to create an opening just large enough to allow entry of the vitreous cutter. Suction tubing is advanced through the retinectomy site and with a gentle cutting action, several samples are removed for analysis. Subretinal aspirates should be put into a cytofixative, such as herpes-glutamic acid buffer mediated organic solvent protection effect (H.O.P.E.) fixative or Cytolyt® (Cytyc Corporation) [25]. In a series of 84 patients who had undergone an initial pars plana vitrectomy without definite diagnosis, additional chorioretinal biopsy with analysis by immunohistochemistry and polymerase chain reaction (PCR) gene rearrangement studies was performed in three patients and confirmed the diagnosis of PVRL in all three [35].

Supplemental techniques can be helpful for diagnostic confirmation of PVRL. Immunohistochemistry is useful for identifying markers for leukocytes (CD45), B-cells (CD20, CD79a, PAX-5), T-cells (CD45RO), and macrophages (CD68) [25]. Additionally, clonal cell populations can be established with antibodies directed against κ and λ light chains [28]. Flow cytometry provides a quantitative means by which to assess the proportion of cells that demonstrate these immunohistochemical markers. PCR gene rearrangement can detect monoclonality of the heavy chain variable (V), diversity (D), and joining (J) immunoglobulin gene segments. While supplementary studies may be helpful in establishing the diagnosis of PVRL, the small volume of vitreous aspirates is frequently inadequate for PCR analysis [36, 37]. PCR may be most successful in tissue specimens in which DNA has been isolated by laser capture microdissection [36]. The measurement of IL-6 and IL-10 in aqueous or vitreous samples can also be helpful in establishing diagnosis, however an elevated IL-10/IL-6 ratio alone is not specific for PVRL [38, 39]. More recently, MYD88 mutations have been shown to be highly associated with PVRL. Identification of this mutation may in the future improve diagnostic accuracy [40].

15.2.8 Systemic Imaging and Evaluation

Due to the association between PVRL and PCNSL, individuals with ophthalmic disease should undergo systemic screening by an oncologist. In confirmed cases of PVRL, MRI of the brain with and without contrast should be performed to exclude central nervous systemic involvement. When CNS involvement is present, the lesions tend to be located in a periventricular distribution; this allows access to the cerebrospinal fluid (CSF) and leptomeninges. Leptomeningeal involvement occurs in 40% of cases [41]. Lumbar puncture may be obtained in selected cases depending upon local practice patterns. CSF samples that are positive typically demonstrate pleocytosis, elevated protein levels, and low or normal glucose. Cytologic identification of malignant lymphoma cells in the CSF is diagnostic. Flow cytometry is the most sensitive and specific marker of PCNSL [42]. Additional diagnostic imaging may include computed tomography scan of the chest, abdomen, and pelvis, testicular ultrasound (in elderly men), and HIV testing in the appropriate setting.

15.2.9 Treatment

PVRL is rare disease and therefore formal treatment consensus guidelines have not been established. Current therapeutic regimens vary depending upon patient factors and local expertise. When disease is limited to the eye and is unilateral, intravitreal therapy with either methotrexate or rituximab (or combination therapy) has been shown to be effective [43, 44]. Prior to the use of intravitreal chemotherapy, external beam radiotherapy (EBRT) was used as first line therapy. At present, the role of EBRT in patients with isolated ocular disease is controversial. EBRT remains a potentially important therapeutic option in patients with bilateral involvement, those who are unable to tolerate intravitreal chemotherapy, and in individuals who are unable return to clinic for multiple injections. In the present era, EBRT is reserved for patients under age 65 years, due to the concern for neurotoxicity in older individuals. In patients with both ocular and CNS disease, the majority are treated with high-dose intravenous chemotherapy. Methotrexate (8 g/m^2) is frequently used, either as monotherapy or as part of a combination regimen. There is consensus that regimens containing high-dose methotrexate, in combination with or without whole brain radiation therapy (WBRT) result in more successful control than regimens that do not contain high-dose methotrexate. Blood–brain barrier disruption (BBBD) has also been used successfully [45].

15.2.10 Prognosis

PVRL is a high-grade, aggressive lymphoma with poor prognosis. The majority of individuals (56–90%) ultimately develop CNS disease [11–13]. In a multicenter, retrospective study of 221 individuals with CNS lymphoma with vitreoretinal involvement, median progression-free survival and overall survival were 18 and 31 months, respectively [30]. Favorable prognostic factors include: age less than 60 years and high initial Karnofsky performance status. Poor prognostic indicators include: involvement of the brainstem and leptomeningeal disease. Vitreoretinal involvement concurrent with CNS disease does not seem to be a prognostic factor [46]. While current retrospective studies have shown that ocular treatment improves disease control and patient symptoms, no survival benefit from ocular therapy has yet been demonstrated [30].

15.3 Primary Uveal Lymphoma

Primary uveal lymphoma is classified based on the site of predominant uveal involvement as: choroidal, iridal, and ciliary body lymphoma. The majority of cases are primary choroidal lymphoma. This is generally a low-grade B-cell lymphoma with an indolent, benign course. Most uveal lymphoma are morphologically similar to extranodal marginal zone lymphoma (EMZL) that involves other systemic sites. Primary iridal lymphoma can be of either B-cell or T-cell origin. These are rare tumors, therefore the incidence of primarily iridal and ciliary body lymphoma is unknown. There are approximately 70–80 case published reports and small series of primary choroidal lymphoma [47].

15.3.1 Clinical Features

Primary uveal lymphoma is most frequently a unilateral disease. When bilateral, the findings may be highly asymmetric. There is a male predominance, and most cases occur in the fifth to seventh decade. Symptoms can include painless, decreased vision, and metamorphopsia due to exudative retinal detachment. In advanced cases, pain and severely decreased vision may result from secondary angle-closure glaucoma. When extraocular extension is present, proptosis and diplopia can occur. A classic fundoscopic finding is the presence of either a placoid choroidal infiltrate, or multiple small, yellow, creamy choroidal infiltrates (Fig. 15.2a). In contrast to PVRL, the vitreous media remains clear. Diffuse thickening of the uveal tract may develop and can be associated with exudative retinal detachment. Occasionally, there may be episcleral extension appearing as a non-mobile "salmon" patch. There is frequent overlap between uveal and ocular adnexal lymphoma [48]. Ocular adnexal lymphoma and uveal lymphoma are similar morphologically and both follow an indolent course in most cases. For this reason, some experts consider uveal lymphoma to be a variant of ocular adnexal lymphoma [49].

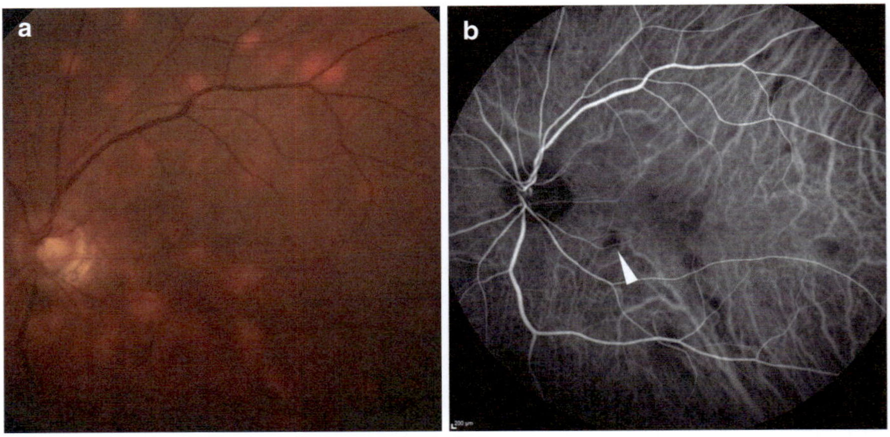

Fig. 15.2 A 72-year-old female was found to have multiple, bilateral, creamy choroidal infiltrates (**a**), which appeared as hypofluorescent foci on ICG (**b**)

15.3.2 Differential Diagnosis

The differential diagnosis of uveal lymphoma is broad and includes: the diffuse form of amelanotic uveal melanoma, uveal effusion syndrome, inflammation such as posterior scleritis, and choroidal metastases. Diffuse uveal melanoma can usually be distinguished based upon its pigmented appearance (although it may be amelanotic in some cases), presence of vascularity, and faster growth rate [50]. Uveal effusion syndrome is frequently bilateral, is associated with dilated episcleral vessels, and tends to occur in individuals with short axial lengths. Posterior scleritis is more common in women and is associated with autoimmune disease. Posterior scleritis also has characteristic ultrasonographic features such as high internal reflectivity and a classic "T-sign" on B-scan. In patients with choroidal metastases, there is frequently a prior history of malignancy. Additionally, B-scan ultrasonography typically confirms medium internal reflectivity.

15.3.3 Fluorescein Angiography (FA)

Fluorescein angiography may be non-specific as an ancillary imaging study for uveal lymphoma as it primarily defines features of the retinal circulation. In some cases, angiography may demonstrate early hypofluoresence with multiple foci of hyperfluorescence and staining in later phases of the angiogram. These angiographic features correlate with the clinically observed choroidal infiltrates.

15.3.4 Indocyanine Green (ICG) Angiography

ICG angiography provides a superior means for characterizing the choroid in comparison to FA, and is therefore the preferred imaging modality for uveal lymphoma. Multiple, round, hypofluorescent lesions (Fig. 15.2b) are typical and correspond to the areas of non-perfusion secondary to the clinically observed space-occupying choroidal infiltrates.

15.3.5 Optical Coherence Tomography (OCT)

OCT, particularly spectral-domain OCT may reveal choroidal thickening, choroidal folds, and an undulating "sea-sick" appearance (Fig. 15.3a, b) of the choroid [51]. Overlying exudative retinal detachment may be apparent on OCT. Enhanced depth imaging (EDI) OCT is particularly useful in characterizing choroidal features.

15.3.6 Ultrasonography

B-scan ultrasonography reveals variable uveal thickening. A-scan ultrasonography demonstrates low internal reflectivity. In addition to characterizing the size and extent of intraocular involvement, ultrasonography is useful in detecting occult extra-scleral extension (Fig. 15.3c). The extra-scleral component may appear as crescentic thickening outside the posterior scleral margin, or as a discrete mass (often near the optic nerve) [48]. Detection of extra-scleral disease is important as this provides a potential site for biopsy to confirm the diagnosis.

15.3.7 Additional Diagnostic Testing

As with other forms of intraocular lymphoma, biopsy remains the gold standard for establishing the diagnosis. Biopsy of the episcleral tumor nodule or choroidal aspirates may confirm diagnosis. Histopathologically, most cases of primary choroidal lymphoma are of the EMZL subtype. The lymphoma cells are usually centrocyte-like, monocytoid, and plasmacytoid type. Dutcher bodies, which are collections of intranuclear immunoglobulin, can be seen. Immunohistochemistry confirms expression of B-cell antigens (CD20 and CD-79a). Gene rearrangement studies or flow cytometry is supportive and can confirm the clonal nature of cell populations.

15.3.8 Systemic Imaging and Evaluation

Neuroimaging, including computed tomography and particularly magnetic resonance imaging of the orbits, may confirm uveal thickening. Neuroimaging is particularly useful for the detection of occult extra-scleral or orbital involvement, which as previously described, may also be observed on ultrasonography.

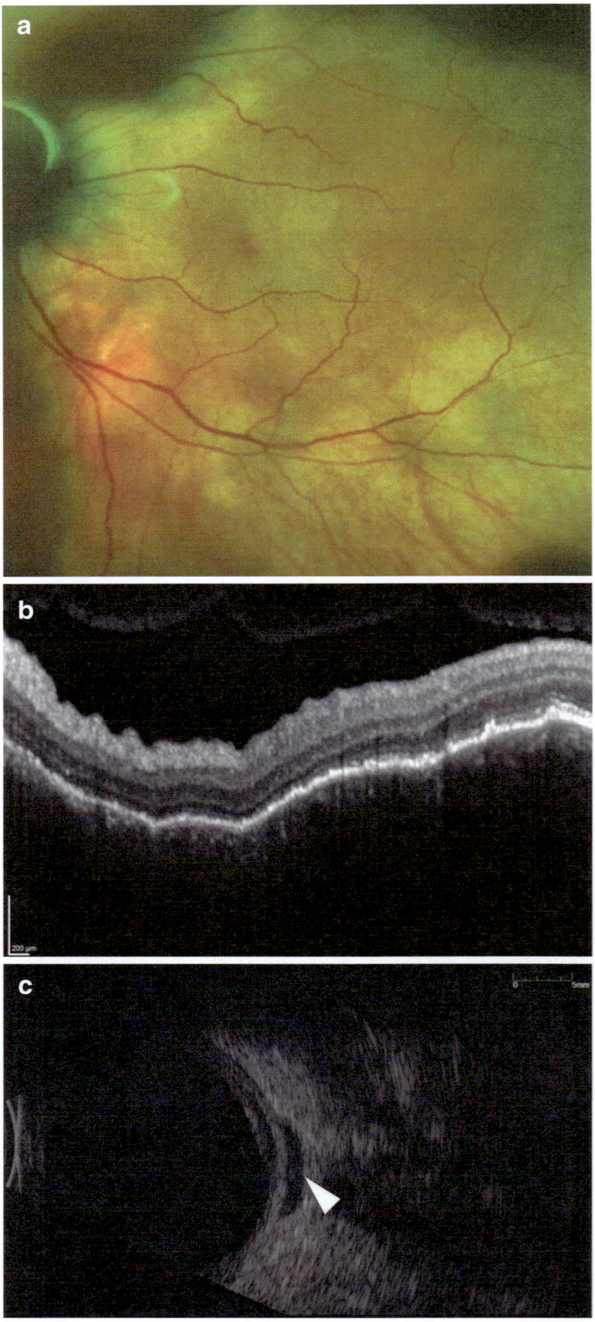

Fig. 15.3 A 67-year-old male with a known history of systemic lymphoplasmacytic lymphoma developed secondary intraocular manifestations. Fundus photograph of the left eye demonstrates a placoid area of amelanotic choroidal thickening (**a**). OCT reveals diffuse choroidal thickening and a "sea-sick" appearance of the choroid (**b**). B-scan ultrasonography detected occult extra-scleral extension (**c**)

Prior to initiation of localized treatment for uveal lymphoma, it is important to perform systemic imaging and laboratory studies to fully evaluate for the possibility of systemic involvement. Systemic evaluation varies by center and local expertise, but imaging studies may include: computed tomography or MRI of the neck, chest, abdomen, and pelvis. Laboratory evaluation may include: complete blood count, and serum protein electrophoresis, among others [52].

15.3.9 Treatment

When disease is limited to the choroid and/or uveal tract, management consists primarily of low-dose intensity-modulated radiotherapy (IMRT) alone (dose ranges from 23–36 Gy). When systemic disease is present, patients can be treated with chemotherapy or monoclonal antibody therapy (rituximab). In some cases, if systemic disease is minimal and asymptomatic, observation may be appropriate. In cases where systemic disease is more widespread, the lymphoma subtype is more aggressive, or the disease burden is causing symptoms, then various systemic therapies are available. Chemotherapy with combination rituximab, cyclophosphamide, doxorubicin, vincristine, and prednisone (RCHOP) is utilized for widespread systemic disease and more aggressive subtypes of lymphoma. Intravenous administration of rituximab may also be useful for cases of bilateral ocular involvement. Staging at the time of initial diagnosis and periodic systemic surveillance are important in monitoring response to therapy. Ideally, patients should be followed by a multidisciplinary team including an ocular oncologist, or ophthalmologist familiar with lymphoma, and a medical oncologist.

15.3.10 Prognosis

While there can be significant ocular morbidity associated with uveal lymphoma, overall mortality related to this condition is quite low and similar to age-matched controls without this disease [48]. Similar to ocular adnexal lymphoma, most uveal lymphoma are of the EMZL subtype. EMZL is typically a slowly progressive, indolent lymphoma which most often demonstrates an excellent response to treatment including radiation, chemotherapy, and monoclonal antibody therapy [48]. In one series of 13 eyes with biopsy proven primary choroidal lymphoma, systemic lymphoma eventually developed in two cases (3 and 7 years after the initial ocular diagnosis) [53].

15.4 Secondary Intraocular Manifestations of Systemic Lymphoma

Intraocular lymphoma secondary to systemic lymphoma most frequently involves the uveal tract. The clinical features are therefore similar to primary uveal lymphoma [54]. Retinal involvement without choroidal infiltration can rarely occur [54]. Other unusual presentations of secondary intraocular lymphoma include: pseudohypopyon (layered lymphoma cells) and iris infiltration [55, 56]. While exceptionally rare, iridal lymphoma secondary to systemic non-lymphoma is probably more common than primary iridal lymphoma [47]. Diffuse large B-cell lymphoma is the most frequent subtype of systemic lymphoma associated with intraocular lymphoma. This is followed by multiple myeloma, extramedullary plasmacytoma, lymphoplasmocytic lymphoma/immunocytoma, and marginal zone B-cell lymphoma [54]. The morphologic and immunophenotypic features of secondary choroidal lymphoma are similar to its primary systemic counterpart. Initial staging evaluation and collaboration with an experienced oncology team are ideal in the management of individuals with systemic lymphoma with intraocular involvement.

15.5 Future Remarks

Intraocular lymphomas are a heterogeneous group of diseases. Each of the major forms: primary vitreoretinal lymphoma, primary uveal lymphoma, and secondary intraocular manifestations of systemic lymphoma are rare disease. Future efforts are needed to characterize these entities, in particular to further understand the relationship between ocular and systemic disease. It has been hypothesized that PVRL may originate from late-germinal center or post-germinal center lymphoid cells, however the neurotropic mechanisms that cause these cells to localize to the CNS is not well understood [57]. Human studies are not well suited for the investigation of intraocular lymphoma pathogenesis or treatment strategies because of the rare nature of the disease. Additionally, the variable presentation, limited volume of available ocular fluids, and fragility of lymphoma cells are challenges in studying these orphan diseases. Animal models have been helpful in the study of lymphoma pathogenesis and investigation of potential therapeutic strategies. The challenge in murine models for intraocular lymphoma is in replicating the clinical features, the behavior of the disease course, molecular profile, systemic immunity, and the microenvironment in humans.

In all fields of oncology, including ophthalmic tumors, there has been a recent trend towards applying standardized staging systems. Among these, a tumor-node-metastasis (TNM) staging system has been developed for ophthalmic neoplasms including ocular adnexal lymphoma and uveal melanoma under the guidance of the American Joint Committee on Cancer (AJCC) [58, 59]. TNM staging has not yet been developed for intraocular lymphoma. Ideally, a universal staging system of this form could be developed in order to facilitate characterization of the clinical and histomorphologic features of these lymphomas that are of prognostic significance, and to assess treatment outcomes.

Key Learning Points

- Intraocular lymphoma can be classified as primary vitreoretinal lymphoma, primary uveal lymphoma, and secondary intraocular manifestations of systemic lymphoma.

- Primary vitreoretinal lymphoma is an aggressive malignancy associated with primary central nervous system lymphoma and poor survival.
- Primary uveal lymphoma most frequently affects the choroid and is generally a low-grade, indolent lymphoma. While there can be significant ocular morbidity associated with this condition, overall survival is generally excellent.
- Secondary intraocular manifestations of systemic lymphoma bear clinical resemblance to uveal lymphoma. The choroid is most frequent affected site. Morphologically, the lymphoma mirrors its primary systemic counterpart.

References

1. Kinney TD, Adam RD. Reticulum cell sarcoma of the brain. Arch Neurol Psychiatr. 1943;50:552–64.
2. Russell DS, Marshall AHE, Smith FB. Microgliomatosis. Brain. 1948;71:1–15.
3. Abrey LE, Ben-Porat L, Panageas KS, Yahalom J, Berkey B, Curran W, et al. Primary central nervous system lymphoma: the Memorial Sloan-Kettering Cancer Center prognostic model. J Clin Oncol. 2006;24(36):5711–5. Epub 2006/11/23.
4. Pe'er J, Hochberg FH, Foster CS. Clinical review: treatment of vitreoretinal lymphoma. Ocul Immunol Inflamm. 2009;17(5):299–306. Epub 2009/10/17.
5. Olson JE, Janney CA, Rao RD, Cerhan JR, Kurtin PJ, Schiff D, et al. The continuing increase in the incidence of primary central nervous system non-Hodgkin lymphoma: a surveillance, epidemiology, and end results analysis. Cancer. 2002;95(7):1504–10. Epub 2002/09/19.
6. Chan CC, Buggage RR, Nussenblatt RB. Intraocular lymphoma. Curr Opin Ophthalmol. 2002;13:411–8.
7. Hochberg FH, Miller DC. Primary central nervous system lymphoma. J Neurosurg. 1988;68(6):835–53. Epub 1988/06/01.
8. Peterson K, Gordon KB, Heinemann MH, DeAngelis LM. The clinical spectrum of ocular lymphoma. Cancer. 1993;72(3):843–9. Epub 1993/08/01.
9. Cassoux N, Merle-Beral H, Leblond V, Bodaghi B, Milea D, Gerber S, et al. Ocular and central nervous system lymphoma: clinical features and diagnosis. Ocul Immunol Inflamm. 2000;8(4):243–50. Epub 2001/03/23.
10. Char DH, Ljung BM, Miller T, Phillips T. Primary intraocular lymphoma (ocular reticulum cell sarcoma) diagnosis and management. Ophthalmology. 1988;95(5):625–30. Epub 1988/05/01.
11. Freeman LN, Schachat AP, Knox DL, Michels RG, Green WR. Clinical features, laboratory investigations, and survival in ocular reticulum cell sarcoma. Ophthalmology. 1987;94(12):1631–9. Epub 1987/12/01.
12. Chan CC, Rubenstein JL, Coupland SE, Davis JL, Harbour JW, Johnston PB, et al. Primary vitreoretinal lymphoma: a report from an International Primary Central Nervous System Lymphoma Collaborative Group symposium. Oncologist. 2011;16(11):1589–99. Epub 2011/11/03.
13. Sagoo MS, Mehta H, Swampillai AJ, Cohen VM, Amin SZ, Plowman PN, et al. Primary intraocular lymphoma. Surv Ophthalmol. 2014;59(5):503–16. Epub 2014/02/25.
14. Rajagopal R, Harbour JW. Diagnostic testing and treatment choices in primary vitreoretinal lymphoma. Retina. 2011;31(3):435–40. Epub 2011/02/22.
15. Gass JD, Trattler HL. Retinal artery obstruction and atheromas associated with non-Hodgkin's large cell lymphoma (reticulum cell sarcoma). Arch Ophthalmol. 1991;109(8):1134–9. Epub 1991/08/01.
16. Michelson JB, Michelson PE, Bordin GM, Chisari FV. Ocular reticulum cell sarcoma. Presentation as retinal detachment with demonstration of monoclonal immunoglobulin light chains on the vitreous cells. Arch Ophthalmol. 1981;99(8):1409–11. Epub 1981/08/01.
17. Lang GK, Surer JL, Green WR, Finkelstein D, Michels RG, Maumenee AE. Ocular reticulum cell sarcoma. Clinicopathologic correlation of a case with multifocal lesions. Retina. 1985;5(2):79–86. Epub 1985/01/01.

18. Purvin V, Van Dyk HJ. Primary reticulum cell sarcoma of the brain presenting as steroid-responsive optic neuropathy. J Clin Neuro-ophthalmol. 1984;4(1):15–23. Epub 1984/03/01.
19. Singh AD, Lewis H, Schachat AP, Peereboom D. Lymphoma of the retina and CNS. In: Singh A, Damato BE, Pe'er J, Murphree AL, Perry JD, editors. Clinical ophthalmic oncology. Philadelphia, PA: Elsevier; 2007. p. 372–7.
20. Velez G, Chan CC, Csaky KG. Fluorescein angiographic findings in primary intraocular lymphoma. Retina. 2002;22(1):37–43. Epub 2002/03/09.
21. Fardeau C, Lee CP, Merle-Beral H, Cassoux N, Bodaghi B, Davi F, et al. Retinal fluorescein, indocyanine green angiography, and optic coherence tomography in non-Hodgkin primary intraocular lymphoma. Am J Ophthalmol. 2009;147(5):886–94. 94 e1. Epub 2009/02/27.
22. Chan CC, Sauer TC. Ocular imaging in primary retinal lymphoma. Am J Ophthalmol. 2009;147(5):764–5. Epub 2009/04/21.
23. Lopez JS, Chan CC, Burnier M, Rubin B, Nussenblatt RB. Immunohistochemistry findings in primary intraocular lymphoma. Am J Ophthalmol. 1991;112(4):472–4. Epub 1991/10/15.
24. Ishida T, Ohno-Matsui K, Kaneko Y, Tobita H, Shimada N, Takase H, et al. Fundus autofluorescence patterns in eyes with primary intraocular lymphoma. Retina. 2010;30(1):23–32. Epub 2009/10/17.
25. Coupland SE. Vitreous biopsy: specimen preparation and interpretation. Monogr Clin Cytol. 2012;21:61–71.
26. Margolis R, Brasil OF, Lowder CY, Singh RP, Kaiser PK, Smith SD, et al. Vitrectomy for the diagnosis and management of uveitis of unknown cause. Ophthalmology. 2007;114(10):1893–7. Epub 2007/05/19.
27. Yeh S, Weichel ED, Faia LJ, Albini TA, Wroblewski KK, Stetler-Stevenson M, et al. 25-Gauge transconjunctival sutureless vitrectomy for the diagnosis of intraocular lymphoma. Br J Ophthalmol. 2010;94(5):633–8. Epub 2010/05/08.
28. Farkas T, Harbour JW, Davila RM. Cytologic diagnosis of intraocular lymphoma in vitreous aspirates. Acta Cytol. 2004;48(4):487–91. Epub 2004/08/07.
29. Whitcup SM, de Smet MD, Rubin BI, Palestine AG, Martin DF, Burnier M Jr, et al. Intraocular lymphoma. Clinical and histopathologic diagnosis. Ophthalmology. 1993;100(9):1399–406. Epub 1993/09/01.
30. Grimm SA, McCannel CA, Omuro AM, Ferreri AJ, Blay JY, Neuwelt EA, et al. Primary CNS lymphoma with intraocular involvement: International PCNSL Collaborative Group report. Neurology. 2008;71(17):1355–60. Epub 2008/10/22.
31. Kim EW, Zakov ZN, Albert DM, Smith TR, Craft JL. Intraocular reticulum cell sarcoma: a case report and literature review. Albrecht von Graefe's Arch Clin Exp Ophthalmol. 1979;209(3):167–78. Epub 1979/01/15.
32. Singh AD, Lewis H, Schachat AP. Primary lymphoma of the central nervous system. Ophthalmol Clin N Am. 2005;18(1):199–207, x. Epub 2005/03/15.
33. Margolis R. Diagnostic vitrectomy for the diagnosis and management of posterior uveitis of unknown etiology. Curr Opin Ophthalmol. 2008;19(3):218–24. Epub 2008/04/15.
34. Bechrakis NE, Foerster MH, Bornfeld N. Biopsy in indeterminate intraocular tumors. Ophthalmology. 2002;109(2):235–42. Epub 2002/02/05.
35. Coupland SE, Bechrakis NE, Anastassiou G, Foerster AM, Heiligenhaus A, Pleyer U, et al. Evaluation of vitrectomy specimens and chorioretinal biopsies in the diagnosis of primary intraocular lymphoma in patients with Masquerade syndrome. Graefe's Arch Clin Exp Ophthalmol. 2003;241(10):860–70. Epub 2003/11/08.
36. Chan CC, Shen D, Nussenblatt RB, Boni R, Zhuang Z. Detection of molecular changes in primary intraocular lymphoma by microdissection and polymerase chain reaction. Diagn Mol Pathol Am J Surg Pathol B. 1998;7(1):63–4. Epub 1998/07/01.
37. Chan CC, Gonzales JA. Classification of lymphomas. In: Primary intraocular lymphoma. 1st ed. Hackensack, NJ: World Scientific Publishing; 2007.

38. Akpek EK, Maca SM, Christen WG, Foster CS. Elevated vitreous interleukin-10 level is not diagnostic of intraocular-central nervous system lymphoma. Ophthalmology. 1999;106(12):2291–5. Epub 1999/12/22.
39. Caraballo JN, Snyder MR, Johnston PB, O Neill BP, Raja H, Kalsanek JG, et al. Vitreoretinal lymphoma versus uveitis: cytokine profile and correlations. Ocul Immunol Inflamm. 2014;22(1):34–41. Epub 2014/02/05.
40. Bonzheim I, Giese S, Deuter C, Susskind D, Zierhut M, Waizel M, et al. High frequency of MYD88 mutations in vitreoretinal B-cell lymphoma: a valuable tool to improve diagnostic yield of vitreous aspirates. Blood. 2015;126(1):76–9. Epub 2015/04/23.
41. Balmaceda C, Gaynor JJ, Sun M, Gluck JT, DeAngelis LM. Leptomeningeal tumor in primary central nervous system lymphoma: recognition, significance, and implications. Ann Neurol. 1995;38(2):202–9. Epub 1995/08/01.
42. Ahluwalia MS, Wallace PK, Peereboom DM. Flow cytometry as a diagnostic tool in lymphomatous or leukemic meningitis: ready for prime time? Cancer. 2012;118(7):1747–53. DOI: 10.1002/cncr.26335. Epub 2011 Oct 24.
43. Kitzmann AS, Pulido JS, Mohney BG, Baratz KH, Grube T, Marler RJ, et al. Intraocular use of rituximab. Eye (Lond). 2007;21(12):1524–7. Epub 2007/04/28.
44. Smith JR, Rosenbaum JT, Wilson DJ, Doolittle ND, Siegal T, Neuwelt EA, et al. Role of intravitreal methotrexate in the management of primary central nervous system lymphoma with ocular involvement. Ophthalmology. 2002;109(9):1709–16. Epub 2002/09/05.
45. Deangelis LM, Hormigo A. Treatment of primary central nervous system lymphoma. Semin Oncol. 2004;31(5):684–92. Epub 2004/10/22.
46. Blay JY, Conroy T, Chevreau C, Thyss A, Quesnel N, Eghbali H, et al. High-dose methotrexate for the treatment of primary cerebral lymphomas: analysis of survival and late neurologic toxicity in a retrospective series. J Clin Oncol Off J Am Soc Clin Oncol. 1998;16(3):864–71. Epub 1998/03/21.
47. Coupland SE. Uveal lymphoproliferative tumors. In: Singh AD, Damato B, Pe'er J, Murphree AL, Perry JD, editors. Clinical ophthalmic oncology. Philadelphia, PA: Elsevier; 2007. p. 316–21.
48. Aronow ME, Portell CA, Sweetenham JW, Singh AD. Uveal lymphoma: clinical features, diagnostic studies, treatment selection, and outcomes. Ophthalmology. 2014;121(1):334–41. Epub 2013/10/23.
49. Fuller ML, Sweetenham J, Schoenfield L, Singh AD. Uveal lymphoma: a variant of ocular adnexal lymphoma. Leuk Lymphoma. 2008;49(12):2393–7. Epub 2008/12/05.
50. Font RL, Spaulding AG, Zimmerman LE. Diffuse malignant melanoma of the uveal tract: a clinicopathologic report of 54 cases. Trans Am Acad Ophthalmol Otolaryngol. 1968;72(6):877–95. Epub 1968/11/01.
51. Arias JD, Kumar N, Fulco EA, Spaide R, Yannuzzi L, Shields CA, et al. The seasick choroid: a finding on enhanced depth imaging spectral-domain optical coherence tomography of choroidal lymphoma. Retin Cases Brief Rep. 2013;7(1):19–22. 2013/01/01.
52. Portell CA, Aronow ME, Rybicki LA, Macklis R, Singh AD, Sweetenham JW. Clinical characteristics of 95 patients with ocular adnexal and uveal lymphoma: treatment outcomes in extranodal marginal zone subtype. Clin Lymphoma Myeloma Leuk. 2014;14(3):203–10. Epub 2014/01/15.
53. Coupland SE, Foss HD, Hidayat AA, Cockerham GC, Hummel M, Stein H. Extranodal marginal zone B cell lymphomas of the uvea: an analysis of 13 cases. J Pathol. 2002;197(3):333–40. Epub 2002/07/13.
54. Coupland SE, Damato B. Understanding intraocular lymphomas. Clin Exp Ophthalmol. 2008;36(6):564–78. Epub 2008/10/29.
55. Shakin EP, Augsburger JJ, Eagle RC Jr, Ehya H, Shields JA, Fischer D, et al. Multiple myeloma involving the iris. Arch Ophthalmol. 1988;106(4):524–6. Epub 1988/04/01.
56. Tranos PG, Andreou PS, Wickremasinghe SS, Brazier JD. Pseudohypopyon as a feature of multiple myeloma. Arch Ophthalmol. 2002;120(1):87–8. Epub 2002/01/25.

57. Aronow ME, Shen D, Hochman J, Chan CC. Intraocular lymphoma models. Ocul Oncol Pathol. 2015;1:214–22.
58. Finger PT, 7th Edition A-UOOTF. The 7th edition AJCC staging system for eye cancer: an international language for ophthalmic oncology. Arch Pathol Lab Med. 2009;133(8):1197–8. Epub 2009/08/06.
59. Coupland SE, White VA, Rootman J, Damato B, Finger PT. A TNM-based clinical staging system of ocular adnexal lymphomas. Arch Pathol Lab Med. 2009;133(8):1262–7. Epub 2009/08/06.

Ocular Manifestations of Closed-Globe (Blunt) Ocular Trauma

16

Judy J. Chen and William F. Mieler

Abstract

Closed-globe blunt ocular trauma is a major medical, epidemiologic, and economic concern due to the high risk of severe vision loss. Types of closed-globe trauma can be divided into two categories: direct and indirect. Direct trauma includes traumatic retinal tear, detachment, and dialysis, traumatic macular hole, commotio retinae, contusion of the retinal pigment epithelium, choroidal rupture, chorioretinitis sclopetaria, and optic nerve avulsion. Indirect ocular trauma includes Valsalva retinopathy, solar and laser-induced retinopathy, Terson syndrome, Purtscher retinopathy, shaken baby syndrome, fat embolism syndrome, and whiplash retinopathy. Awareness of these conditions may help increase early detection and prevent reversible vision loss.

16.1 Introduction

Ocular trauma is a major epidemiologic concern due to the highly dependent nature of our society on visual information and interaction. Studies estimate that there are close to 2.5 million eye injuries per year [1] in the United States and over 55 million eye injuries restricting activities for more than one day world-wide [2], with the cumulative lifetime presence of eye injuries estimated at 1,400 per 100,000 population [3]. Even more devastatingly, a study utilizing data from the United States Eye Injury Registry (USEIR) found that the median age of patients with legal blindness (defined as worse than 20/200 vision) from trauma was 26 years of age [4]. This condition therefore affects people during the most productive years of their lives with lasting consequences.

J.J. Chen • W.F. Mieler (✉)
Department of Ophthalmology, University of Illinois at Chicago, Chicago, IL, USA
e-mail: wfmieler@gmail.com

J. Chhablani et al. (eds.), *Retinal and Choroidal Imaging in Systemic Diseases*,
https://doi.org/10.1007/978-981-10-5461-7_16

Table 16.1 Closed-globe (blunt) ocular injuries

Direct ocular or periocular trauma
Traumatic retinal tears, detachment, and dialysis
Traumatic macular hole
Commotio retinae (Berlin's edema)
Contusion of the retinal pigment epithelium
Choroidal rupture
Chorioretinitis sclopetaria
Optic nerve avulsion
Indirect ocular trauma
Valsalva retinopathy
Solar (and laser-induced) retinopathy
Terson syndrome
Purtscher retinopathy
Shaken baby syndrome
Fat embolism syndrome
Whiplash retinopathy

Of all ocular injuries, approximately 40% are closed-globe (blunt) injuries. Although closed-globe injuries are associated with an overall better prognosis than open-globe injuries (penetrating, perforating, and intraocular foreign body), Kuhn et al. found that 23.1% of patients suffering an ocular contusion had a final visual acuity less than 20/200. The high burden of disease and the severity of visual impairment make it imperative for eye physicians to educate themselves and their communities about this preventable condition. Additionally, ophthalmologists should learn to recognize the manifestations of closed-globe ocular trauma, in order to facilitate appropriate treatment and prevent further visual loss.

The various types of closed-globe (blunt) ocular trauma, direct and indirect, are listed in Table 16.1.

16.2 Closed-Globe Trauma (Direct Ocular or Periocular)

16.2.1 Traumatic Retinal Tears, Detachment and Dialysis

One of the most common manifestations of closed-globe ocular trauma is a retinal tear, detachment, and/or dialysis. It is estimated closed-globe ocular trauma accounts for 10–19% of all phakic detachments [5–7].

Several studies have demonstrated that ocular trauma occurs primarily in younger patients and is more common among males. Goffstein and Burton's review of 586 primary phakic detachments reported that the mean age of trauma-associated detachments was 28 years whereas non-traumatic cases had a mean age of onset of 53 years [7]. Seventy eight percent of traumatic detachments occurred in males compared to 48% of spontaneous cases. Cox et al. [8] reported a similar age and gender distribution. In addition, myopic eyes appeared to have a particular predisposition to retinal detachment following trauma.

Retinal dialyses are the most common form of retinal break leading to a traumatic retinal detachment. Such dialyses occur when ocular contusion produces a sudden anteroposterior compression of the globe, which results in a lateral expansion of the equatorial region and disinsertion or tearing of the retina. Clinically, traumatic dialyses most commonly occur in the inferotemporal or superonasal quadrants. Cox found that superonasal dialysis was the most common, followed by inferonasal dialysis, and occurred in 38% and 27% of 143 affected eyes, respectively [8]. Goffstein and Burton's study reported that dialyses occurred in the inferotemporal quadrant in 31% of 111 traumatized eyes and only 22% in other quadrants [7].

Other types of retinal defects can also lead to traumatic retinal detachment. Goffstein and Burton reported flap tears in 11% of cases (Fig. 16.1), tears in regions of lattice degeneration in 8%, and giant retinal tears in 16% [7] (Fig. 16.2). Cox and Schepens discovered retinal holes without apparent vitreous attachments in 36% of eyes [8], as well as avulsion of the vitreous base in 26% of eyes, which the authors considered pathognomonic for ocular trauma. High contact sports such as boxing can predispose patients to retinal breaks and detachments, with the reported incidence of retinal tears in boxers as high as 24% [9, 10].

Determination of whether trauma was the cause of a retinal detachment can oftentimes be difficult, especially since there may be a significant delay between the insult and detection of the detachment. Johnston reported that the retinal break or detachment was diagnosed within 24 hours in only 31% of cases, while 64% were diagnosed within the first 6 weeks; overall the retinal detachment rate was 84% in patients with contusion related breaks [11]. Factors that suggest a traumatic etiology for a retinal detachment include: (1) objective evidence of trauma, (2) unilateral pathology, (3) age less than 40 years, (4) giant retinal tear or dialysis, and (5) a latent interval of less than 2 years.

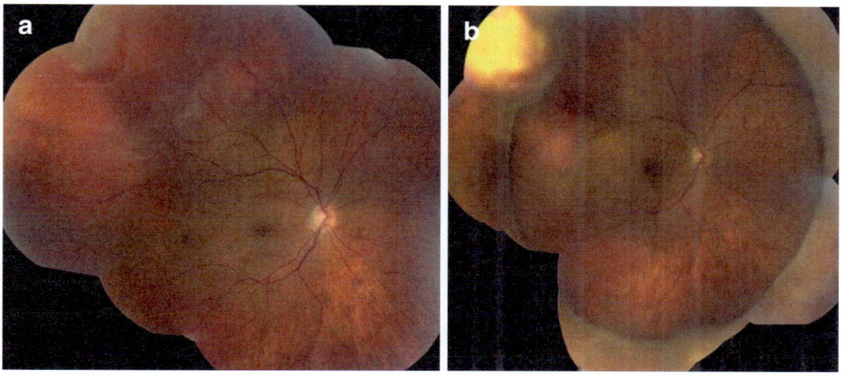

Fig. 16.1 Color photograph (right eye) showing a superotemporal peripheral retinal tear/detachment (**a**), which was subsequently treated with a scleral buckle (**b**) (Courtesy of Steven G Schwartz, MD, Naples, FL)

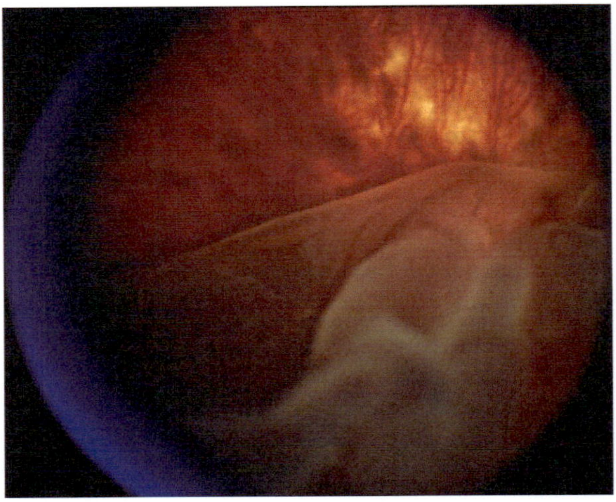

Fig. 16.2 Color photograph (right eye) revealing a 210° giant retinal tear following a closed-globe injury. The retina was repaired via a pars plana vitrectomy, with restoration of vision to 20/60

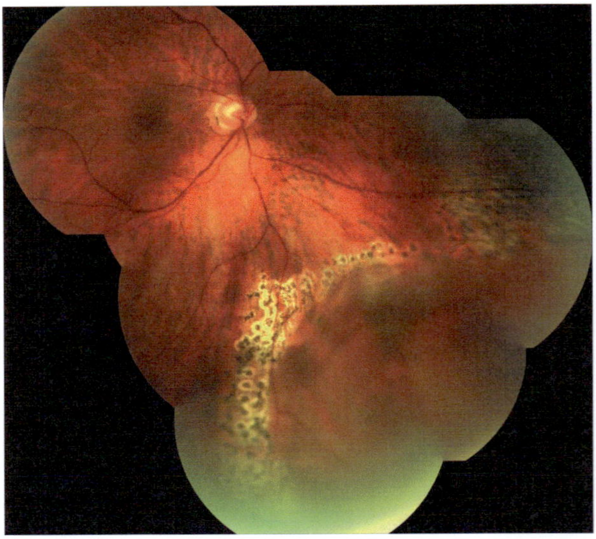

Fig. 16.3 Color photograph (right eye) showing a localized inferonasal peripheral retinal tear/detachment, demarcated by photocoagulation (Courtesy of Steven G Schwartz, MD, Naples, FL)

Treatment of traumatic retinal tears includes standard laser and cryopexy (Fig. 16.3). Retinal detachments may be treated with scleral buckling (Fig. 16.1), vitrectomy with air/gas tamponade (Fig. 16.2) or silicone oil, or pneumatic retinopexy. Overall the anatomic success rate and final visual acuity for traumatic retinal detachments are similar to non-traumatic cases, except in the case of giant retinal tears, where the anatomic success rate is lower, with published rates between 66% and 89% [12, 13].

16.2.2 Traumatic Macular Hole

Trauma is a well-recognized etiology for full-thickness macular holes, accounting for 9% of all macular holes and having been found in up to 6% of traumatized eyes [8] (Fig. 16.4). Unlike age-related macular holes in which tangential vitreofoveal traction leads to hole formation, the mechanism of traumatic macula hole formation is less well understood. It is thought that the unique anatomical arrangement of the normal fovea devoid of inner retinal layers and capillaries predisposes the area to the development of a full-thickness hole after trauma. A combination of mechanisms such as contusion related necrosis, vitreous traction, and subfoveal hemorrhage have also been proposed as possible causes [14].

The natural history of traumatic macular holes is well documented in various case series. Yamashita et al. [15] described a series of 18 patients with traumatic macular holes in which eight achieved spontaneous closure of the hole within 4 months after trauma with associated visual acuity improvement (Fig. 16.5). More recently, Miller et al. [16, 17] at the Massachusetts Eye and Ear Infirmary reported a series of 28 patients with traumatic macular holes in which 11 (39.3%) closed spontaneously, with median time to hole closure of 5.6 weeks (range 1.7–67.3 weeks). They found that younger patients with smaller holes were more likely to achieve spontaneous closure. Based on this data, they recommend observation for 3 months after presentation before surgical intervention.

In patients who do not achieve spontaneous closure of traumatic macular holes, several series have reported favorable results from surgical intervention. A few earlier studies described the use of adjuvants to encourage hole closure. Rubin et al. [18] reported a series of 12 patients managed with vitrectomy and TGF-B2. In this series,

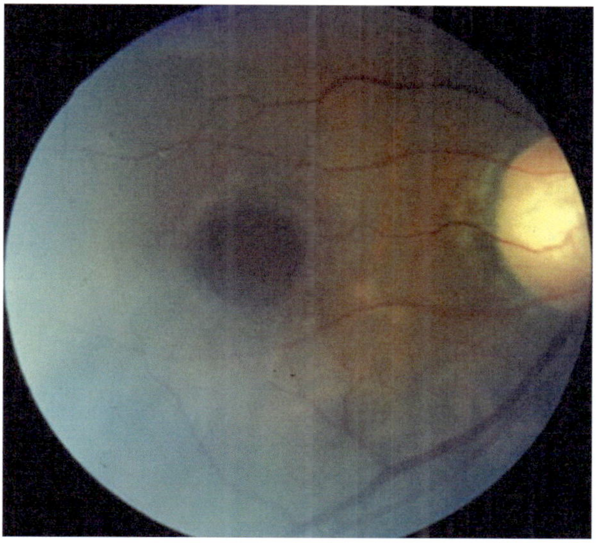

Fig. 16.4 Color photograph (right eye) documenting a large traumatic macular hole, surrounded by a cuff of subretinal fluid. Traumatic macular holes tend to be larger than age-acquired macular holes

Fig. 16.5 Color photograph and SD-OCT (right eye) of a patient (**a**) with an acute closed-globe injury where he sustained a large macular hole with subretinal hemorrhage and a peripheral retinal dialysis. VA was hand motions. The macular hole was observed and by 1 week (**b**), the hole had spontaneously closed. With additional time (**c**), the subretinal hemorrhage also resorbed, and vision improved to 20/100

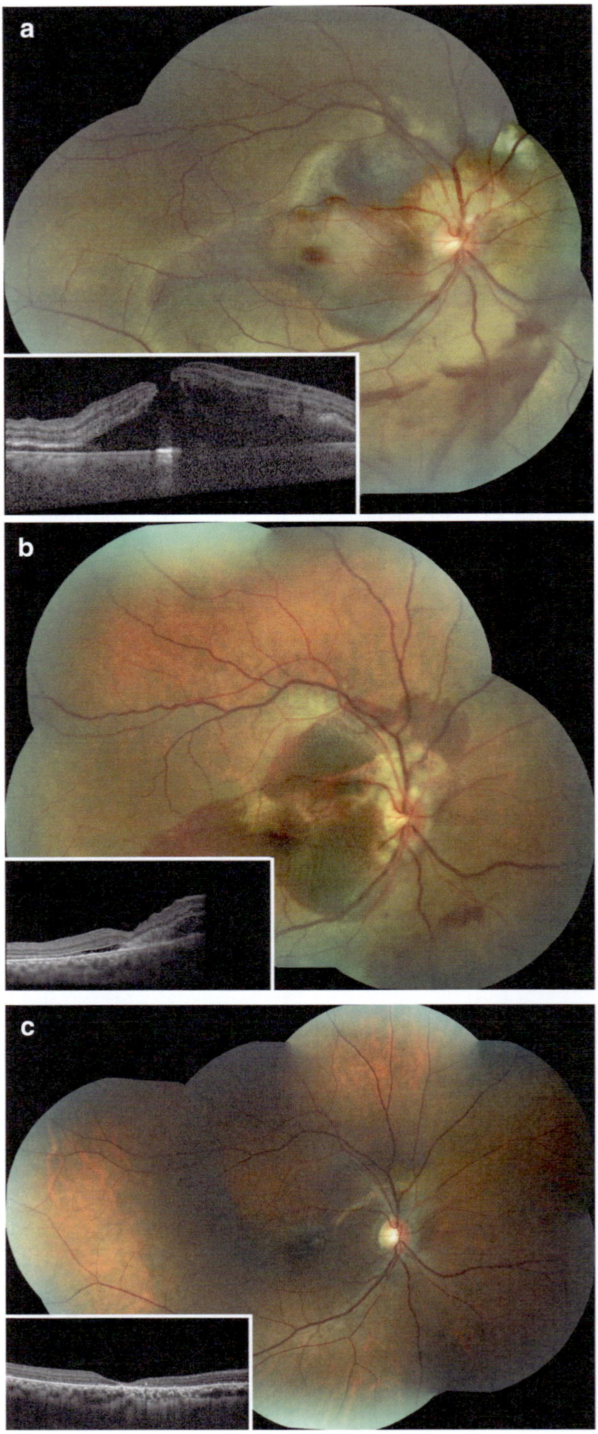

eight (67%) were closed after one procedure and 11 (92%) were successful with additional intervention. Visual acuity improved by two or more lines in eight (67%) patients, with six (50%) achieving a visual acuity of 20/40 or better. Using platelet concentrate, Garcia-Arumi et al. [19] treated eyes with a mean pre-operative visual acuity of 20/80 and achieved closure in 13 of 14 eyes (93%), with improvement of four or more lines of vision in successful cases and a final mean visual acuity of 20/30.

More recent studies have shown excellent outcomes without the use of adjuvants, including several that have reported a >90% closure rate of traumatic macular holes with standard pars plana vitrectomy and gas tamponade, and greater than 80% improvement of two or more lines in visual acuity [20, 21] (Fig. 16.6). While C_3F_8 is more frequently used, one study by Amari et al. [22] using SF_6 tamponade

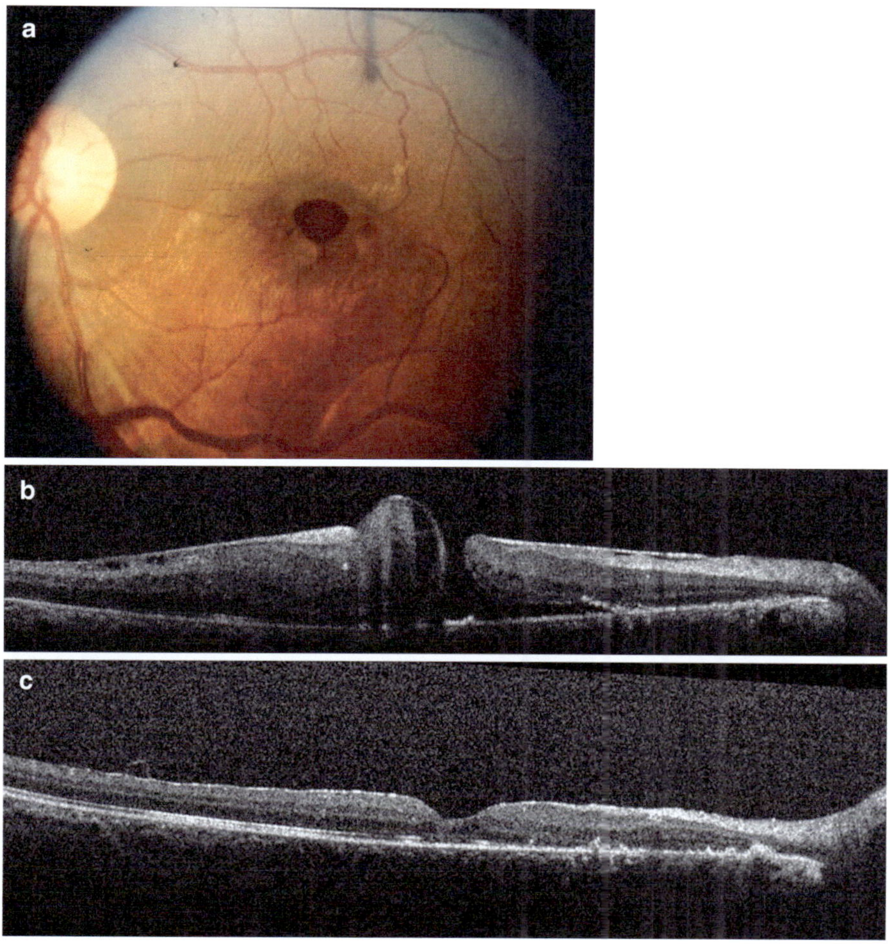

Fig. 16.6 Color photograph (left eye) of a traumatic macular hole (**a**), with a mild amount of retinal hemorrhage as well (**a**, **b**). After 2 months of observation, the macular hole was surgically repaired via pars plana vitrectomy surgery, with peeling of the ILM (**c**), and visual acuity improved to 20/80

reported a similar mean visual acuity improvement albeit with a lower initial anatomic hole closure rate of 70% (16/23). Another study comparing silicone oil tamponade and C_3F_8 gas found a significantly lower hole closure rate with oil (66.67% vs. 92.3%) [23].

Surgical treatment of traumatic macular holes, like that of age-related macular holes, appears to be highly successful and should be considered after a short period of observation (Fig. 16.6). Since these patients are typically young in age, the surgeon should be prepared to address a firmly adherent posterior hyaloid.

16.2.3 Commotio Retinae (Berlin's Edema)

Commotio retina (Berlin's edema) was first reported by Berlin in 1873 [24] to describe a grayish-whitening that primarily affects the outer retina after closed-globe ocular trauma (Fig. 16.7). There may also be varying degrees of retinal hemorrhage. Using an elastic stick, Berlin was able to produce commotio-like lesions in rabbits experimentally and concluded that the retinal changes were from extracellular retinal edema [24]. It most commonly occurs following direct blunt trauma to the globe, such as with a paintball [25] or soccer ball [26].

Early histopathologic data suggested that the injury from commotio retinae was related to disruption of the outer retina. Different authors have published data demonstrating disruption of photoreceptor outer segments [27], intracellular edema within glial cells [28], and fluid filled spaces in outer retinal layers [29]. Mansour et al. [30] examined an enucleated eye less than 24 hours post injury and found only photoreceptor outer segment disruption and apical RPE cell damage without damage to intercellular junctions or the rest of the retina. Minimal intraretinal albumin was seen, suggesting only slight breakdown in the blood–retinal barrier.

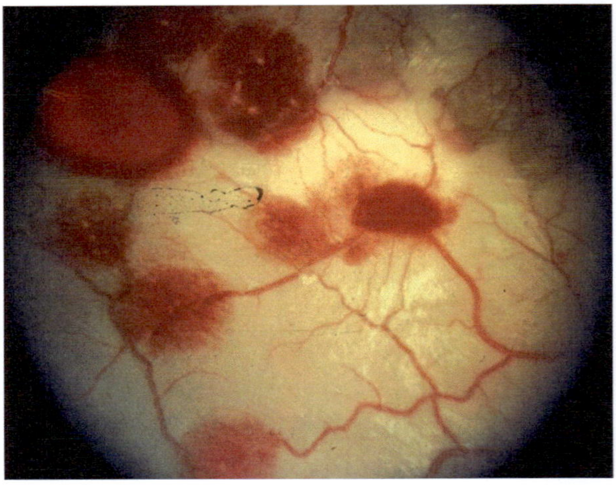

Fig. 16.7 Color photograph (left eye) of a patient who sustained a closed-globe injury, with resultant extensive retinal whitening, intraretinal and pre-retinal hemorrhage, compatible with commotio retinae. The findings gradually normalized, and as the macula was not involved, the patient did well visually

The clinicopathologic progression of commotio was further elucidated by Sipperly et al. [31]. Using experimentally traumatized owl monkeys, they found that retinal opacification occurred within 4–12 hours following injury and correlated histopathologically with disruption of photoreceptor outer segments. Twenty-one hours post injury, the outer segments were phagocytosed by the RPE and the inner segments demonstrated severe mitochondrial degeneration. Migration of RPE cells into the outer retina was seen at 48 hours and eventually multiple layers of RPE formed on Bruch's membrane. In areas of severe injury, outer segments did not regenerate and inner segments were in direct apposition to the RPE. Generalized thinning of the outer nuclear and plexiform layers followed. At no point did any discernible extracellular or intracellular edema occur. Pulido and Blair [32] also found no evidence of blood–retina barrier disruption in their evaluation of ten affected patients with vitreous flouorophotometry.

Clinically, the retinal changes of commotio may affect any part of the retina, from the posterior pole to extensive areas of peripheral retina. These findings may also be associated with choroidal rupture and pre-retinal, intra-retinal, or sub-retinal hemorrhages [33]. Visual acuity may range from 20/20 to 20/400 and does not correlate with the degree of retinal whitening, which may be so severe as to give the appearance of a cherry red spot in the macula [34] (Fig. 16.8). On fluorescein angiography, regions of opaque retina block the background choroidal pattern, exhibiting intact capillary perfusion without leakage [35]. Over several days, the retinal whitening clears spontaneously (Fig. 16.8).

Visual prognosis depends upon the extent of the injury. If only the photoreceptor outer segments are involved, these will often regenerate, restoring normal retinal structure and function [30, 31]. In other cases, permanent visual decrement may occur despite a normal appearing retina, or in the setting of cystic macular changes, partial or full thickness macular hole, or secondary to traumatic retinal pigmentary

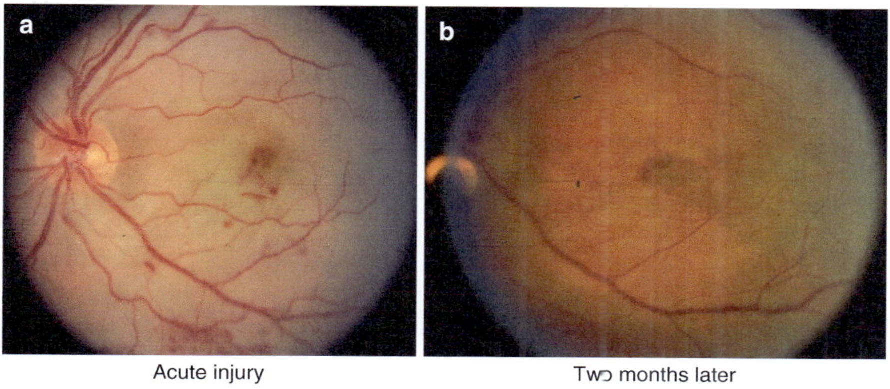

Fig. 16.8 Color photograph (left eye) of a patient (**a**) who was involved in a motor vehicle accident, where there was deployment of an air bag. Acutely, retinal whitening and hemorrhages were seen, compatible with commotio retinae. After 2 months, the commotio had resolved (**b**), leaving behind mild macular pigment epithelial mottling

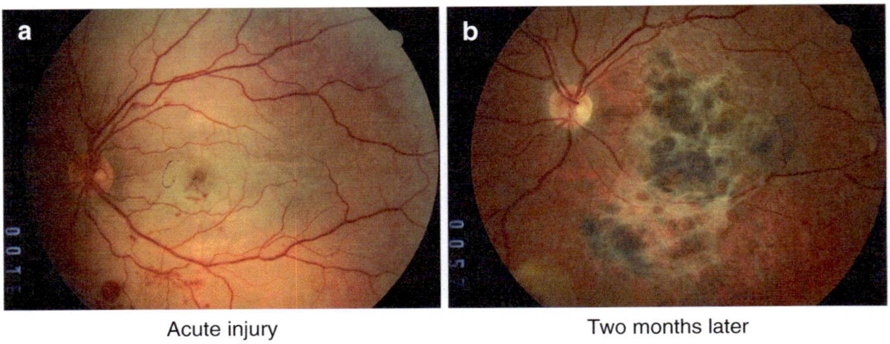

Fig. 16.9 Color photograph (left eye) of a patient (**a**) who sustained a hockey stick injury, with resultant commotio retinae. By 2 months, significant reactive hyperplastic retinal pigmentary changes had developed (**b**), which limited vision on a permanent basis

disruption (Fig. 16.9). In general, areas of commotio retinae are observed and monitored for resolution, and intervention is only recommended for complications such as development of a macular hole.

Clinical examination with optical coherence tomography (OCT) imaging reaffirms that commotio retinae is associated with disruption of photoreceptors rather than true retinal edema, and may be used to follow recovery. Souza-Santos et al. [36] performed OCT imaging on 11 eyes and found that mild lesions with good visual outcome showed transient hyperreflectivity of the outer retina while those with severe trauma and poor visual prognosis exhibited acute disruption of the inner/outer segment junction in addition to hyperreflectivity of the overlying retina. Therefore, OCT imaging in these cases may not only be useful in describing the extent of the initial trauma, but also in follow-up during recovery and in estimating final visual outcome.

16.2.4 Contusion of the Retinal Pigment Epithelium

Blunt ocular trauma may cause RPE contusion and tears in association with other retinal findings, as part of the spectrum of posterior segment manifestations of non-penetrating ocular trauma.

Patients will develop retinal pigment epithelial cell edema and an overlying serous retinal detachment acutely, as reported by Friberg [37] (Fig. 16.10). Forty-eight hours after the injury, there was noted to be a cream colored discoloration. Fluorescein angiography demonstrated late RPE staining without retinal or pigment epithelial elevation in association with a transmission defect corresponding to a macular hole. Within 2 weeks, the areas of pigment epithelial staining began to depigment and 5 months after injury, pigment clumping and RPE atrophy were notable clinically, with corresponding transmission defects without leakage seen on repeat angiography (Fig. 16.11).

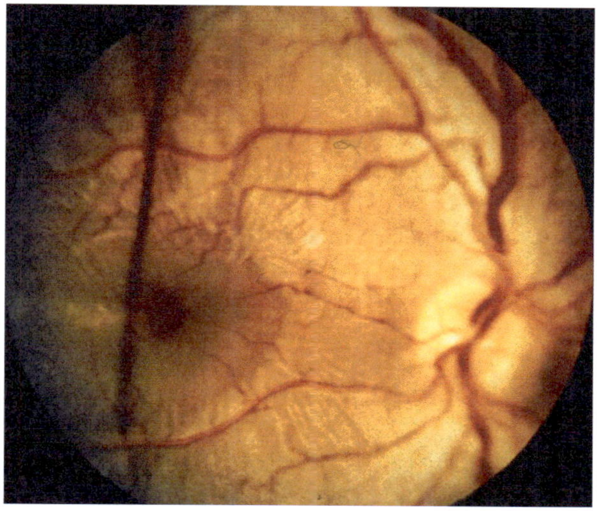

Fig. 16.10 Color photograph (right eye) of a patient who sustained a closed-globe injury, and developed a shallow serous detachment, which gradually subsided spontaneously

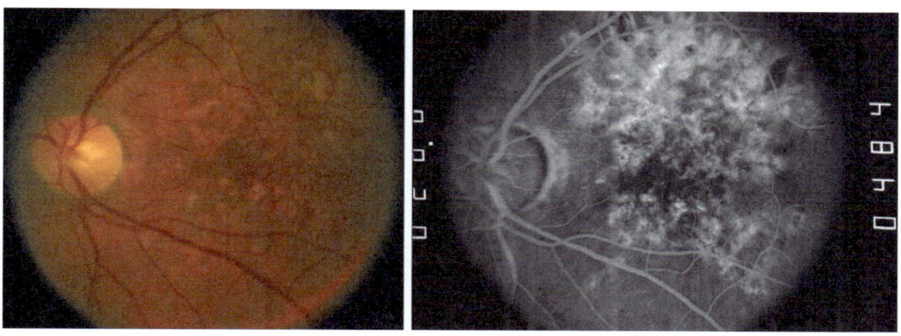

Fig. 16.11 Color photograph (**a**) and fluorescein angiogram (left eye) (**b**) documenting a contusive injury to the eye, with resultant retinal pigment epithelial mottling, as seen clinically and angiographically

Histologic and microscopic examinations of animal and human models of RPE contusion further help elucidate the changes caused by blunt trauma. Blight and Hart [27] examined the eyes of experimentally traumatized pig eyes and reported that, in addition to disrupted photoreceptor outer segments, electron microscopy revealed ruptures in the inner membranes of the RPE cells with associated intracellular edema. In their examination of a human case, Mansour et al. [30] noted that RPE damage was manifested by loss of apical processes, disruption of the plasma membrane and formation of multiple microcystic spaces. The damage was localized along the apical surface with no visible damage to the intercellular junctions or remainder of the cell. The observation that serous retinal detachment may sometimes accompany acute RPE injury probably relates to associated RPE dysfunction [38].

RPE tears may also occur following blunt trauma. Levin et al. [39] reported horizontal parafoveal RPE tears in two patients without evidence of pre-existing RPE detachments. Fluorescein angiography revealed mottled window defects in the region of the tears with associated blocking defects from the rolled up RPE. The authors proposed that the tears were caused by rapid spherical expansion of the globe creating forces sufficient to tear the RPE while sparing Bruch's membrane.

Visual outcome in patients affected with RPE contusions is variable, based on severity of injury and areas of the retina involved. No treatment has been shown to be effective for this condition.

16.2.5 Choroidal Rupture

Choroidal rupture, first described by von Graefe [40] in 1854, is a tear in the choroid, Bruch's membrane, and retinal pigment epithelium (RPE). They have been reported in up to 5–10% of cases of closed-globe blunt ocular trauma [41, 42] and while they can occur with open globe injuries, the majority (72% in one study) [42] are due to closed globe injuries. While the majority of reports are due to sports-related injuries [43], other projectiles including a human fist [44], a stone [45, 46], a champagne cork [47], or even a car airbag [48] have been reported to cause choroidal ruptures.

Choroidal ruptures may be either direct or, more commonly, indirect. Direct choroidal ruptures occur at a site of contusive impact, are anteriorly located, and tend to be oriented parallel to the ora serrata. Indirect choroidal ruptures, also known as *contrecoup* injuries, are posteriorly located away from the site of impact, crescent shaped, and concentric to the optic nerve, typically involving the inner choroid. The retina is spared due to its elasticity and the sclera is spared due to its rigidity [41]. In up to 25% of cases, ruptures may be multiple [49]. Other manifestations of ocular injury, such as commotio retina, may accompany choroidal ruptures and subretinal or vitreous hemorrhage may initially obscure the rupture site [38]. Mechanical deformation of the globe is believed to result in tearing of the choroid, Bruch's membrane, and retinal pigment epithelium [50], although other possibilities such as pressure necrosis and vascular injury have been proposed [51].

Clinically, a choroidal rupture is detected as a curvilinear or crescent-shaped yellow line, which is oftentimes obscured acutely by subretinal hemorrhage (Fig. 16.12). At presentation, visual acuity can vary from 20/20 to light perception, depending on the location of the choroidal rupture, amount of associated hemorrhage, or other manifestations of ocular trauma [43]. Fibroblastic activity usually occurs between 6 and 14 days leading to a well-developed scar by 3–4 weeks [50] (Fig. 16.13). Ruptures are more commonly located temporal to the optic nerve [52]. Ament and colleagues reported a case series of 111 cases of choroidal rupture, of which 68% occurred in the macula (37% foveal and 31% extrafoveal) and 32% were peripheral

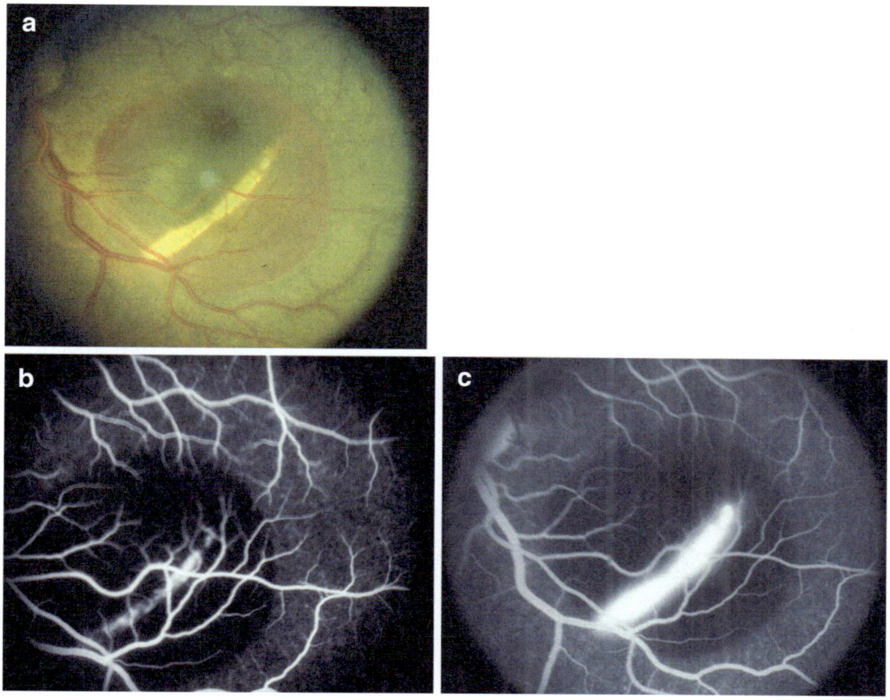

Fig. 16.12 Color photograph (**a**) and fluorescein angiogram (left eye) (**b** early, **c** late) documenting an acute choroidal rupture, with localized serosanguinous fluid in the macular region

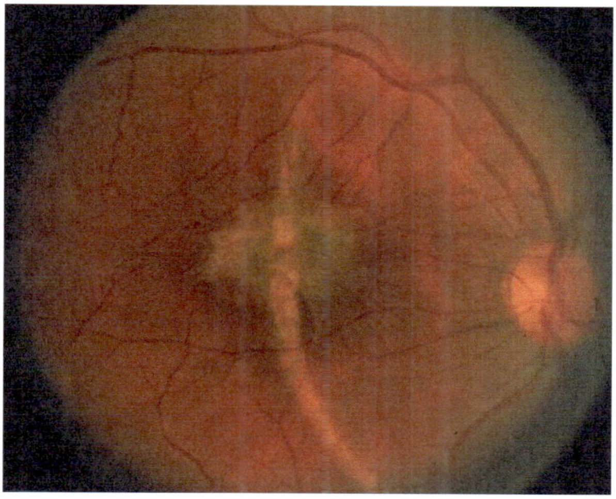

Fig. 16.13 Color photograph (right eye) revealing a choroidal rupture through the fovea with early fibroblastic proliferation. VA was limited to 20/400

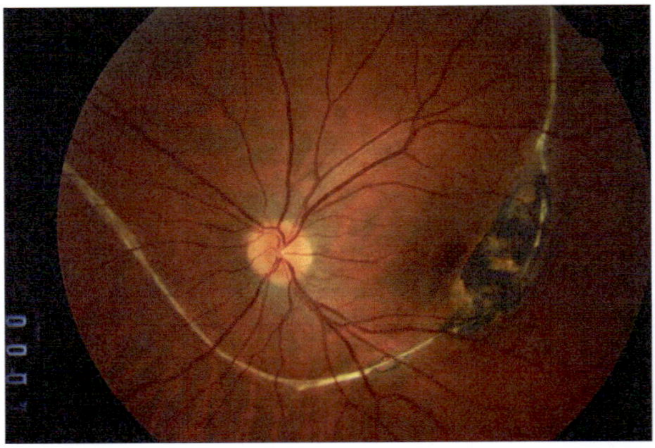

Fig. 16.14 Color photograph (left eye) demonstrating a very prominent choroidal rupture, curvilinear to the optic nerve, and virtually extending completely around the eye

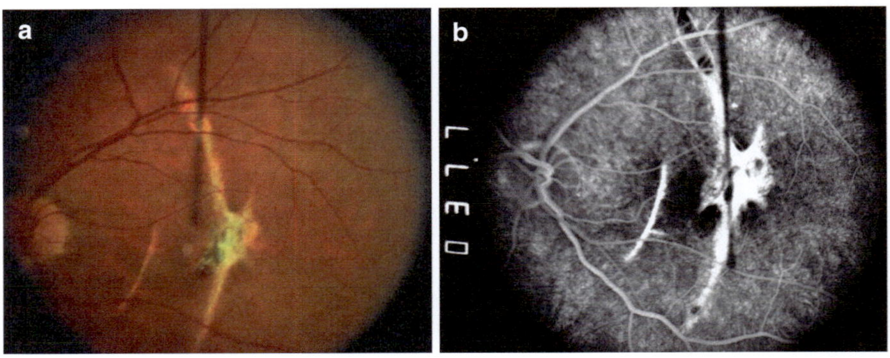

Fig. 16.15 Color photograph (**a**) and fluorescein angiogram (left eye) (**b**) documenting a double choroidal rupture with choroidal neovascularization (CNV) and scarring as well

[42] (Fig. 16.14). They also noted that while most patients had only one rupture, 21% had two ruptures, 11% had three ruptures, and 7% had four or more ruptures [42] (Fig. 16.15).

Fluorescein angiography may be helpful to reveal choroidal ruptures partly obscured by blood. Early hypofluorescence due to disruption of the choroid, late dye leakage at the rupture site, or large vessels seen traversing the choroidal defect in partial ruptures have all been described as typical FA findings [43]. More recently, use of ICG angiography has been described to identify hypofluorescent areas corresponding to choroidal ruptures not initially revealed by fluorescein angiography [53]. This latter modality may be the more sensitive way of detecting choroidal ruptures in the acute phase.

Late complications of choroidal rupture include choroidal neovascularization (CNV), optic atrophy [54], and chorioretinal anastomosis [55]. Ament and colleagues reported a 10% incidence of CNV occurring 1–18 months after trauma, and noted that longer ruptures, ruptures within the arcades, and older age all predisposed patients to CNV [42]. Visual field changes including nasal steps [56], baring of the blind spot, central and paracentral scotomas, and generalized constriction have all been described [14].

Visual outcome following choroidal rupture is variable. Since most ruptures are temporal to the nerve, involvement of the fovea may result in severe visual loss. Wood and Richardson [57] reviewed 30 cases of indirect choroidal rupture retrospectively and noted visual improvement to 20/40 or better in 17 (57%) cases. Visual loss was attributable to choroidal neovascularization in five eyes while the remainder demonstrated either a pigmentary maculopathy, had evidence of inner retinal injury, or optic nerve atrophy. Ament's group also noted that patients with CNV tended to have a worse visual outcome [42].

Choroidal ruptures do not require treatment, but patients should be monitored closely for development of CNV. Initially, laser photocoagulation and photodynamic therapy (PDT) were used for CNV but they quickly fell out of favor when it was demonstrated that the resolution was short-lived and recurrence was common [43]. Anti-vascular endothelial growth factor (VEGF) agents are now the preferred initial treatment for the treatment of CNV due to choroidal rupture, with studies reporting regression of CNV and improvement of vision at up to 9 months [58, 59]. There have also been reports of success with submacular surgery. Gross et al. [60] reported three cases complicated by subfoveal neovascularization treated with submacular surgery who achieved final visual acuities of 20/30 or better. Histologically, these membranes demonstrated reactive pigment epithelium lining one surface of the membrane without photoreceptors [61], suggesting that choroidal ruptures develop type 2 subretinal CNV, which tends to portend a better prognosis after surgery than type 1 CNV.

To summarize, choroidal ruptures may result in immediate or delayed visual loss. Secondary CNV may develop, though it oftentimes responds well to anti-VEGF therapy.

16.2.6 Chorioretinitis Sclopetaria

Chorioretinitis sclopetaria is a term originally used by Goldzieher in 1901 to describe a simultaneous defect of the retina and choroid resulting from a high velocity missile passing close to the eye without direct scleral injury [62]. The most common causes of chorioretinitis sclopetaria are bullets or BB pellets [63–69], although there have also been reports of sclopetaria resulting from unusual etiologies such as fishing line sinkers [70]. This type of injury represents a form of periocular closed-globe ocular injury.

The pathogenesis of sclopetaria relates to the viscoelastic properties of the involved tissues. Rapid deformation of the globe, caused by the concussive-like force of the missile as it impacts surrounding orbital tissue, induces sufficient stress to rupture the choroid and retina while the more compliant posterior hyaloid remains intact [71]. The choroid, which is under constant physiologic stress, retracts because it lacks attachments to the sclera between the equator and ora serrata [72], revealing an area of bare sclera often associated with marked retinal and vitreous hemorrhage [41] (Fig. 16.16). With time, a loose and dense connective tissue fills the defect resulting in a white scar, which attaches the surrounding tissues firmly to the sclera

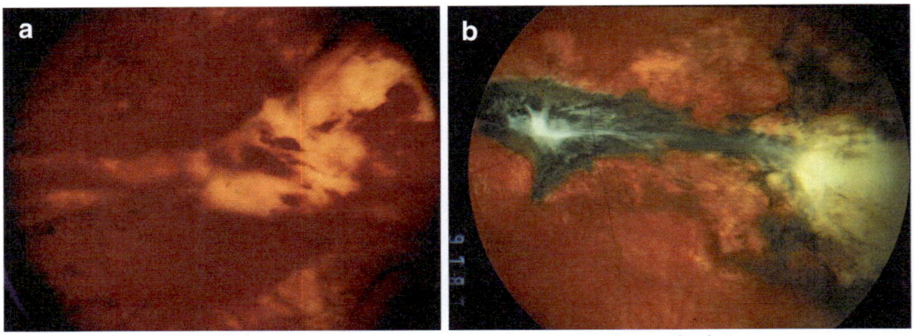

Fig. 16.16 Color photographs (left eye) from a patient who sustained a bullet injury to his left orbit. Acutely, there is extensive intraretinal, preretinal, and vitreous hemorrhage (**a**). After 3 months (**b**), the hemorrhage has resorbed, and the patient is left with an organized fibrotic scar posteriorly, with chorioretinal atrophy in the temporal periphery

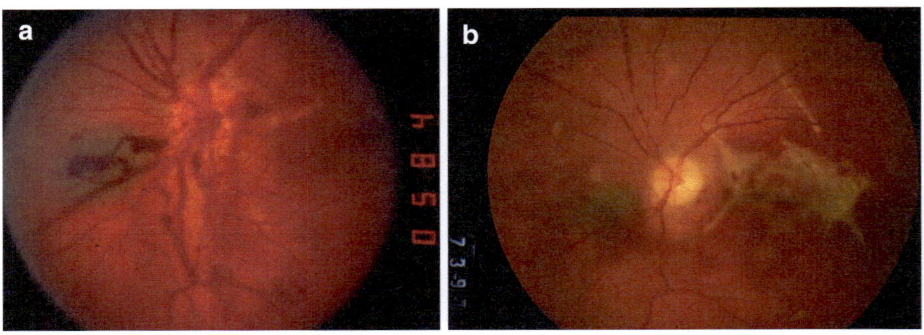

Fig. 16.17 Color photographs (left eye) from a patient who sustained a pellet injury to his left orbit. Acutely, there is moderate subretinal, intraretinal, and vitreous hemorrhage (**a**). With time, the hemorrhage resorbed (**b**), though vision was limited by development of a macular fibrotic scar along with probable choroidal ruptures

[73]. Retinal detachment is unusual since the retina and choroid remain apposed with an overlying intact posterior hyaloid in younger patients.

The condition is unusual and visual prognosis is guarded, as suggested by a few small series. Martin et al. [71] published one case series of eight eyes of seven patients with sclopetaria resulting from high-speed missile injuries. Seven of eight were initially observed; the other was treated with prophylactic scleral buckle. The retina remained attached for six months in all eyes. Late retinal detachments occurred in two eyes as a result of retinal tears unrelated to the area of sclopetaria. Two eyes developed vitreous hemorrhage associated with posterior vitreous separation. Visual acuity recovered to 20/20 in four observed eyes whereas traumatic maculopathy, macular hole, traumatic optic neuropathy, vitreous hemorrhage, and retinal detachment caused visual loss in the remainder (Fig. 16.17). Ahmadabadi et al. [64] published another case series of 13 eyes with sclopetaria, which were followed for a mean of 37 months. Two patients required vitrectomy for dense vitreous hemorrhage and suspected retinal detachment, although only one required retinal detachment repair. Final visual acuities ranged from 20/1200 to no light perception, despite the retina remaining attached in all patients. These results suggest that observation of these patients is reasonable while maintaining a high level of vigilance for other trauma-related complications.

16.2.7 Optic Nerve Avulsion

Although uncommon, optic nerve avulsion is a devastating and often irreversible consequence of ocular trauma, and it may be seen in virtually any type of trauma. Salzman first described avulsion of the optic nerve due to injury in 1903 [74]. Subsequent reports involved war injuries from severe concussive or penetrating orbital injuries [75, 76], but more recently it has been reported after seemingly minor sports injuries as well [77, 78].

The underlying mechanism of optic nerve avulsion involves the vulnerability of the axons at the level of the lamina cribosa, where relatively elastic myelinated nerve fibers lose their protective sheath. Various causes for optic nerve avulsion, based on this mechanism, have been reported in the literature including: (1) direct optic nerve traction from an object, such as a finger, causing extreme rotation and anterior displacement of the globe until rupture of the non-myelinated nerve fibers occurs; [79, 80] (2) an abrupt increase in intraorbital pressure from orbital injury or transmitted orbital shock waves, pushing the globe anteriorly and stretching the optic nerve; [81, 82] or (3) a dramatic intraocular pressure rise, which pushes the nerve out of the scleral canal [75, 83].

Clinically, a patient with optic nerve avulsion typically presents with an immediate, profound loss of vision [84, 85]. If the avulsion is partial, some visual function may be retained [86]. On examination, the optic nerve will appear empty and non-perfused, with varying amounts of peripapillary and vitreous hemorrhage (Fig. 16.18).

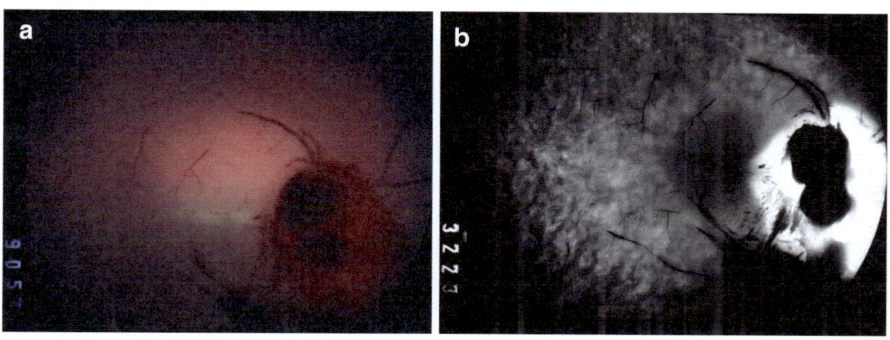

Fig. 16.18 Color photograph (**a**) and fluorescein angiogram (right eye) (**b**) from a patient who sustained a relatively minor injury in that he was struck on the right side of his head while playing baseball. He immediately lost all vision in the right eye, and ocular findings were compatible with avulsion of his optic nerve. CT scanning was unable to absolutely document the findings

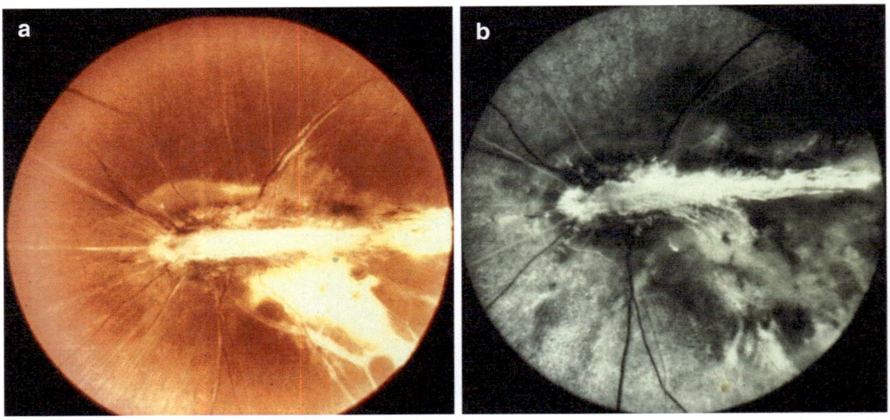

Fig. 16.19 Color photograph (**a**) and fluorescein angiogram (right eye) (**b**) from a patient who experienced an avulsed optic nerve several months earlier. The region of the optic nerve appears atrophic and fibrotic, and there is only very minimal restoration of perfusion seen angiographically. VA remains NLP

In mild cases, the nerve may have the appearance of an optic nerve pit [83]. Fluorescein angiography will often demonstrate a partial [86] or complete absence [85] of filling of the retinal vasculature, although the degree of perfusion will depend on the extent of injury. CT or MRI studies will often times demonstrate an apparently intact optic nerve [41], although fat stranding and a linear hypodensity corresponding to the avulsed nerve [87] may also be seen. With time, fibroglial tissue fills the cavity left by the evulsion and may mimic the appearance of a developmental optic nerve defect [88] (Fig. 16.19). There are no known treatments for optic nerve avulsion.

16.3 Indirect Ocular Trauma

16.3.1 Valsalva Retinopathy

Valsalva retinopathy occurs when there is a sudden rise in intrathoracic or intra-abdominal pressure against a closed glottis. This causes a rapid rise in intravenous pressure within the eye, causing spontaneous rupture of intra-retinal capillaries or veins [89]. Commonly reported causes of Valsalva retinopathy have included heavy lifting [90], prolonged coughing, vomiting [91], straining at stool, sexual activity [92], or childbirth [93, 94]. There have even been reports of Valsalva retinopathy due to bleeding diathesis [95], handstands [96], from airbag trauma [97], or as a complication of general anesthesia [98]. On funduscopic examination, a well-circumscribed round or dumbbell-shaped collection of sub-internal limiting membrane (ILM) hemorrhage is typically present in the macula area (Fig. 16.20). With time, vision typically returns to normal as the hemorrhage resorbs or formed elements of the blood settle inferiorly, sometimes resulting in a fluid level within the area of hemorrhage (Fig. 16.21).

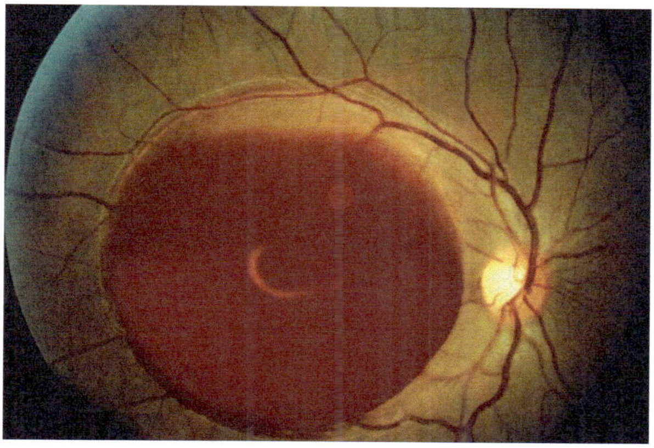

Fig. 16.20 Color photograph (right eye) in a patient who noted central visual loss OD immediately after lifting several heavy objects. This eye was observed and the sub-ILM hemorrhage slowly cleared without intervention

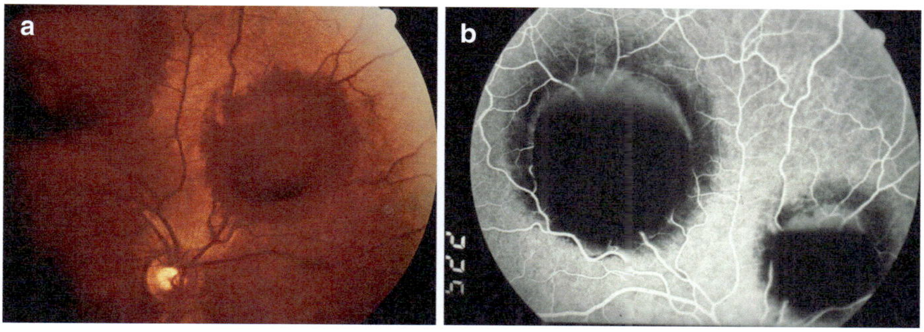

Fig. 16.21 Color photograph (**a**) and fluorescein angiogram (right eye) (**b**) demonstrates two areas of sub-ILM hemorrhage with fluid layers, in a prison inmate who lost vision when he was nearly choked to death by a fellow inmate several weeks earlier. Central vision was fine. No follow-up could be obtained

In recalcitrant cases where dense hemorrhage is present, visual recovery may be achieved through intravitreal drainage by opening the overlying ILM with argon or, preferably, a neodymium: yttrium-garnet (YAG) laser (Fig. 16.22). One study of 17 patients found 100% restoration of 20/20 vision with YAG laser treatment [99]. Reported complications of this procedure include macular hole and retinal detachment although further study is needed to define the risks associated with this procedure. Goel et al. [100] utilized SD-OCT to investigate evolution of the premacular hemorrhage following YAG laser; they found that the laser caused formation of a premacular cavity which persisted despite successful drainage of hemorrhage and may be responsible for metamorphopsias in some patients. Vitrectomy may be performed for those patients who fail to respond to laser or in cases where breakthrough vitreous hemorrhage has occurred [101, 102].

In addition, disorders such as diabetes, hypertensive retinopathy, and congenital retinal vessel (arterial or venous) tortuosity can lead to a similar clinical picture in the absence of abnormal physical activity. In these cases, visual prognosis is limited by the degree of coexisting retinal disease.

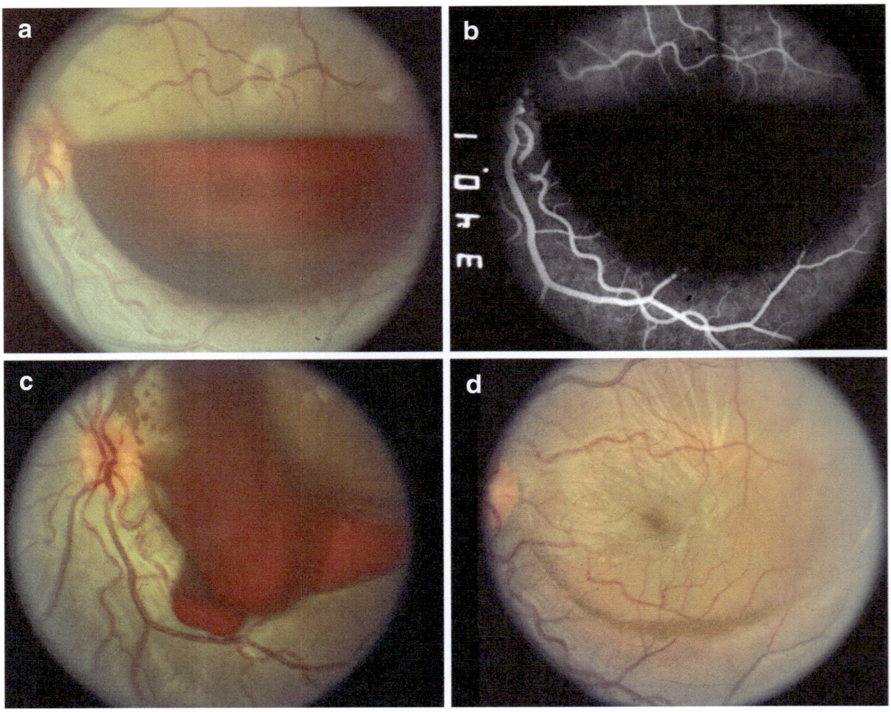

Fig. 16.22 Color photographs (**a**) and fluorescein angiogram (left eye) (**b**) in which there was minimal initial clearing of a pocket of sub-ILM hemorrhage after several weeks. A Yag:laser was therefore employed to "drain" the hemorrhage (**c**). The goal was accomplished, and only fine striae remain in the posterior hyaloid (**d**) (Courtesy of Susan M Malinowski, MD, Detroit, MI)

16.3.2 Solar Retinopathy

Solar retinopathy is a phototoxic reaction in the fundus caused by directly staring at a light source. Virtually any source of light can produce it, but most cases are caused by direct sun gazing during a solar eclipse, religious rituals, or directly viewing a laser pointer. It is also known in the literature as photic maculopathy, eclipse burns, and foveomacular retinitis [103, 104].

The reaction is photochemical in nature, and generally juxtafoveal, usually bilateral and asymmetric, with more severe disease in the dominant or fixation eye. Gass [103] postulated that the photochemical injury was mediated by highly reactive free radicals [105], through light-induced damage to the apical melanosomes of the RPE by blue-light wavelengths [106]. The severity of the reaction is dependent upon numerous factors including: (1) duration, intensity, and spectral content of the light, (2) clarity of the ocular media, (3) amount of ocular pigmentation, (4) body temperature, and (5) environmental conditions [105].

In general, patients will either be completely asymptomatic or present with a small central scotoma. In the acute setting, fundus examination may show a small yellow or reddish spot in the fovea, surrounded by faint gray granular pigmentation [103] (Fig. 16.23). These changes may be made especially obvious on autofluorescence or fluorescein angiography [106]. As the condition becomes chronic, the yellow discoloration will fade and leave a pathognomonic reddish spot [103] (Fig. 16.24). SD-OCT and multi-modal imaging has now shown that red spot correlates to an outer retinal hole, which is often square-shaped and usually spans from the RPE layer to the external limiting membrane [107]. This is consistent with loss of the inner and outer segments. These OCT findings are not specific to solar retinopathy, however, and can also be seen in tamoxifen retinopathy, juxtafoveal telangiectasia, foveolar vitreomacular traction, etc. [107].

Streaks of damaged retinal pigment epithelium can be seen after repetitively intentionally staring into a laser pointer (Fig. 16.25). Damage in this scenario can be extensive.

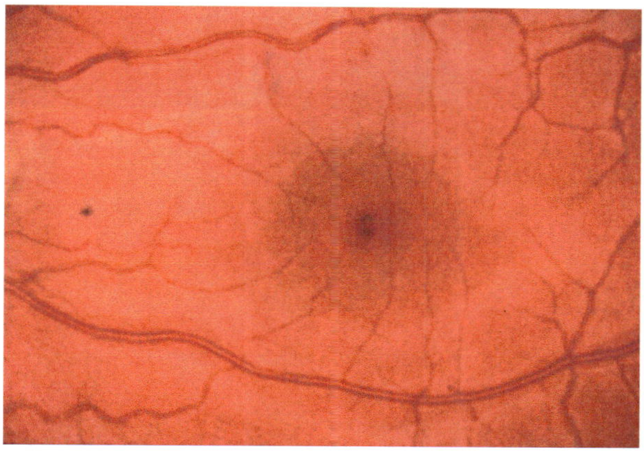

Fig. 16.23 Color photograph (left eye) demonstrating a reddish macular reflex following an episode of sun gazing. The reflex gradually normalized, though was eventually replaced by a small spot of hypopigmentation. VA was 20/40

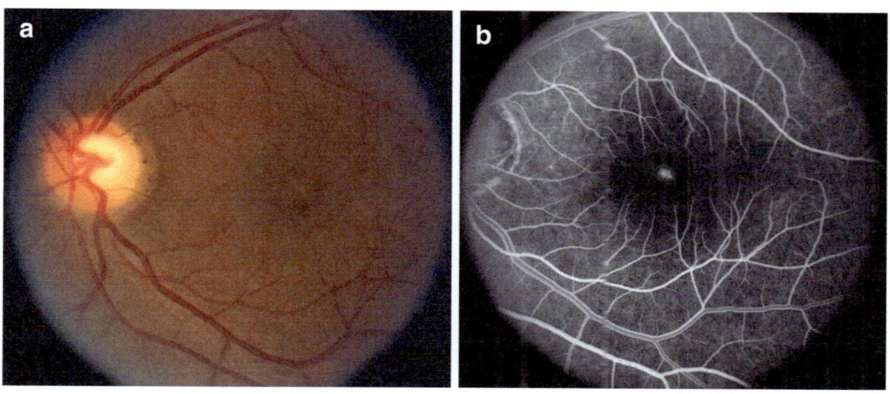

Fig. 16.24 Color photograph (**a**) and fluorescein angiogram (left eye) (**b**) document a small central zone of hypopigmentation in a patient seen 2 months after several episodes of sun gazing. Angiographically, a small transmission defect is seen. VA was 20/30

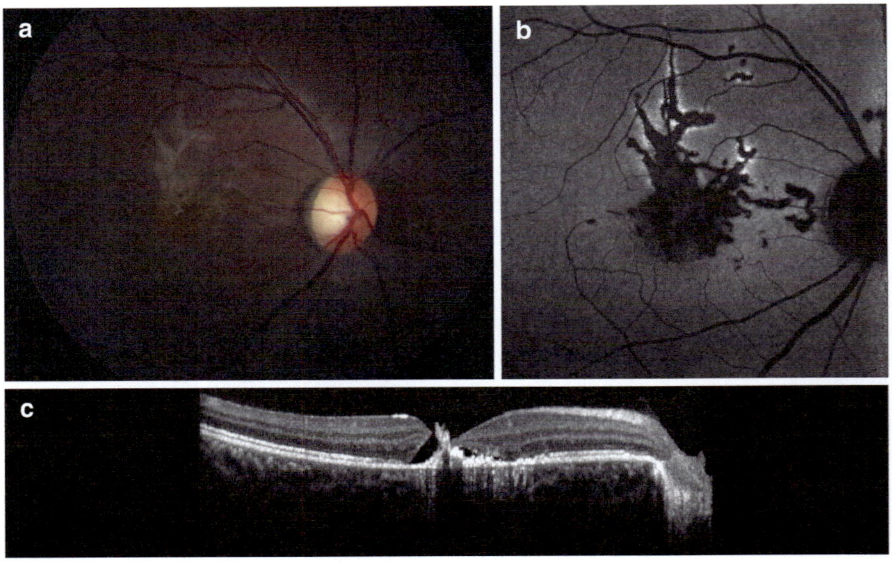

Fig. 16.25 Color photograph (**a**), fundus autofluorescence (**b**), and an SD-OCT (**c**) from a patient who intentionally pointed a laser into his eye(s). The irregular, linear streaks are quite diagnostic. While VA improved once the laser abuse was stopped, the vision never fully recovered (Courtesy of Amani Fawzi, MD, Chicago, IL)

There is no known treatment for solar retinopathy, however the condition can often improve with observation, with some regeneration of the outer retina.

16.3.3 Terson Syndrome

The association of vitreous hemorrhage with sub-arachnoid hemorrhage was reported by Litten [108] in 1881 and Terson [109] in 1900. Considered rare before the 1960s [110], it is now estimated that 20% of patients with either sub-arachnoid or sub-dural hemorrhage will develop intraocular hemorrhages. Furthermore, the presence of intraocular findings has been associated with a higher death rate from subarachnoid hemorrhage [111]. Typically, retinal hemorrhages are scattered in a peripapillary distribution and located in the subretinal, intraretinal, as well as sub-ILM or sub-hyaloid spaces (Fig. 16.26); the sub-hyaloid blood may break through into the vitreous cavity and cause vitreous hemorrhage [112].

The pathogenesis of Terson syndrome is not well established. Early reports suggested that the hemorrhage dissected through the optic nerve sheath from the arachnoid space [113]. However, the lack of an anatomic communication in a normal eye and the absence of an association between the hemorrhages and the optic nerve make this explanation unlikely [41]. Rather the hemorrhages more likely to be a

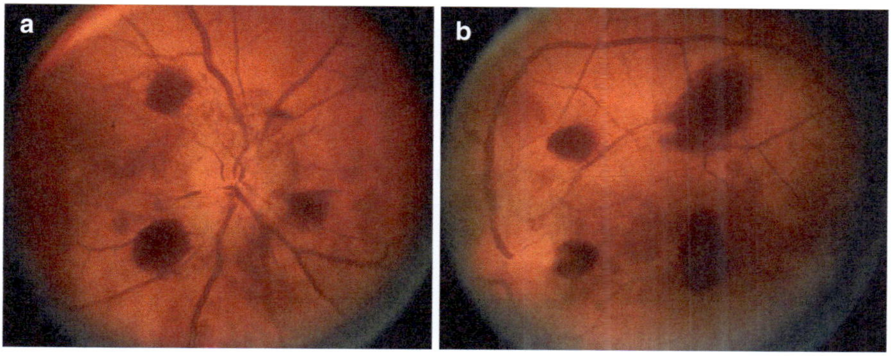

Fig. 16.26 Color photographs (both eyes) from a patient with traumatic subarachoid hemorrhage (**a**, **b**). In addition to the juxtapapillary hemorrhage, there is also mild optic disc edema. The patient did well with observation

secondary effect of increased intracranial pressure. Terson postulated that a sudden rise in venous pressure resulting from increased intracranial pressure caused ruptures of epiretinal and peripapillary capillaries [109]. Miller et al. [114] have attributed the findings to compression of the central retinal vein and its choroidal anastomosis.

The most common sequelae of Terson syndrome is epiretinal membrane (ERM) formation. Subhyaloid hemorrhage provides a scaffold for cellular proliferation and the formation of a dome shaped ERM. Histologically, these membranes are due to the proliferation of glial cells and their basement membrane, overlying an intact ILM [115]. Other complications associated with Terson syndrome include perimacular retinal folds [116], similar to those of shaken baby syndrome, and retinal detachments [117].

Overall, the visual outcome of Terson syndrome is favorable. Schultz et al. [118] found that 25 of 30 eyes achieved 20/50 or better vision with an average of four years of follow-up. Fourteen eyes in this series were treated with pars plana vitrectomy to clear dense vitreous hemorrhages and severe epiretinal membranes, while the rest were observed. There was no difference in visual outcome between the two groups, however visual recovery was more rapid with vitrectomy. Seventy-eight percent of eyes in this series developed ERMs. Therapeutically, pars plana vitrectomy can be considered in visually significant ERMs or non-clearing vitreous hemorrhages, particularly in children at risk for amblyopia [119].

16.3.4 Purtscher Retinopathy

In 1910, the clinical findings now known as Purtscher retinopathy were described by Omar Purtscher in a patient who suffered head trauma and was subsequently noted to have multiple areas of retinal whitening and hemorrhage in the posterior pole [120]. Purtscher hypothesized that the retinal whitening resulted from lymphatic extravasions secondary to increased intracranial pressure [121]. Later reports described similar retinal findings in a variety of conditions including acute pancreatitis [122], compressive trauma to the trunk or extremities [123], fat embolism syndrome [124], and renal failure [125], which has been deemed "Purtscher-like retinopathy."

Patients will complain of a decline in visual acuity, ranging from mild deficits to hand motions vision [126]. Usually the visual changes will occur 24–48 h after the trauma. On examination, an afferent pupillary defect may be present in the more severely affected eye. Characteristically, the retina will exhibit multiple discrete patches of superficial retinal whitening, known as Purtscher flecken, cotton wool spots (Fig. 16.27), and hemorrhage concentrated around a normal or edematous optic nerve head [127, 128]. Purtscher flecken are classically polygonal, variable in size, and should exhibit a clear zone between the affected retina and an adjacent arteriole. The fundus abnormalities are usually limited to the posterior pole within the macula and nearly always bilateral, although unilateral cases have been reported [129, 130]. Fluorescein angiography may demonstrate impaired retinal artery and capillary perfusion with late leakage, venous staining, and optic disc edema [129]. Indocyanine green angiography has noted choroidal hypofluorescence, suggesting choroidal ischemia as well [131]. Histopathologic examination of an eye demonstrated inner retinal atrophy consistent with retinal artery occlusion [132].

Clinical resolution may take several months and can be associated with permanent visual loss when concomitant optic atrophy or retinal pigment epithelial changes are present [131] (Fig. 16.28). One study of 23 cases found spontaneous improvement of two or more Snellen lines in 50% of patients [133]. Possible factors associated with a poor outcome include optic disc swelling or leakage on fluorescein angiography, choroidal hypoperfusion with outer retinal involvement, retinal capillary non-perfusion, prior episodes of Purtscher retinopathy, duration of retinal changes, and massive Purtscher flecks on presentation [126, 133].

The pathogenic mechanisms that lead to Purtscher retinopathy are unclear. Purtscher originally hypothesized that the retinal whitening was a result of increased

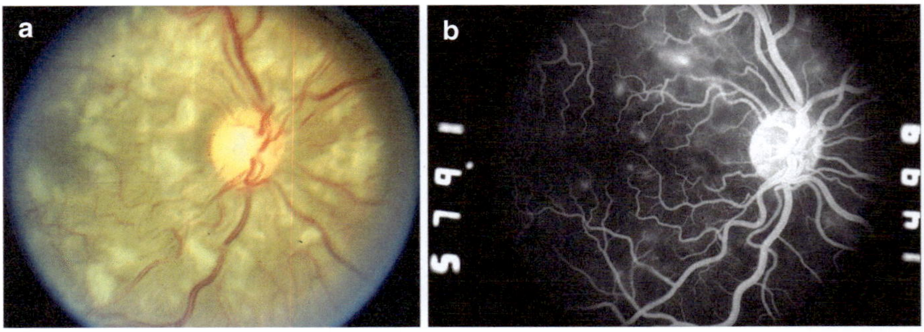

Fig. 16.27 Color photograph (**a**) and fluorescein angiogram (right eye) (**b**) from a patient with Purtscher retinopathy. Multiple areas of peripapillary ischemia are seen, and the angiogram documents mild vascular leakage

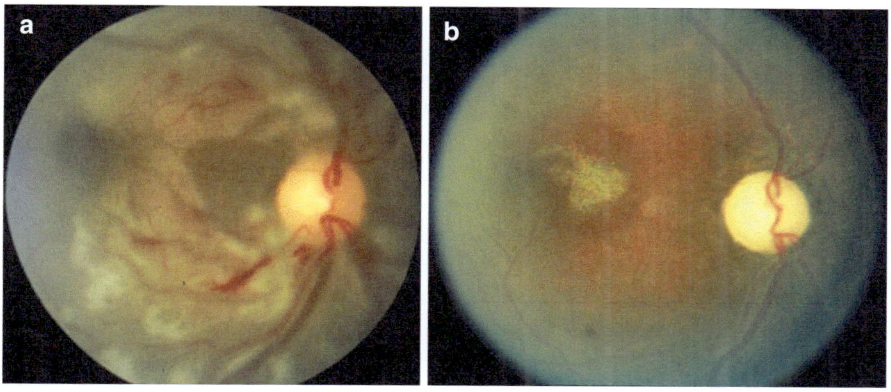

Fig. 16.28 Color photographs (right eye) in a patient (**a**) who was run over by an automobile sustaining primarily chest trauma. The acute findings of Purtscher retinopathy gradually resolved, though the patient was left with diminished visual function (**b**) due to a combination of optic nerve atrophy and macular pigment scarring

intracranial pressure causing lymphatic extravasion [121] but various other mechanisms have been subsequently proposed, including intravascular coagulopathy and granulocyte aggregation resulting from traumatic endothelial injury [134] and air embolism resulting from chest compression [129]. Experimentally, similar retinal changes have been created by infusion of fibrin clots within the ophthalmic artery [135] or glass microbeads in the carotid artery [136, 137]. Some of these laboratory studies have provided evidence of compliment activation in Purtscher retinopathy, which is consistent with the observation that both trauma and pancreatitis activate the complement pathway [41, 138].

No treatment has been demonstrated to be consistently effective for this condition. There are isolated cases of success with high-dose intravenous corticosteroids [133, 139], which is felt to work through inhibition of granulocyte aggregation secondary to complement activation in a dose dependent manner [126]. However, Agarwal and McKibbin in their case series noted a similar incidence of visual improvement between patients who were treated and those who were observed [132]. There have also been occasional reports of hyperbaric oxygen in the treatment of Purtscher retinopathy with mixed results [140]. Therefore, despite the existence of papers citing the reported benefits of treatment, there is no consensus that any intervention is superior to observation alone in Purtscher retinopathy.

16.3.5 Shaken Baby Syndrome

Child abuse occurs in 1% of children in the United States annually [141] and according to World Health Organization statistics, a quarter of all adults report having been physically abused as children [142]. Indeed, 10% of traumatic injuries of children under 5 years old are non-accidental and between 5% and 20% of these injuries are lethal [143]. Of those children who survive child abuse, 15% will have permanent physical abnormalities. Because 30–40% of abused children and up to 95% of patients with shaken baby syndrome (SBS) will have funduscopic evidence of injury, the ophthalmologist can play a critical role in diagnosis, especially since there may be few outward signs of abuse [144–146].

The pathogenesis of SBS is related to the repetitive angular acceleration–deceleration motion that occurs in shaking, which causes high gravitational forces to be exerted on an infant's head [147]. Most other forms of injury involve translational linear acceleration–deceleration forces, which reach their peak force only for a moment during impact and the force is disseminated through the skull, the body, and the object of impact [147]. In contrast, angular acceleration–deceleration forces are sustained, self-perpetuating forces and there is no protective mechanism for the brain from these magnified gravitational forces. As a result, biomechanical studies show that the magnitude of the acceleration and deceleration in SBS is 50 times greater than when the head is hit forcefully against a surface [148].

Anterior and posterior segment findings may result from violent shaking, direct ocular injury, head injury, chest injuries, or choking. While no finding is pathognomonic for shaking injury, the most common and characteristic finding of retinal hemorrhage is present in 64–89% of cases and may involve all layers of the retina [149] (Fig. 16.29). The retinal hemorrhages are deep, extensive, and mainly located in the posterior pole. Eisenbry [150] reported that 64% of abused children less than 3 years old manifested retinal hemorrhages whereas only 3% had such hemorrhages after accidental head injury. Odom et al. [143] prospectively evaluated 43 patients who underwent at least one minute of cardiopulmonary resuscitation (CPR). Despite the presence of clotting abnormalities and prolonged CPR in the

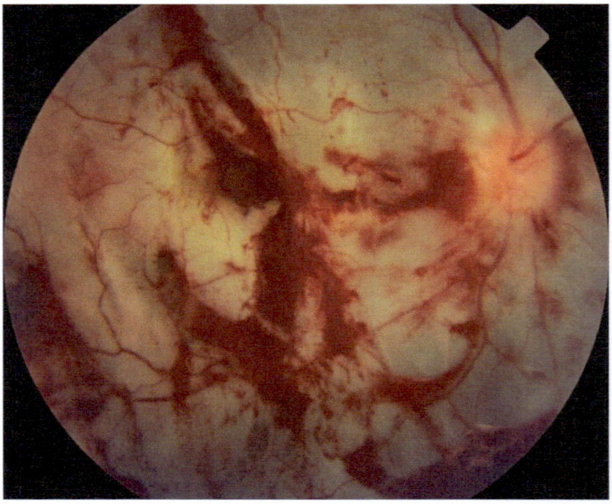

Fig. 16.29 Color photograph (right eye) from a baby who endured severe shaking from her caregiver, with resultant subretinal, intraretinal, and preretinal hemorrhages. Fortunately, the infant survived, was placed in a safe environment, and the ocular abnormalities cleared

majority of patients, only one patient manifested slight punctate retinal hemorrhages [143]. Therefore, while retinal hemorrhages may be present in exceptional cases, it is not characteristic of other forms of trauma and therefore is highly specific for child abuse [148].

In addition to retinal hemorrhage, perimacular folds [151], retinoschisis, cotton wool spots, retinal vessel engorgement, and papilledema may be present [152]. The overall clinical picture may simulate Purtscher retinopathy syndrome, Terson syndrome, or central retinal vein occlusion [153]. Vitreous hemorrhage, retinoschisis, retinal detachment, and chorioretinal atrophy may also occur [149, 153, 154]. The presence of dense vitreous hemorrhage in infants has been associated with poor visual and neurological prognosis [152]. In many cases of shaken baby syndrome, there will also be associated intracranial hemorrhage or contusion, which essentially assures the diagnosis. Wilkinson et al. [155] found that a subhyaloid hemorrhage greater than two disc diameters in size, vitreous hemorrhage, or diffuse hemorrhage involving the peripapillary and peripheral retina was associated with a high initial neurologic injury score.

Computed tomography immediately following shaking injury may demonstrate only subtle intracranial abnormalities despite the presence of retinal hemorrhages. In these patients, close monitoring of neurologic status, fontanelles, head circumference, and CT scans is critical as evidence of subdural hemorrhage may be delayed following injury [156, 157]. A midline shift on CT and non-reactive pupils at presentation has been recently associated with infant mortality [158].

Treatment should be administered according to the severity of injury. External ocular injuries such as eyelid injuries or open-globe injuries should be addressed first [147]. Most of the intraocular and posterior segment manifestations are managed best by observation in the acute phase, as most hemorrhages will clear spontaneously. Even simple retinal folds or detachments are rarely routine surgeries and may lead to complications and poor outcomes. However, patients should be closely monitored since deprivation amblyopia can occur within four weeks [147]. In cases of non-clearing vitreous hemorrhage or hemorrhage obscuring the macula, pars plana vitrectomy may be considered. Alternatively, intravitreal tPA and gas has been proposed as an alternative to vitrectomy to clear subhyaloid blood in selected cases [159]. Retinal detachments may be repaired with barrier laser with or without scleral buckle, although encircling buckles should be avoided and the buckle may need to be released at a later date [160]. Retinoschisis can be treated with laser or cryotherapy at the borders to prevent extension; flattening of the schisis with surgery or pneumatic retinopexy is usually not successful and does not improve vision. If traumatic damage to the optic nerve is suspected, a trial of intravenous corticosteroids may be considered [161].

Overall ocular prognosis is related to how much damage has been done to the macula. A series by Kivlin et al. [162] found that one-fifth of survivors retained poor vision, but this was mostly related to cortical blindness. Extensive retinal injury, especially retinal folds and retinoschisis, and non-reactive pupils were associated with a higher mortality rate while good visual reaction and reactive pupils were related to a good visual prognosis and higher survival rate.

16.3.6 Fat Embolism Syndrome

Fat embolism syndrome (FES) was first reported in 1861, describing a clinical syndrome that affects many organ systems following medullated long bone fractures [163]. Patients with FES present with variable degrees of pulmonary insufficiency, mental deterioration associated with thrombocytopenia, and petechiae of the upper extremities and conjunctiva [164]. Some may even become critically ill and, in severe cases, mortality rates may be as high as 20% [165]. Subclinical affliction can be detected by abnormal arterial blood gas findings [166].

About half of all patients with clinical FES will present with retinal lesions [135, 167]. The most common findings are cotton wool spots and retinal hemorrhages [136, 137], but intravenous fat and central retinal artery occlusions have also been described [168] (Fig. 16.30). Similar to the systemic clinical findings, the retinal lesions may appear and resolve successively. On histologic examination, the retinal lesions appear as microinfarcts in the inner retina and uveal tract [169].

Fat emboli and microinfarcts in the retina as a result of long bone fractures can be seen in the absence of systemic findings. One study by Chuang et al. [170] examined 100 consecutive patients admitted to a hospital with long bone or pelvic fractures. The study excluded patients with hypertension, diabetes, or other conditions associated with vascular retinopathy. Four patients were found to have retinal findings consistent with FES, including cotton wool spots and blot hemorrhages, in the absence of pulmonary, neurologic, or dermatologic findings. This study demonstrates that the retina may be involved even in subclinical cases of FES, and therefore retinal screening and evaluation even in the absence of systemic findings is warranted. The visual prognosis in most patients with FES is favorable, but some patients may develop permanent paracentral scotomas [170].

It should be noted however, that these types of findings are seen much less commonly today, as rehabilitation and mobilization of the patient is instituted much more rapidly in the setting of bony fractures.

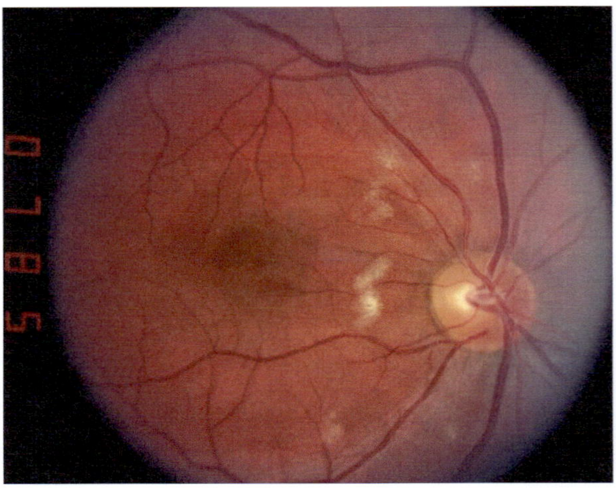

Fig. 16.30 Color photograph (right eye) from a patient with a fractured femur (and chest injuries) sustained in a skiing accident. Following rather prolonged immobilization, mild ocular features of fat emboli syndrome were seen. The findings resolved spontaneously over time

16.3.7 Whiplash Retinopathy

Whiplash retinopathy is an uncommon cause of vision loss in the setting of a traumatic flexion-extension injury to the head and neck. Typically, there is an immediate mild reduction in visual acuity, usually no worse than 20/30, with development of gray swelling of the foveal region and a 50–100 micron foveolar pit [171]. Fluorescein angiography in the acute phase may be normal or may show slight focal areas of pigmentary disturbance [172]. Vision usually returns to normal, leaving a pit with whitish borders and a subtle disturbance of the RPE [173].

It has been speculated that any insult, whether toxic or physical, may result in selective photoreceptor loss and give rise to the appearance of a foveolar pit [173–175]. Identical foveolar pits may be seen in the setting of sun gazing, mild foveomacular retinitis, toxic medications, and direct ocular trauma. In whiplash retinopathy, the foveolar pit is believed to result from vitreomacular traction. Other trauma-induced alterations of the vitreomacular interface include prefoveal vitreous wisps, opercula, full thickness macula holes, and posterior vitreous detachment [176]. There is no known treatment for whiplash retinopathy but surgery may be considered if a full thickness macular hole develops.

Conclusion

Closed-globe (blunt) ocular trauma results in a variety of overlapping ocular findings, which have been frequently described in the literature. The effects of trauma may result from direct ocular injury, or be indirect, developing secondary to injury from a distant site. These conditions can be difficult to diagnose due to the variability of visual impairment, and in some situations significant time may elapse before the effects of trauma are fully manifest. For many of these conditions, there is no specific treatment.

An understanding and awareness of the ocular findings and anticipatory management may limit further complications and visual decline in select cases. Additionally, ophthalmologists should work to educate the community about the appropriate precautions that should be undertaken, such as safety glasses and avoidance of risky activities, in order to minimize or prevent ocular injury. Only in this fashion can the overall burden of closed-globe injuries be decreased.

References

1. Morris R, Kuhn F, Witherspoon CD, Stevens D. Counseling the patient and the family. In: Kuhn F, Pieramici D, editors. Ocular trauma: principles and practice. New York: Thieme; 2002. p. 22–6.
2. Negrel A-D, Thylefors B. The global impact of eye injuries. Ophthalmol Epidemiol. 1998;5:143–69.
3. National Society to Prevent Blindness. Visual problems in the U.S. data analysis definitions. Data sources, detailed data tables, analysis, interpretation. New York: National Society to Prevent Blindness; 1980. p. 25–6.

4. Kuhn F, Morris R, Witherspoon CD, Mann L. Epidemiology of blinding trauma in the united states eye injury registry. Ophthalmol Epidemiol. 2006;13:209–16.
5. Dumas JJ. Retinal detachment following contusion to the eye. Int Ophthalmol Clin. 1967;7:19–38.
6. Schepens CL, Marden D. Data on the natural history of retinal detachment. Further characterization of certain unilateral nontraumatic cases. Am J Ophthalmol. 1966;61:213–26.
7. Goffstein R, Burton TC. Differentiating traumatic from nontraumatic retinal detachment. Ophthalmology. 1982;89:361–8.
8. Cox MS, Schepens CL, Freeman HM. Retinal detachment due to ocular contusion. Arch Ophthalmol. 1966;76:678–85.
9. Bianco M, Vaiano AS, Colella F, Coccimiglio F, Moscetti M, Palmieri V, Focosi F, Zeppilli P. Ocular complications of boxing. Br J Sports Med. 2005;39:70–4.
10. Giovinazzo VJ, Yannuzzi LA, Sorenson JA, Delrowe DJ, Cambell EA. The ocular complications of boxing. Ophthalmology. 1987;94:587–96.
11. Johnston PB. Traumatic retinal detachment. Br J Ophthalmol. 1991;75:18–21.
12. Aylward GW, Cooling RJ, Leaver PK. Trauma-induced retinal detachment associated with giant retinal tears. Retina. 1993;13:136–41.
13. Nacef L, Daghfous F, Chaabini M, Azaiez A, Ayed S. Ocular contusions and giant retinal tears. J Fr Ophtalmol. 1997;20:170–4.
14. Hart JC, Nitikos E, Raistrick ER, Doran RML. Indirect choroidal tears at the posterior pole: a fluorescein angiographic and perimetric study. Br J Ophthalmol. 1980;64:59–67.
15. Yamashita T, Uemara A, Uchino E, Doi N, Ohba N. Spontaneous closure of traumatic macular hole. Am J Ophthalmol. 2002;133:230–5.
16. Miller JB, Yonekawa Y, Eliott D, Kim IK, Kim LA, Loewenstein JI, Sobrin L, Young LH, Mukai S, Vavvas DG. Long-term follow-up and outcomes in traumatic macular holes. Am J Ophthalmol. 2015;160:1255–8.
17. Miller JB, Yonekawa Y, Eliott D, Vavvas DG. A review of traumatic macular hole: diagnosis and treatment. Int Ophthalmol Clin. 2013;53:59–67.
18. Rubin JS, Glaser BM, Thompson JT, Sjaarda RN, Pappas SS, Murphy RP. Vitrectomy, fluid-gas exchange and transforming growth factor-beta-2 for the treatment of traumatic macular holes. Ophthalmology. 1995;102:1840–5.
19. Garcia-Arumi J, Corcostegui B, Sararols L. The role of vitreoretinal surgery in the treatment of posttraumatic macular hole. Retina. 1997;17:372–7.
20. Chow DR, Williams GA, Trese MT, Margherio RR, Ruby AJ, Ferrone PJ. Successful closure of traumatic macular holes. Retina. 1999;19:405–9.
21. Johnson RN, McDonald HR, Lewis H, Grand MG, Murray TG, Mieler WF, Johnson MW, Boldt HC, Olsen KR, Tornambe PE, Folk JC. Traumatic macular hole: observations, pathogenesis, and results of vitrectomy surgery. Ophthalmology. 2001;108:853–7.
22. Amari F, Ogino N, Matsumura M, Negi A, Yoshimura N. Vitreous surgery for traumatic macular holes. Retina. 1999;19:411–3.
23. Ghoraba HH, Ellakwa AF, Ghali AA. Long-term result of silicone oil versus gas tamponade in the treatment of traumatic macular holes. Clin Ophthalmol. 2012;6:49–53.
24. Berlin R. Zur sogenannten commotio retinae. Klin Monatsbl Augenheilkd. 1873;1:42–78.
25. Baath J, Ells AL, Kherani A, Williams RG. Severe retinal injuries from paintball projectiles. Can J Ophthalmol. 2007;42:620–3.
26. Kent JS, Eidsness RB, Colleaux KM, Romanchuk KG. Indoor soccer-related eye injuries: should eye protection be mandatory? Can J Ophthalmol. 2007;42:605–8.
27. Blight R, Hart JCD. Structural changes in the outer retinal layers following blunt mechanical blunt mechanical non-perforating trauma to the globe: an experimental study. Br J Ophthalmol. 1977;61:573–8.
28. Hart JCD, Blight R. Electrophysiological and pathological investigation of concussional injury. Trans Ophthalmol Soc UK. 1975;95:326–34.
29. Yanoff M, Fine B. Surgical and nonsurgical trauma. In: Ocular pathology. 7th ed. Hagerstown: Harper & Row; 2014. p. 132–3.

30. Mansour AM, Green WR, Hogge C. Histopathology of commotio retinae. Retina. 1992;12:24–8.
31. Sipperly JO, Quigley HA, Gass JDM. Traumatic retinopathy in primates: the explanation of commotio retinae. Arch Ophthalmol. 1978;96:267–73.
32. Pulido JS, Blair NP. The blood-retinal barrier in Berlin's edema. Retina. 1987;7:233–6.
33. Agarwal A, JDM G. Traumatic retinopathy. In: Gass' atlas of macular diseases. 5th ed. Philadelphia: Saunders; 2012. p. 714–6.
34. Benson WE. The effects of blunt trauma on the posterior segment of the eye. Trans Penn Acad Ophthalmol Otolaryngol. 1982;2:26–33.
35. Hart JCD, Frank HJ. Retinal opacification after blunt non-perforating concussional injuries to the globe: a clinical and retinal fluorescein angiographic study. Trans Ophthalmol Soc UK. 1975;95:94–100.
36. Sousa-Santos F, Lavinsky D, Moraes NS, Castro AR, Cardillo JA, Farah ME. Spectral-domain optical coherence tomography in patients with commotio retinae. Retina. 2012;32:711–8.
37. Friberg TR. Traumatic retinal pigment epithelial edema. Am J Ophthalmol. 1979;88:18–21.
38. Agarwal A, JDM G. Traumatic retinopathy. In: Gass' atlas of macular diseases. 5th ed. Philadelphia: Saunders; 2012. p. 716–8.
39. Levin LL, Seddon JM, Topping T. Retinal pigment epithelial tears associated with trauma. Am J Ophthalmol. 1991;112:396–400.
40. Von Graefe A. Zwei Falle von Ruptur der Choroidea. Graefe's Arch Ophthalmol. 1854;1:402.
41. Williams DF, Mieler WF, Williams GA. Posterior segment manifestations of ocular trauma. Retina. 1990;10(Suppl 1):S35–44.
42. Ament CS, Zacks DN, Lane AM, Krzystolik M, D'Amico DJ, Mukai S, Young LH, Loewenstein J, Arroyo J, Miller JW. Predictors of visual outcome and choroidal neovascular membrane formation after traumatic choroidal rupture. Arch Ophthalmol. 2006;124(7):957–66.
43. Patel MM, Chee YE, Eliott D. Choroidal rupture: a review. Int Ophthalmol Clin. 2013;53:69–78.
44. Wyszynski RE, Grossniklaus HE, Frank KE. Indirect choroidal rupture secondary to blunt ocular trauma. A review of eight eyes. Retina. 1988;8:237–43.
45. Carrim ZI, Simmons IG. Traumatic choroidal rupture. Emerg Med J. 2009;26:880.
46. Abri A, Binder S, Pavelka M, Tittl M, Neumüller J. Choroidal neovascularization in a child with traumatic choroidal rupture: clinical and ultrastructural findings. Clin Exp Ophthalmol. 2006;34:460–3.
47. Hilton GF. Late serosanguineous detachment of the macula after traumatic choroidal rupture. Am J Ophthalmol. 1975;79:997–1000.
48. Kim JM, Kim KO, Kim YD, Choi GJ. A case of air-bag associated severe ocular injury. Korean J Ophthalmol. 2004;18:84–8.
49. Godtfredson E. Re-examination of central ruptures of the choroid. Acta Ophthalmol. 1942;20:337–50.
50. Aguilar JP, Green WR. Choroidal rupture: a histopathologic study of 47 cases. Retina. 1984;4:269–75.
51. Siegrist MH. Traumatische Ruptur von Ciliararterien. Klin U Med Inst der Schweie. 1895;3:554.
52. Secretan M, Sickenberg M, Zografos L, Piguet B. Morphometric characteristics of traumatic choroidal ruptures associated with neovascularization. Retina. 1998;18:62–6.
53. Kohno T, Miki T, Shiraki K, Kano K, Hirabayashi-Matsushita M. Indocyanine green angiographic features of choroidal rupture and choroidal vascular injury after contusion ocular injury. Am J Ophthalmol. 2000;129:38–46.
54. Glazer LC, Han DP, Gottleib MS. Choroidal rupture and optic atrophy. Br J Ophthalmol. 1993;77:33–5.
55. Goldberg MF. Chorioretinal vascular anastomoses after blunt trauma to the eye. Am J Ophthalmol. 1976;82:892–5.
56. Maberly AL, Carvounis EP. The visual field in indirect traumatic rupture of the choroid. Can J Ophthalmol. 1977;12:147–52.

57. Wood CM, Richardson J. Indirect choroidal ruptures: aetiological factors, patterns of ocular damage, and final visual outcome. Br J Ophthalmol. 1990;74:208–11.
58. Yadav NK, Bharghav M, Vasudha K, Shetty KB. Choroidal neovascular membrane complicating traumatic choroidal rupture managed by intravitreal bevacizumab. Eye. 2009;23:1872–3.
59. Chanana B, Azad RV, Kumar N. Intravitreal bevacizumab for subfoveal choroidal neovascularization secondary to traumatic choroidal rupture. Eye. 2009;23:2125–6.
60. Gross JG, King LP, de Juan E, Powers T. Subfoveal neovascular membrane removal in patients with traumatic choroidal rupture. Ophthalmology. 1996;103:579–85.
61. Gotzaridis EV, Vakalis AN, Sethi CS, Charteris DG. Surgical removal of sequential epiretinal and subretinal neovascular membranes in a patient with traumatic choroidal rupture. Eye. 2003;17:790–1.
62. Goldzieher W. Bietrag zur pathologie der orbitalen schussverletzungen. Z Augenheilkd. 1901;6:277.
63. Papakostas TD, Yonekawa Y, Skondra D, Vavvas DG. Traumatic chorioretinal rupture (sclopetaria). Int Ophthalmol Clin. 2013;53:119–25.
64. Ahmadabadi MN, Karkhaneh R, Roohipoor R, Tabatabi A, Alimardani A. Clinical presentation and outcome of chorioretinitis sclopetaria: a case series study. Injury. 2010;41:82–5.
65. Taban M, Taban M, Sears JE. Ocular findings following trauma from paintball sports. Eye (Lond). 2008;22:930–4.
66. Otto CS, Nixon KL, Mazzoli RA, Raymond WR 4th, Ainbinder DJ, Hansen EA, Krolicki TJ. Chorioretinitis sclopetaria from BB ex memoria. Ophthalmic Surg Lasers. 2001;32:152–5.
67. Brown GC, Tasman WS, Benson WE. BB-gun injuries to the eye. Ophthalmic Surg. 1985;16:505–8.
68. Hart JC, Natsikos VE, Raistrick ER, Doran RM. Chorioretinitis sclopetaria. Trans Ophthalmol Soc UK. 1980;100(pt 2):276–81.
69. Perry HD, Rahn EK. Chorioretinitis sclopetaria: choroidal and retinal concussion injury from a bullet. Arch Ophthalmol. 1977;95:328–9.
70. Katsumata S, Takahashi J, Tamai M. Chorioretinitis sclopetaria caused by fishing line sinker. Jpn J Ophthalmol. 1984;28:69–74.
71. Martin DF, Awh CC, McCuen BW, Jaffe GJ, Slott JH, Machemer R. Treatment and pathogenesis of traumatic chorioretinal rupture. Am J Ophthalmol. 1994;117:190–200.
72. Moses RA. Detachment of the ciliary body. Anatomical and physical considerations. Invest Ophthalmol. 1965;4:935.
73. Dubovy SR, Guyton DL, Green WR. Clinicopathologic correlation of chorioretinitis sclopetaria. Retina. 1997;17:510–20.
74. Salzman M. Die Ausrissing des Sehnersen (avulsio nervi optica). Z Augenheilkd. 1903;9:489.
75. Lister W. Some concussion changes met with in military practice. Br J Ophthalmol. 1924;8:305–18.
76. Caiger MH. Ocular injuries resulting from the war. Trans Ophthalmol Soc UK. 1941;61:54–73.
77. Chow AY, Goldberg MR, Frenkel M. Evulsion of the optic nerve in association with basketball injuries. Ann Ophthalmol. 1984;16:35–7.
78. Chong CC, Chang AA. Traumatic optic nerve avulsion and central retinal artery occlusion following rugby injury. Clin Exp Ophthalmol. 2006;31:88–9.
79. Duke-Elder WS, MacFaul P. Injuries. In: System of ophthalmology, vol. 14. St. Louis: CV Mosby; 1972. p. 187–94.
80. Williams DF, Williams GA, Abrams GW, Jesmanowicz A, Hyde JS. Evulsion of the retina associated with optic nerve evulsion. Am J Ophthalmol. 1987;104:5–9.
81. LaGrange F. Les Fractures de l'orbite par les Projectiles de Guerre. Libraires de L'académie de médecine. Paris: Masson; 1917.
82. Rones B, Wilder HC. Non perforating ocular injuries in soldiers. Am J Ophthalmol. 1947;30:1142–60.
83. Park JH, Frenkel M, Dobbie JG, Choromokos E. Evulsion of the optic nerve. Am J Ophthalmol. 1971;72:969–71.

84. Buchwald HJ, Otte P, Lang GE. Evulsion of the optic nerve following blunt bulbar trauma. Klin Monatsbl Augenheilkd. 2003;220:303–8.
85. Morris WR, Osborn FD, Fleming JC. Traumatic evulsion of the globe. Ophthal Plast Reconstr Surg. 2002;18:261–7.
86. Hart JCD, Pilley SFJ. Partial evulsion of optic nerve. Fluorescein angiographic study. Br J Ophthalmol. 1970;54:781–5.
87. Modjtahedi BS, Fortenbach CR, Lorch AC. Optic nerve head avulsion: clinical, radiographic, and sonographic correlations. Ophthalmology. 2015;122:2442.
88. Stanton-Cook L. Injury simulating congenital anomaly. Br J Ophthalmol. 1953;37:188–9.
89. Duane TD. Valsalva hemorrhagic retinopathy. Trans Am Ophthalmol Soc. 1972;70:298.
90. Liu Z, Pan X, Bi H. Treatment of valsalva retinopathy. Optom Vis Sci. 2014;91(11):e278–81.
91. Ramskold LAH, Asaria RH. Valsalva retinopathy secondary to hyperemesis gravidarum. Eur J Obstet Gynecol Reprod Biol. 2012;162:118–9.
92. Michaels L, Tint NL, Alexander P. Postcoidal visual loss due to valsalva retinopathy. BMJ Case Rep. 2014;2014:bcr2014207130.
93. Eneh A, Almeida D. Valsalva hemorrhagic retinopathy during labor: a case report and literature review. Can J Ophthalmol. 2013;48:e145–7.
94. Ladjimi A, Zaouali S, Messaoud R, Ben Yahia S, Attia S, Jenzri S, Khairallah M. Valsalva retinopathy induced by labour. Eur J Ophthalmol. 2002;12:336–8.
95. Karagiannis D, Gregor Z. Valsalva retinopathy associated with idiopathic thrombocytopenic purpura and positive antiphospholipid antibodies. Eye. 2006;20:1447–9.
96. Oliphant H, Holmes C, Hassan A, Baddeley P. Handstand induced visual loss: valsalva retinopathy. BMJ Case Rep. 2014;2014:bcr2014206733.
97. Manche EF, Goldberg RA, Mondino BJ. Air bag-related ocular injuries. Ophthalmic Surg Lasers. 1997;28:246–50.
98. Honemann C, Brandt L. Valsalva retinopathy: a rare complication after general anesthesia. A&A Case Rep. 2015;5:231–3.
99. Durukan AH, Kerimoglu H, Erdurman C, Demirel A, Karagul S. Long-term results of Nd:YAG laser treatment for premacular subhyaloid haemorrhage owing to Valsalva retinopathy. Eye. 2008;22:214–8.
100. Goel N, Kumar V, Seth A, Raina UK, Ghosh B. Spectral-domain optical coherence tomography following Nd:YAG laser membranotomy in valsalva retinopathy. Ophthalmic Surg Lasers Imaging. 2011;42:222–8.
101. De Maeyer K, Van Ginderdeuren R, Postelmans L, Stalmans P, Van Calster J. Sub-inner limiting membrane haemorrhage: causes and treatment with vitrectomy. Br J Ophthalmol. 2007;91:869–72.
102. Ubig MW, Mangouritsas G, Rothbacher HH, Hamilton AM, McHugh JD. Long-term results after drainage of premacular subhyaloid hemorrhage into the vitreous with a pulsed Nd:Yag laser. Arch Ophthalmol. 1998;116:1465–9.
103. Agarwal A, JDM G. Traumatic retinopathy. In: Gass' atlas of macular diseases. 5th ed. Philadelphia: Saunders; 2012. p. 738–41.
104. Mainster MA, Turner PL. Retinal injuries from light: Mechanisms, hazards, and prevention. In: Ryan SJ, Hinton DR, Schachat AP, Wilkinson P, editors. Retina. 4th ed. Philadelphia: Elsevier/Mosby; 2006. p. 1857–70.
105. Yannuzzi LA, Fisher YL, Slakter JS, Krueger A. Solar retinopathy: a photobiologic and geophysical analysis. Retina. 1989;9:28–43.
106. Brue C, Mariotti C, Franco ED, Fisher Y, Guidotti JM, Giovannini A. Solar retinopathy: a multimodal analysis. Case Rep Ophthalmol Med. 2013;2013:1–5.
107. Comander J, Gardiner M, Loewenstein J. High-resolution optical coherence tomography findings in solar maculopathy and the differential diagnosis of outer retinal holes. Am J Ophthalmol. 2011;152:413–9.
108. Litten M. Ueber einige vom allgemein-klinishen Standpunkt aus interessante, Augenveranderungen. Berl Klin Wochnschr. 1881;18:23–7.

109. Terson A. De l'hemorrhagie dans la corps vitre au cours de l'hemorrhagie cerebrale. Clin Ophthalmol. 1900;6:309.
110. Paunoff F. Glaskörperblutungen bei Subarachnoidalblutung (Terson-Syndrome). Klin Monatsbl Augenheilkd. 1967;141:625.
111. Shaw HE, Landers MB III, Sydnor CF. The significance of intraocular hemorrhages due to subarachnoid hemorrhage. Ann Ophthalmol. 1977;9:1403–5.
112. Agarwal A, JDM G. Traumatic retinopathy. In: Gass' atlas of macular diseases. 5th ed. Philadelphia: Saunders; 2012. p. 724–7.
113. Daubler FH, Marlow SB. A case of hemorrhage into the optic nerve sheaths as a direct extension from a diffuse intrameningeal hemorrhage caused by rupture of aneurysms of a cerebral artery. Arch Ophthalmol. 1917;46:553–6.
114. Miller AJ, Cuttino JT. On the mechanism of massive preretinal hemorrhage following rupture of a congenital medial-defect intracranial aneurysm. Am J Ophthalmol. 1948;31:15–24.
115. Weingeist TA, Goldman EJ, Folk JC, Packer AJ, Ossoinig KC. Terson's syndrome: clinicopathologic correlations. Ophthalmology. 1986;93:1435–42.
116. Keithahn MAZ, Bennett SR, Cameron D, Mieler WF. Retinal folds in Terson syndrome. Ophthalmology. 1993;100:1187–90.
117. McRae M, Teasell RW, Canny C. Bilateral retinal detachments associated with Terson's syndrome. Retina. 1994;14:467–8.
118. Schultz PN, Sobol WM, Weingeist TA. Long-term visual outcome in Terson Syndrome. Ophthalmology. 1991;98:1814–9.
119. Clarkson JG, Flynn HW, Daily MJ. Vitrectomy in Terson's syndrome. Am J Ophthalmol. 1980;90:549–52.
120. Purtscher O. Noch unbekannte befunde nach schadeltrauma. Ber Dtsch Ophthalmol Ges. 1910;36:294–301.
121. Purtscher O. Angiopathia retinae traumatic. Lymphorrhagien des Augengrundes. Albrecht von Graefes Arch Klin Exp Ophthalmol. 1912;82:347–71.
122. Sanders RJ, Brown GC, Brown A, Gerner EW. Purtscher's retinopathy preceding acute pancreatitis. Ann Ophthalmol. 1992;24:19–21.
123. Kelly JS. Purtscher's retinopathy related to chest compression by safety belts. Fluorescein angiographic findings. Am J Ophthalmol. 1972;72:278–83.
124. Mellor A, Soni N. Fat embolism. Anaesthesia. 2001;56:145–54.
125. Stoumbos VD, Klein ML, Goodman S. Purtscher's-like retinopathy in chronic renal failure. Ophthalmology. 1992;99:1833–9.
126. Agarwal A, McKibbin MA. Purtscher's and Purtscher-like retinopathy: a review. Surv Ophthalmol. 2006;51:129–36.
127. Agarwal A, JDM G. Traumatic retinopathy. In: Gass' atlas of macular diseases. 5th ed. Philadelphia: Saunders; 2012. p. 722–5.
128. Burton TC. Unilateral Purtscher's retinopathy. Ophthalmology. 1980;47:1096–105.
129. Kocak N, Kaynak S, Kaynak T, Oner HF, Cingil G. Unilateral Purtscher-like retinopathy after weight-lifting. Eur J Ophthalmol. 2003;13:395–7.
130. Gomez-Ulla F, Fente B, Torreiro MG, Salorio MS, Gonzalez F. Choroidal vascular abnormality in Purtscher's retinopathy shown by indocyanine green angiography. Am J Ophthalmol. 1996;122:261–3.
131. Pratt MV, de Venecia G. Purtscher's retinopathy: a clinicohistopathological correlation. Surv Ophthalmol. 1970;14:417–23.
132. Agarwal A, McKibbin MA. Purtscher's retinopathy: epidemiology, clinical features and outcome. Br J Ophthalmol. 2007;91:1456–9.
133. Holak HM, Holak S. Prognostic factors for visual outcome in Purtscher retinopathy. Surv Ophthalmol. 2007;52:117–8.
134. Jacob HS, Craddock PR, Hammerschmidt DE, Moldow CF. Complement-induced granulocyte aggregation; an unsuspected mechanism of disease. N Engl J Med. 1980;302:789–94.
135. Gossling HR, Pelligrini VD. Fat embolism syndrome: a review of pathophysiology and physiological basis of treatment. Clin Orthop Relat Res. 1982;165:68–82.

136. Czerny V. Ueber die Klinische Bedeutung der Fettembolie. Berl Klin Wschr. 1875;12:593–5.
137. Urbanek J. Uber Fettembolie des Auges. Graefes Arch Ophthalmol. 1933;131:147–73.
138. Lai JC, Johnson MW, Martonyi CL, Till GO. Complement induced retinal arteriolar occlusions in the cat. Retina. 1997;17(3):239–46.
139. Wang AG, Yen MY, Liu JH. Pathogenesis and neuroprotective treatment in Purtscher's retinopathy. Jpn J Ophthalmol. 1998;42:318–22.
140. Lin YC, Yang CM, Lin CL. Hyperbaric oxygen treatment in Purtscher's retinopathy induced by chest injury. J Chin Med Assoc. 2006;69:444–8.
141. Mayer BW, Burns P. Differential diagnosis of abuse injuries in infants and young children. Nurse Pract. 2000;25:15–37. 15–8,21,25–26 passim; quiz 36–37.
142. WHO factsheets: child maltreatment. Factsheet N150, updated 2/2014.
143. Odom A, Christ E, Kerr N, Byrd K, Cochran J, Barr F, Bugnitz M, Ring JC, Storgion S, Walling R, Stidham G, Quasney MW. Prevalence of retinal hemorrhages in pediatric patients after in-hospital cardiopulmonary resuscitation: a prospective study. Pediatrics. 1997;99(6):E3.
144. Friendly DS. Ocular manifestations of physical child abuse. Trans Am Acad Ophthalmol Otolaryngol. 1971;75:318–32.
145. Jensen AD, Smith RE, Olson MI. Ocular clues to child abuse. J Pediatr Ophthalmol Strabismus. 1971;8:270–2.
146. Harley RD. Ocular manifestations of child abuse. J Pediatr Ophthalmol Strabismus. 1980;17:5–13.
147. Tsao K, Kazlas M, Weiter JJ. Ocular injuries in shaken baby syndrome. Int Ophthalmol Clin. 2002;42:145–55.
148. Duhaime AC, Christian CW, Rorke LB, Zimmerman RA. Nonaccidental head injury in infants – the "shaken-baby syndrome". N Engl J Med. 1998;338:1822–9.
149. Kaur B, Taylor D. Fundus hemorrhages in infancy. Surv Ophthalmol. 1992;37:1–17.
150. Eisenbry AB. Retinal hemorrhage in the battered child. Childs Brain. 1979;5:40–4.
151. Massicotte SJ, Folberg R, Torczynski E, Gilliland MG, Luckenbach MW. Vitreoretinal traction and perimacular folds in the eyes of deliberately traumatized children. Ophthalmology. 1991;98:1124–7.
152. Matthews GP, Das A. Dense vitreous hemorrhages predict poor visual and neurological prognosis in infants with shaken baby syndrome. J Pediatr Ophthalmol Strabismus. 1996;33:260–5.
153. Greenwald MJ, Weiss A, Oesterle CS, Friendly DS. Traumatic retinoschisis in battered babies. Ophthalmology. 1986;93:618–25.
154. Harcourt B, Hopkins D. Permanent chorioretinal lesions in childhood of suspected traumatic origin. Trans Ophthalmol Soc UK. 1988;95:295–9.
155. Wilkinson WS, Han DP, Rappley MD, Owings CL. Retinal hemorrhage predicts neurologic injury in the shaken baby syndrome. Arch Ophthalmol. 1989;107:1472–4.
156. Giangiacomo J, Khan JA, Levine C, Thompson VM. Sequential cranial computed tomography in infants with retinal hemorrhages. Ophthalmology. 1988;95:295–9.
157. Dias MS, Backstrom J, Falk M, Li V. Serial radiography in the infant shaken impact syndrome. Pediatr Neurosurg. 1998;29:77–85.
158. McCabe CF, Donahue SP. Prognostic indicators for vision and mortality in shaken baby syndrome. Arch Ophthalmol. 2000;118:373–7.
159. Conway MD, Peyman GA, Recasens M. Intravitreal tPA and SF6 promote clearing of premacular subhyaloid hemorrhages in shaken and battered baby syndrome. Ophthalmic Surg Lasers. 1999 Jun;30:435–41.
160. Wilkenson CP, Rice TA. Other causes of retinal detachment. In: Wilkenson CP, Rice TA, editors. Michel's retinal detachment. 2nd ed. St Louis: Mosby; 1997. p. 208–10.
161. Levin LA, Beck RW, Joseph MP, Seiff S, Kraker R. The treatment of traumatic optic neuropathy: the International Optic Nerve Trauma Study. Ophthalmology. 1999;106:1268–77.
162. Kivlin JD, Simons KB, Lazoritz S, Ruttum MS. Shaken baby syndrome. Ophthalmology. 2000;107:1246–54.

163. Zenker FA. Beltrage zur Anatomie und Physiologie der Lunge. Dresden: J Braunsdorf; 1861. p. 20.
164. Kumar V, Abbas AK, Aster JC. Hemodynamic disorders, thromboembolic disease, and shock. In: Robbins & Cotran pathologic basis of disease. 9th ed. Philadelphia: Saunders; 2015. p. 128.
165. Beck JP, Collins JA. Theoretical and clinical aspects of posttraumatic fat embolism syndrome. In: Calandruccio RA, editor. American Academy of Orthopedic Surgeons instruction course lectures, vol. 22. St Louis: CV Mosby; 1973. p. 38–87.
166. McCarthy B, Mammen E, LeBlanc LP, Wilson RF. Subclinical fat embolism: a prospective study of 50 patients with extremity fractures. J Trauma. 1973;13:9–16.
167. Adams CBT. The retinal manifestations of fat embolism. Injury. 1971;2:221–4.
168. Evans JJ. Cerebral fat embolism with recovery and involvement of the central retinal artery. Br J Ophthalmol. 1940;24:614–6.
169. DeVoe AG. Ocular fat embolism. A clinical and pathologic report. Trans Am Ophthalmol Soc. 1949;47:254–62.
170. Chuang EL, Miller FS, Kalina RE. Retinal lesions following long bone fractures. Ophthalmology. 1985;3:370–4.
171. Agarwal A, JDM G. Traumatic retinopathy. In: Gass' atlas of macular diseases. 5th ed. Philadelphia: Saunders; 2012. p. 722–3.
172. Kelley JS, Hoover RE, George T. Whiplash maculopathy. Arch Ophthalmol. 1978;96:834–5.
173. Grey RHB. Foveo-macular retinitis, solar retinopathy, and trauma. Br J Ophthalmol. 1978;62:543–6.
174. Grey RHB. Macular and vitreal disturbances produced by traumatic vitreous rebound. South Med J. 1970;63:1197–8.
175. Abebe MT, De Laey JJ. Foveomacular retinitis as a result of ocular contusion. Bull Soc Belge Ophtalmol. 1992;243:171–5.
176. Daily L. Further observations on foveolar splinter and macular wisps. Arch Ophthalmol. 1973;90:102–3.

MIX
Papier aus verantwortungsvollen Quellen
Paper from responsible sources
FSC® C105338

If you have any concerns about our products,
you can contact us on
ProductSafety@springernature.com

In case Publisher is established outside the EU,
the EU authorized representative is:
Springer Nature Customer Service Center GmbH
Europaplatz 3, 69115 Heidelberg, Germany

Printed by Libri Plureos GmbH
in Hamburg, Germany